Short Textbook of Community Health Nursing

Dr. G.N. Prabhakara
Principal and Professor of PSM
SDM College of Medical Sciences and Hospital
Dharwad, Karnataka, India

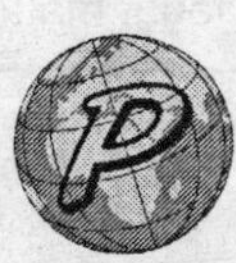

PEEPEE
PUBLISHERS AND DISTRIBUTORS (P) LTD.

Short Textbook of Community Health Nursing

Published by:
Pawaninder P. Vij
Peepee Publishers and Distributors (P) Ltd.
Head Office: 160, Shakti Vihar, Pitam Pura, New Delhi-110 034
Corporate Office: 7/31, Ansari Road, Daryaganj, Post Box-7243, New Delhi-110002 (India)
Ph: 65195868, 23246245, 9811156083
e-mail: peepee160@yahoo.co.in
e-mail: peepee160@rediffmail.com
e-mail: peepee160@gmail.com
www.peepeepub.com

First Edition: **2007**
Reprint: 2008

ISBN: 81-8445-004-4

Printed at:
Lordson, C-5/19, Rana Pratap Bagh, Delhi-110 007

Preface

Now a time has come that without nursing profession Medical profession is incomplete. It is one of the noblest jobs in health care services.

The purpose of this book is to provide Theory and Practice of Community Health Nursing to General Nursing students/Midwifery Students who intend to have their diploma and B.Sc Nursing students who intend to have their degree in nursing. They will be Registered Nurses with these recognized diploma or degree in nursing.

Recommendations of nursing syllabus in community health nursing are followed.

Areas like Sociology, Psychology, Health Statistics, RCH, Human Sexuality, Mental Health, and Home Visiting are emphasised with practical approach.

Omission or inclusion of points in the text is solely based on author's personal experience as teacher over a period of 34 years at teaching nursing in Central Government colleges, State Government colleges.

I trust this book will serve the students and faculty of Community Health Nursing in General Nursing/Midwifery and B.Sc.Nursing.

G.N. Prabhakara

Acknowledgements

Nursing students in my walk of life to whom I taught are responsible for bringing out my experiene in the form of **Short Textbook of Community Health Nursing.**

Initiation, motivation, guidance, proof reading and specific appropriations are from my wife Mrs. Malathi Prabhakara, Former Scientist CFTRI, CSIR, Mysore and my son Dr. Bharat MP, Post Graduate and Tutor in Radiodiagnosis and Imaging, SDM College of Medical Sciences and Hospital, Dharwad, India.

Heartfelt thanks to my colleagues Dr. JV Chowti, Dr. KR Pravin Chandra, Dr. R Venkatesh, Dr. MS Shivaswamy, Dr. Mayur Sherkhane, Dr. Pushpa Patil, Dr. BF Appannavar, Dr. T Sadashivappa, Dr. SR Kakhandaki, Dr. JG Chimmalgi, Dr. Sushma J Chowti, Dr. Jyothi Hiremath, Dr. Juliet Pinheiro, Dr. Manjula S Pujari and Dr. Maya Kakhandki, Sri YB Inganalli and Mrs. Uma P for review and proof reding of the title.

High appreciations and heartfelt thanks to Mr. Pawaninder P Vij, Director, Peepee Publishers and Distributors (P) Ltd., New Delhi in giving a good commendable shape to my modest work.

Contents

CHAPTER ONE

Introduction

Progress of nursing has reflected the social outlook of present century, so also health care centres, district hospitals and teaching hospitals have adapted this change.

The beginner nurse has to adjust, at her entry, to new surroundings and should not get bewildered by many aspects of hospital life. Preconceived idea by nursing student about hospital and about nursing may bear little resemblance to reality; hence the need for understanding the structure and function of hospital.

Health care especially nursing care is a continuous exercise to be carried out day and night without interruption; for the sick there is no time interval. All departments are geared to serve the sick; units and disciplines like various specialities, dispensary, laboratory, X-ray, physiotherapy and ancillary staff like orderly, porter, domestic workers who have to work in a coordianted manner to offer health care services in a most effective and efficient manner. Hospital is a complex institution/organization which demands your attention that is not equated in many other spheres.

Hospital serves as an in-house training centre to doctors, radiographers, physiotherapists, midwives, social workers, medical postgraduates as well as undergraduate students including nursing students. Nursing profession has a greater role to play not only in curative treatment/arresting of disease, but also to restore the patient as far as possible to full activity. The co-operation of patient is required so that he takes interest in recovery and subsequent welfare; nursing profession has a great role to play in getting the patient's co-operation as well.

Nursing has its role in hospital research. Experience and observation has helped health staff to give a confidence based specific treatment. Joseph Lister's "Antiseptic Surgery" has opened the door to great surgical advances. Such great examples are available to mitigate sufferings of mankind and truly are part of hospital services.

Nurse and Patient

"Do the sick no harm": This is from none other than Florence Nightingale. Constant vigilance is needed in nursing procedures in order that these may be carried out with the highest degree of competence.

Monitoring administration of dangerous drugs, measures to prevent cross infection, care of elderly, care of child, care of woman in labour pain need substantial attention which are available only from nursing profession.

Anxiety and stress of patient need attention to overcome distressing effect on family life. To watch an experienced and sympathetic ward sister set about the task of allaying the fears of anxious relatives and establishing their confidence in the hospital and the staff is a valuable lesson in good human relationships.

Health is influenced by an array of demographic, socio-economic, political and environmental factors that are constantly changing. Major obstacles to health are poverty and deteriorating economic conditions. The demand for trained nurses has been increasing due to: social and political crises, ageing process of the population and deteriorating environmental factors. Despite improvement in health care, there is a wide gap between health service givers and consumers; more so between trained nurses and the needy population. Hence, effective use of human resources, intersectoral cooperation and community participation which builds up partnership between individual and community is called for, to bridge the gap (Fig. 1.1).

Nursing is the key component of health care in all socio-economic setting. It ranges from carrying out high technology investigations like aortogram to low technology first contact care like O.R.S. preparation.

HISTORICAL ASPECT

Nursing in Early Centuries

Many illnesses of today are found recorded in early centuries and history has shown the existence of these illnesses. Ancient India is first to give a place of honour to 'VAIDYA' who treats and to 'SUSHRUSHA' who nurses. Nurse at that time was an attendant. There is no mention of any specially trained attendant or skilled nursing. Other countries notable in history are Egypt, Assyria and Greece, where honouring in civil life those who cared for the sick was common practice. However attending to the sick was inextricably mingled with religious practices. Sickness was thought of as the work of evil spirits and due to wrath of Gods.

There was a transition in the attitude from attributing illness to the work of evil spirits with the birth of Greek physician "Hippocrates" in fourth century B.C. who pointed out that illness is due to disorder function of the body and is due to disobeying the laws of health. This still serves as a model in nursing profession. His pupils, assistants, women of the household and women of slaves used to assist in nursing care of the sick.

In late early centuries the word "Midwife" was coined. It was a hereditary family profession. During seventeenth century the word "Man Mid-Wife" came into existence.

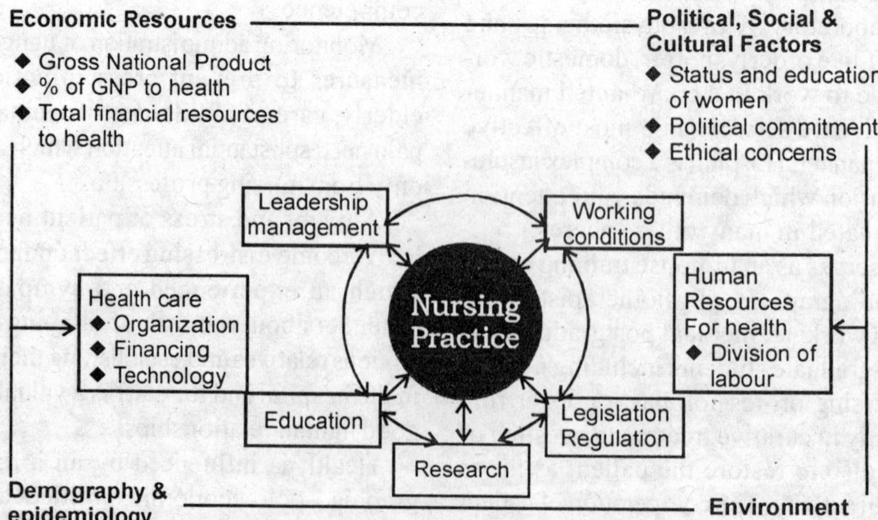

Fig. 1.1: Influencing factors in nursing practice

Nursing in Christian Era

Biblical notation gave the very humblest living creature's nursing equal to service to God. It connotes the duty and privilege of strong, to bear the burdens of the weak. Here we see the spiritual need of the sick was met with. We see the first organised visiting service to the sick by the order of Deaconesses, working with the Deacons under the Bishops. During fourth century St. Jerome's followers included nursing among Christian duties and were not an order. Many monasteries had houses for nuns and monks. It was under the control of Abbess (Elderly Christian woman). Their wide knowledge and able administration is found recorded in the history.

In 12th century we come across famous order of "the Knights Hospitallers" of St. John of Jerusalem. This lead to hospital maintenance in Jerusalem, Rhodes and Malta. "Serving Brothers" were named for nursing. Below this hierarchy, "Subsidiary women" found nursing in "Hospitallers langue".

In 16th century nursing profession was totally suppressed. Traditional Healers predominated and no nursing care takers are observed in the history.

In 19th century, there was rejuvenation of nursing activities with group activity particularly with "St. John Ambulance Association" and "Voluntary Nursing Corps".

French Connection

"Augustinian Sisters", the most important order is seen in seventeenth century in France. Paris Hospital which was called "Hotel-Dieu" was managed by these sisters. Their nursing care was an overcrowded regimen involving nursing of patients, domestic work of washing and attending religious duties. A big cot used to have 5-6 patients which did not allow proper nursing care. They were controlled by priests who did not allow them to know about human body, since it was not considered suitable that celibate nurse should know much about their patient's bodies or their illness. This made nursing inefficient.

The Nursing Community grew with First Superior of the Sisters of Charity "Mile. Le Gras". She helped Vincent DePaul (French priest) to take a house in Paris, gathered country girls to train nursing. Thus a voluntary visiting service by influential ladies formed "Dames de charite". These ladies nursed the sick at home, at hospital, at home for aged, home for insane and even in battlefield. There is a record of teaching instructions, by reading, by writing and use of arithmetic.

Dark Age of Nursing

After "Dames de charite" in 17th century nearly for 150 years there was little progress which is called Dark Age of Nursing. In early 19th century, progressive leaders in science and profession awakened public conscience to "Nurse care of the sick". With great advance in medicine, surgery and science during later half of 19th century, real nursing service was started.

Pre Nightingale Reformation

Upbringing to be Deaconesses by training young women of good character is recorded in history of nursing which was by a German pastor and his wife (Theodore and Frederica Fliedner). Duties of nurse included care of young children and religious visiting. Pastor's wife gave practical instructions; pastor gave ethical lectures and physician gave instruction in their professional duties. *Florence Nightingale* who received this practical training clearly saw that nursing and hygiene could be improved. Many activities are found in 1840 by protestant Nursing Sisters. In 1845 St. John house started a Nursing Training School.

Era of Florence Nightingale (Fig. 1.2)

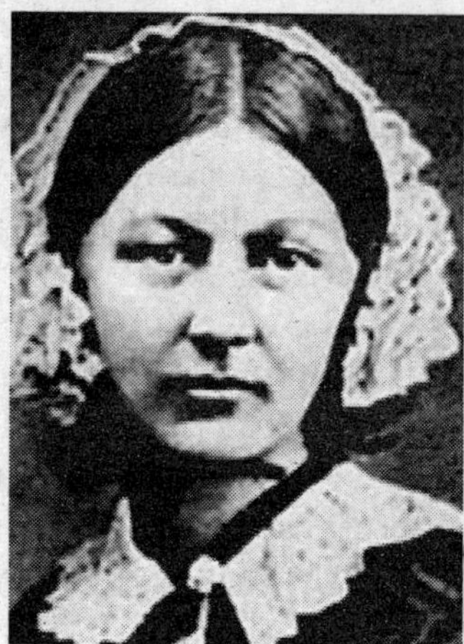

Fig. 1.2: Miss Florence Nightingale
Pioneer of Modern Nursing
Born on : 12th May, 1820
Died on : 13th August, 1910

A great opportunity of a life of preparation for task of care to soldiers came to Nightingale when she was asked the help by War Secretary, Sidney Herbert. She then took a band of nurses out to the *Crimea* to give nursing care to soldiers. She had good education and from high social strata. She had great opposition from home for the above task. She set standards of practical nursing, hospital administration, which still serves as a model.

NURSING ORGANISATIONS

"British Nurse Association" was the first organised body of trained nurses in 1887. The Founder was Miss Gorden Manson (Matron of St. Bartholomew's Hospital. She is widely known under the name Mrs. Bedford Fenwick (after marrying Dr. Bedford Fenwick).

In 1894 Matron's Council of Great Britain and Matron's Council of Ireland were formed. In 1901, First International Congress of Nurses was held at Buffalo.

Leaders of nursing profession started college of nursing in 1916. A new bill was sponsored by Health Ministry and became "the Nurses Registration Act", in 1919.

In India, with the establishment of "Lady Reading Health School" (in 1918) preparation of nursing workers started. Bhore Committee appointed by British Government (1946) and Mudaliar Committee appointed by Indian Government (1961) recommended replacement of untrained and partially trained nurses by trained nurses. As first model in Nursing Education, a College of Nursing was established in Delhi in 1946. It is well-known as R.A.K. College of Nursing in post-Independent India.

Importance of nursing care in the community was thus visualised in India and following chronological progress is seen:

1947 – The Indian Nursing Council Act, 1947 was promulgated in December 1947.
– The Indian Nursing Council was constituted.

1951 – A Special Subcommittee of Council, 1949, was appointed to study syllabus for General Nursing and Midwifery.

1953 – A guide for teachers and examiners in relation to health subject was approved by the council.

1954 – Special provision for Male Nurse was made with (2/6) prescribed course of duration of 3 months in place of Nursing for Women.
– Integration of Public Health in Nursing done.
– Minimum standards were laid down for recognition of Nursing Colleges.

1956 – Curriculum was developed for Nursing Colleges.
– Resolutions by Florence Nightingale Committee of trained nurses association of India was accepted.

1963 – Revision of syllabus done.
– Guidance for School of Nursing by W.H.O. made available.

1982 – Second Revision of syllabus done.
– Workshop reports of syllabus were accepted for national uniformity.

a. Staff
b. Extension service
c. Physical facility
d. Clinical facility
e. Hostel
f. Number of hours of teaching.

Nursing under W.H.O.

Attainment of Health by all—a set out preamble of the constitution of WHO gave a starter to nursing services all over the world. Positive health demarcated the line of action by nurse to serve both well and ill in the community. Right to Medical care and Right to nursing care are implied in the Fundamental Human Rights.

A changing trend in community care (from individual care) gave birth to Community Health Nursing. It ranged from Speciality Hospital, Teaching Hospital, District Hospital, Taluka Hospital, Community Health Centres, Primary Health Centres and sub centres in the nation and nursing service started as team approach to health care.

W.H.O. approved the goal of Primary Health care and Health For All. International Council of Nurses made these as priority issues. These concepts restructured the health services. (Both urban and rural) M.P.W. (female) for a sub centre to cover a population of 5000 was made mandatory. The Nursing Council of India revised the curriculum for training of A.N.M. A scheme of Village Health Guides to provide first contact care to a population of 1000 was started. Training of Indigenous Dais for safe deliveries was emphasised. Thus nursing care had gone beyond the horizon to serve the community for promotion of health and care of the people wherever they live and wherever they work.

First, Second and Third level of care (Primary, Secondary and Tertiary Care) brought the nurses to home, school, health centres and varied (other) centres across the country.

NURSING EDUCATION IN INDIA

Basic Nursing

Diploma in General Nursing and Midwifery	3½ years
B.Sc. Nursing	4 years
Community Health Nursing (MPW female)	1 year 6 months

Post Basic Nursing

B.Sc. Nursing	2 years
M.Sc. Nursing	2 years
PhD Nursing	3 years
Public Health Nursing	10 months
Health Assistants (female)	6 months
B.Sc. in MCH	2 years
M.Sc. in Public Health Nursing	2 years
PhD in Public Health	3 years.

CHAPTER TWO

Sociology and Psychology

SOCIOLOGY

The word sociology is derived from *socios* meaning society and *logos* meaning study.

Sociology along with human anthropology, psychology and psychiatry form Behavioural Sciences since they determine and influence human behaviour or how he conducts himself in the society.

Definition

A study of sociology, thus, provides an insight into the understanding of activities that concern our society, our family, our hospital (organisation) etc.

The word sociology was coined by French author Auguste Compte (1798-1857) from his original work "Social Physics". His law was that human efforts to understand world in ordinary words, always pass through theological, metaphysical and positive stage as they are supernatural stage, natural stage and scientific stage.

He defined sociology as "the investigation of the laws of action and reaction of different parts of social system or social institutions and analysis of society as a unit for progress, change and development."

Emeile Durkheim defined sociology "as the study of social facts".

Karl Marx points out that sociology is a science that deals with social changes primarily by economic influences. Max Weber (1864-1920) points out "the study of organisation of social and economic life according to the principles of efficiency and on the basis of technical knowledge". Thus broader definition of sociology includes four elements viz., (i) Social institutions, (ii) Interaction between these institutions, (iii) Family forms a unit of study in sociology, (iv) Focuses attention on social acts and social relationships.

Nature and Scope

Medical sociology in the field of sociology has areas of interest for the study of health, disease, health behaviour and social-medical interactions. We have many social diseases like tuberculosis, leprosy, sexually transmitted diseases, AIDS. Though they are caused by biological agents, we are turning our interests to study social, behavioural and cultural factors in disease occurrence. A nurse needs to be appraised of both biological and behavioural causation of well-being or ill-being in human beings.

Sociology can help to improve health service facility by:

a. Awareness of cultural differences
b. Assessment of effects by national policies, and
c. Can lead to self enlightenment or increased self understanding.

Further scopes are:

a. Rights of individual is understood
b. Responsibility for health increases
c. Family pattern influencing health is understood.

d. Cultural pattern influencing health and disease is perceived
e. Role of social structure is made visible
f. Social problems are analysed
g. Social agencies that are available become visible.

Man and Society

Health or disease in man is determined by his social environment. Social and structural factors have direct bearing on the nature of illness. Social problems like poverty, poor sanitation, illiteracy affects man's positive health. A patient whether in a hospital or at home has his own habits, customs and beliefs. This new outlook has brought a closer link to man and society (Fig. 2.1).

Individual

Constitution of India has given guarantee of fundamental rights of individual:

a. The right to equality
b. The right to freedom and expression
c. The right against exploitation
d. The right to freedom of practice and propagation of religion
e. The right of minorities to conserve their culture
f. The right to property
g. The right to constitutional remedies for the enforcement of fundamental rights.

Responsibility for Health

This involves mutual adjustment and understanding by individual, his society, his community and his state.

Though society assures availability of services, it is the individual who should be responsible for personal health. They include healthy habits in terms of diet, rest, care of skin, care of teeth, immunisation, reporting of sick and service utilisation.

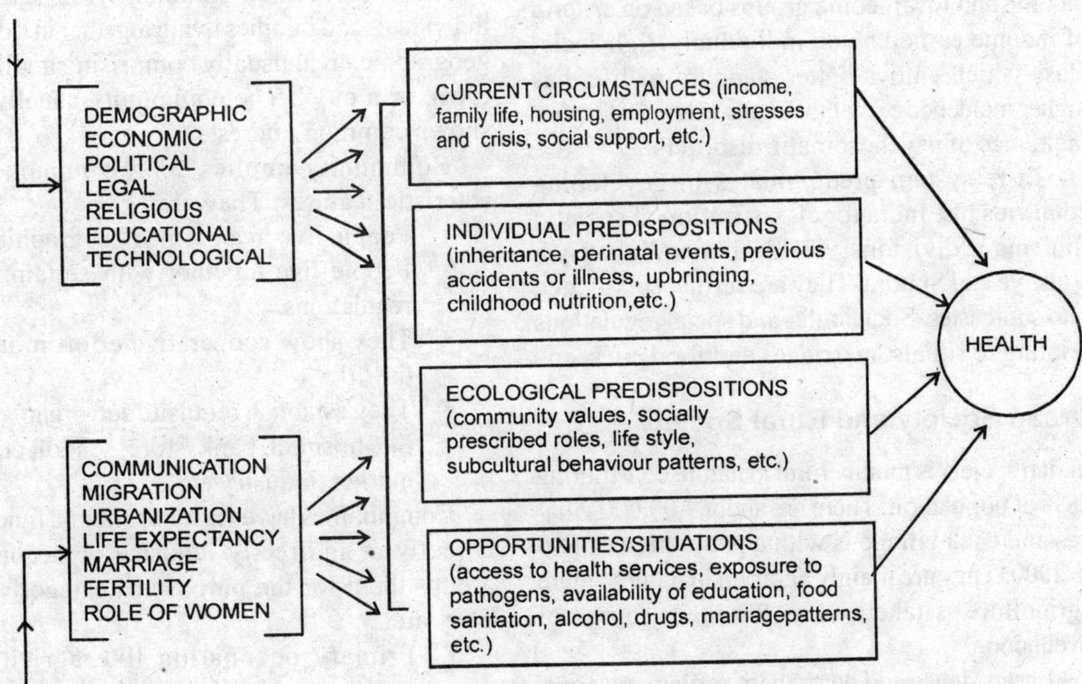

Fig. 2.1: Social factors in health

SOCIETY

Man has always lived in group which is partially or fully organised, which we call as society. Man cannot live without society. It maintains standard or laid down principles. Every individual maintains a social relationship which regulates the human behaviour. Here we notice social regulation, Law and Customs. Effort of an individual is either motivated or is hindered by social norms which stipulate either right or wrong.

Structure of Society

There is no satisfactory classification of the society according to occupation. In developed countries classifications like skilled workers, unskilled workers, professionals, labourers etc., are adopted which do not provide uniformity in classification.

Income is used as an economic factor to classify the society into high income, middle income and low income groups based on criteria of income earned by an individual. High social class which enjoys better standard of life, has higher incidence of metabolic disorders and higher incidence of psychosomatic disorders.

Caste system predominates in developing countries like India for classification of society; four main divisions viz. Brahmin, Kshatriya, Vaishya and Shudra. They are further subdivided into sub-castes. Social rules and social regulations relating to rituals, marriages and food are seen.

Urban Society and Rural Society

Indian society is mainly rural in nature constituting 78% of population. There are about 7,00,000 villages and each village is with a population of 500 to 2000. They are mainly agrarian in nature where agriculture is taken up as the main source of livelihood.

Large, dense and permanent settlements form urban areas which account for 22% of population. According to 2001 census there are 8637 towns and cities. Now there are 300 mega cities indicating extent of urbanisation. We come across occupational diversity and impersonal social life.

There is wide difference between urban and rural society in terms of health aspect, like disease pattern, socio-economic characteristics, demography and availability of health man power, health status and nature of health problem (Table 2.1).

Social Mobility

Indian society is a "closed-class" system. There is restricted movement of social ladder. People changing their religion, caste and race are not commonly found. Recently, urbanisation and civilisation is making people accept social mobility on the basis of gaining wealth or on the basis of achievement.

COMMUNITY

W.H.O. has defined community as "group of individuals and families living together in a defined geographic area, usually comprising a village, a town, or a city". The community usually have shown common interests.

Community implies some common characteristic features. They are:

- People live in a defined geographic area.
- People live together with certain social regulations.
- They show cooperative effort in day-to-day life.
- They establish requisite sub organisations like hospital, bank, store, school, college, market, industry etc.

Communities have varied economic functions. Directly or indirectly industry or occupation groups them for the purpose of categorisation. They are:

- Primary occupation like agriculture, forestry, fishing, mining etc.
- Secondary occupation like Fabrication, Auto industry, Food processing, etc.

Table 2.1: Showing difference between urban and rural society

Disease Pattern	*Rural Society*	*Urban Society*
	Infections	*Metabolic diseases* *Cancer diseases*
Socio-economic characteristics		
Domicile	Rural	Urban
Family	Joint family	Single family
Occupation	Mainly agriculture	Mainly industry
Per capita income	Low	High
Literacy	Low	High
Standard of living	Low	High
Medical care	Low	High
Demography		
Population	Young more	Older more
Problem	Of paediatric age	Of old age
Birth rate	High	Low
Death rate	High	Low
Growth rate	High	Low
I.M.R.	High	Low
M.M.R.	High	Low
Life expectancy	Low	High
Health problems	Infection Malnutrition	Obesity Non communicable disease
Health manpower	Shortage of manpower	More than adequate

- Tertiary occupation like education, health services, recreation club etc.

Community is also grouped under following categories:

a. *Rural community:* Villages form a specified boundary, specified independent occupation, specified administrative setup.
b. *Standard urban area:* A town with a population of 50,000 having encroachment of rural community with mutual socio-economic link.
c. *Urban agglomeration:* A few cities with good growth with delineated boundary.
d. *Urban community:* Population density is seen more than 400 people per square kilometre and is declared urban area by Government.
e. *Cosmopolitan community:* Mega Cities with above 3 lakh population, specified geographic boundary, defined under city corporations.

SOCIAL PROBLEMS

All of us follow social norms which is the outcome of socialisation, which we are used to doing so. All social norms are accompanied by sanctions that promote conformity and protect against non-conformity. A sanction is any reaction from others to the behaviour of an individual or a group that is meant to ensure compliance with a given norm. There are some individuals who refuse to live by the rules that majority of us follow. We come across alcoholism, drug users, S.T.D. Juvenile delinquency, prostitution, violent criminals. These people do not conform to a given set of norms that are accepted by significant number of people in a community. Some have health implications in the community.

Alcoholism

It is a global problem; over the past 50 years production, consumption and abuse has grown to such an extent to cause civil unrest. With the changes in social order alcohol is being considered a symbol of civilisation resulting in high alcoholism. Mild to serious health problems resulting from alcoholism are:

- Loss of balance by poor reasoning due to alcohol content in the blood
- Peptic ulcer and gastritis
- Cirrhosis of liver
- Hypertension
- Heart failure
- Urinary disturbance
- Impotence and sterility
- Foetal damage.

  Social implications of alcoholism are as under:
  - Crime
  - Murder
  - Prostitution
  - Neglect of family
  - Unemployment
  - Indebtedness
  - Malnutrition
  - Delinquent child
  - Traffic accidents
  - Other psychosocial problems.

Health education and awareness programme can check the menace due to alcoholism. There are de-addiction centres to rehabilitate alcoholics. Simultaneously they need good and continued counselling.

Drug Users

Repeated intake of habit forming drugs causes drug addiction (now it is called substance abuse). Patient shows violent behaviour, nausea, vomiting and other severe allergic manifestations if a given drug is not made available. This is called physical dependence. Gradually drug users increase their dose intake indicating the development of tolerance. Finally they even commit crime (compulsion) to procure drug.

Social factors which seem to influence drug abuse are:

- Accessibility to young generation
- Broken homes
- Disturbed home environment
- Escapism from tense life and frustrated life.

Common drugs to produce drug abuse are:

Narcotics	–	Morphine Heroin Codeine Opium
Marijuana	–	Hashish Ganja Bhang
Hallucinogens	–	LSD Mescaline
Hypnotics	–	Barbiturates
Tranquillisers	–	Chlorpromazine Equanil
Stimulants	–	Amphetamine Cocaine

Case management includes:

- Drug identification
- Detoxication in hospital environment
- Counselling
- Rehabilitation
- Change of environment in some cases
- Psychotherapy in some cases.

Social therapy includes:

- Individual health education
- Target group awareness

Legislative procedure available:

- Narcotic drug and psychotropic substance Act, 1985 to combat source.

S.T.D.

This is associated with development of slum and shanty town. Industrialisation influences sexually transmitted diseases.

S.T.D. and prostitution are interrelated. In early days 5 classical venereal diseases viz. syphilis, gonorrhoea, chancroid, lymphogranuloma venereum and granuloma inguinale used to top the list. Now more than 20 different entities are included in the list of S.T.D. Among new entrants Genital Chlamydial infection, Genital herpes, Genital human papilloma infection, and A.I.D.S. found to be predominating.

Social causes of STD are many and following are commonly seen in pre-disposing to infection:

- Prostitution
- Possible high financial return
- Conducive lifestyle of urbanisation
- Idea of independence leading to behavioural change
- Alcoholism
- Broken homes.

Case detection by screening, full course of treatment of diagnosed cases, health education of the community seem to be practicable intervention strategies.

Juvenile Delinquency

Delinquent means any person who deviates from his or her normal behaviour, thus committing theft, sexual offence, murder, burglary, etc.

Juvenile delinquency refers to problem with children. Broken homes, poverty, feeble minded children precipitate the child to commit an offence. Here juvenile crime is confined to a boy below 16 years and a girl below 18 years of age.

Social measures like improving family life, free schooling for education, child guidance and other social welfare services are aimed at preventing juvenile delinquency. The Children Act 1960, provides legislative measures through orphanage, foster home, adoption, borstals and remand homes. Of late Juvenile Justice Act 1986, has made provision for rehabilitation of juvenile delinquent.

Prostitution

It is one of the old known social evils very commonly involving broken homes, illegitimate love making and easy money as sex worker. Poverty seems to lead a woman to prostitution.

This is closely related to sexually transmitted diseases and AIDS.

Social regulation and a good culture in the family can reduce its incidence. The suppression of Immoral Traffic Act in women and girls (SITA) 1956, now called as the Immoral Traffic (Prevention) Act 1986, covers men and women who are exploited for commercial purpose.

Violent Criminals

Various causes including lack of social regulations in the family and mental illness due to organic lesions found to produce violent criminals. A little different to crime, we have Deviant. The concept of deviance is much broader than that of crime which refers to non-conformist conduct that breaks the law.

Unmarried Mothers

It is insignificant in developing countries like India. But teenage mothers without wedlock issues are becoming social problems.

They require guidance, counselling and nursing care.

Physically Challenged

This category comprising blind, deaf, physically handicapped, crippled with leprosy, mental retardation is included under social problem.

Rehabilitation services with health care, education of blind, deaf, physical rehabilitation, vocational training are being undertaken to meet the above social challenges.

Difference Between Society and Community

Society is group of people who settle down permanently and organise themselves. This shows a social system with demonstrable social relationships between individuals. Here behaviour of individual is regulated by social regulations.

Society changes from time to time as a dynamic process. It incorporates one or more communities.

Community is a social group determined by a markable boundary. It shows common values and common interests. It demarcates a geographical area to map out a village, a town, a city or a nation. Community is a network of human relationships; it is a major functioning unit of society; our house is located in a community our children are educated in a community. Human basic needs are met in the community.

Role, Status, Race

Role

In the social system we have many roles to play like son, daughter, brother, sister, teacher, lecturer, priest, mother, father, grandfather, grandmother and the like. These roles demarcate our relationships within a social system. Role confirms the behaviour of an individual to differentiate with others in the group. When it is given by virtue of age, sex, etc., it is called "Ascribed Role". By virtue of education, job experience when done it is "Achieved Role". We play our role as nurses and doctors in health care services. When training is given to a nurse it is called "Role Induction".

Status

Status is an Achieved Role or Ascribed Role in the community or society. It can be head of the family, head of the state and head of the country. This is possible by social selection and is demarcated with political activity. Status gives power to produce or to modify norms, values and customs. It is also called a social honour or prestige accorded to a person by society. Such status groups follow their normal life style and behavioural pattern. According to sociologists status may be positive or negative. Group leader is a positive status; outcast is negative status.

Race

On the basis of biologically grounded features, many competencies are assigned to a group or to individuals who demonstrate a set of social relationships. Many attributes of biological origin help to differentiate a group which is called Race.

SOCIALISATION

It is a social process where man inducts his role as an individual in a family, society or community. He gains the knowledge of norms, values, sanctions and customs in the process of socialisation.

Types of Socialisation

Primary Socialisation

A child on developing awareness of social norms and values achieves a sense of self. This infant and childhood process is first time socialisation. The child gets easily influenced and hence its development of sense of self determines the culture it gets.

Secondary Socialisation

This is achieved by man when he gets exposed to outside family environment like school, neighbourhood etc., where he gets the second chance to achieve sense of self. This further ties him up to the future social norms and values.

Re-Socialisation

When a person has to mix with other culture, other race that have customs other than his primary or secondary level, he starts acquiring that culture to become a member of that group. This is a needed sociological call. Typical example is when a boy or a girl from India goes to U.S.A. for higher studies, first few weeks of his or her adaptation to acquire new culture.

Process of Socialisation

It is a life long process in man. It allows individuals to develop themselves and their potential to learn and to make adjustments.

Sigmund Freud has postulated that dependency, fear; need for sympathy and love takes the child to social process of socialisation where he/she may replicate the values and culture of parents and other relatives.

Principle of socialisation is used in nursing training where we do "role induction". During nursing training, set of norms are achieved by the student nurse.

Social Control

Human social behaviour is regulated by many factors. At family level we come across social regulations and in a society we see law and enactment. These are to regulate social behaviour towards normal. This has the control over deviation from normal.

Rewards and *punishments* control behaviour. Standardised social interactions become *customs.* Among them a few are stringent and are called *mores.* They become *social regulations* when we observe them as formal ones. Cultural standards in a society are termed as value orientation. *Fashion* is a typical example of value orientation in social control. Right way of doing things in society is called *folkway.* Most of the occasions, folkways are done by reflex and do not carry vital importance.

In nursing profession we have many social controls for an effective training. Code of conduct and dress code is a formal social control enforced in nursing college. Similarly, nurses take an oath in an oath-taking ceremony which can be regarded as formal social control of the institution.

Social Group

A number of individuals when they interact, when they perceive creating a sense of "we" or "they", social group is formed. There are many uses of social group.

Crowd, Public, Audience

These are temporary without commonness. They are just emotional and do not have goal oriented activities. Colloquially it is called "mob" and mob mentality is described when there is no need for interaction in a group.

FAMILY

Definition

"It is a group of individuals who are biologically related and live together, and eat from a common kitchen." House and social environment are shared by them and hence a family is called a "Social unit" or a "Cultural unit". By removing the word "biologically related", the unit becomes a "household".

Types of Family

Nuclear family: This is an elementary family of married couple and their unmarried children.

Joint family: This has more than one married couple and their children, who live together in the same household.

Three generation family: When married sons or daughters live with parents along with their children.

Extended family: When old generations live, unmarried children live, polyandrous and polygamous couple live, married daughters live in father's house (matrilocal), married sons live in in-laws house (patrilocal) extended family is formed.

Family Cycle

There are four stages:

Stage 1 : Stage of formation when couple marry.

Stage 2 : Stage of growth when children are born.
Stage 3 : Stage of retraction when children marry and go away.
Stage 4 : Stage of disintegration when death of one or both parents occurs.

Functions of the Family

- Child birth and child rearing
- Sexual gratification
- Primary socialisation of individual occurs
- Social and mental stress are overcome
- Social and economic support is obtained
- Social interaction brings about new knowledge
- Each member has a role play and a job responsibility.

Family Problems

- Infertility, sterility
- Adoption
- Egoism
- Marital disharmony
- Broken family
- Poor social interaction
- Divorce
- Economic problem
- Malnutrition
- Alcoholism
- Conflict due to non adaptation of culture
- Susceptibility to diseases
- Chronic illness in the family.

Marriage

It is a socially approved relation which allows sexual relationship between two individuals of opposite sex. Marriage forms basis of a family of procreation with an expectation that married couple will produce and bring up children.

Deviant marriage: Modern families are seen with homosexual marriages which do not serve the purpose of marriage. Similarly polygamy or polyandry is deviant marriage which forms extended families as seen in certain religions.

Modern Families

Pattern of family is getting changed due to accessibility and availability of social and economic sanctions. When both couple are earning members, child rearing is by a contract worker. Marriage is a permanent bond and leaving to separate and no longer living together is legally permitted by the Act of Divorce. Following outcomes are seen in modern families:

- Lone parent household
- Remarriage
- Female partner to head the family
- Violence and abuse in the family
- Low accordance to family values.

Change in Indian Family

Slowly, size of the family, type of the family and composition of the family are changing due to varied social interactions and progressive urbanisation and civilisation. Slowly, there has been reduction in joint family or three generation family. Average size of the family has come down from 6.3 to 4.7.

This change has led to loosening of social regulation, and decreasing role of family in health and disease. Indian women, like western culture, face difficulty in reproductive and child health period, which used to be taken care of by elderly women at home. Kinship in the family is slowly deteriorating. Nuclear family is predominant mainly because of industrialisation of societies. Divorce rate is increasing. Thus there is considerable diversity in family norms.

Legislation on Indian Marriage and Family

Family law, Hindu law cover the legal implications of divorce, remarriage, property dispute and caretaker of offspring, which regulate the social problems from time to time.

As a policy measure age at marriage for a boy and girl have been fixed at 18 and 21 years respectively. This dictum is given as a family planning measure.

Civil marriage and registered marriage are allowed as per Marriage Act in India. As per Registration of Births, Deaths and Marriage Act, Registration of Marriage (even after civil marriage) is made mandatory.

Since social regulation is no longer found useful in social control over family issues, legislation on Indian marriage is put into action for allowing smooth and effective family pattern.

The Urban Families

Since population is getting concentrated in urban areas due to industrialisation with varied occupation, urban family has moulded to a pattern which needs consideration in a social system. This has led to "urban crisis" which is a direct impact of increased exponential urban growth (now it is 3.09%).

Following table gives urban rural contrast (Table 2.2):

Table 2.2: Urban-Rural contrast for families

Item	*Rural*	*Urban*
Population	Thin	Dense
Occupation	Agriculture	Varied
Social dependence	Self-reliant	Dependent
Social interaction	Primary	Secondary
Caste system	Dominant	Not dominant
Geographic boundary	Small	Big
Residence area	Not planned	Planned

Urban families are facing following economic, social and health problems:

- *Health problems:* Diarrhoea, STD, Hepatitis, skin infection, malignancy.
- *Social problems:* Alcoholism, drug use, prostitution.
- *Environmental problems:* Road accidents, atmosphere pollution (Air, water, soil pollutions).
- *Economic problems:* Poverty.
- *Psychological problems:* Stress, anxiety, neurosis, suicides.

Above family problems are mainly (a) Poverty induced or (b) Prosperity induced.

Healthy family movement is determined by social interactions and civic amenities.

They are: Small family norm.
Quality and quantity of food.
Healthy environment.
Slum improvement measures.

Social Stratification

Social inequality is present in all types of communities. In some it may be by race, while in others it may be by caste.

Ranking of social activities according to values are age old phenomenon. This is a requirement for functioning of society. Another cause of social classification seems to be to hold position and power in a society.

Health Implications

a. Social class is related to certain types of diseases; malnutrition among low socio-economic, hypertension among high socio-economic group illustrate the relation.
b. Susceptible or risk group identification is possible.
c. Health service planning is possible.

Social Classification

By Occupation

We come across this classification in Britain (Registrar General of England) (Table 2.3).

Table 2.3: Socio-economic classification by occupation

Social Class	*Occupation*
I	Professional
II	Managerial
III	Skilled
IV	Semiskilled
V	Unskilled

By Education

By educational status social stratification is done in the society.

By Income

Income alone is not considered for social classification. It gives value of socio-economic grouping. However with other variables many methods are adopted in research methodology.

Rural Community in India

About 71.6% of population live in rural community in over 700,000 villages. Govt. of India has 3-tier system of health care for primary health care through village health guide, Anganwadi worker and traditional birth attendant.

Health Profile of Villages

- Health problems—infection, malnutrition, poor sanitation, shortage of health personnel.
- Demography picture—more young people with paediatric problem, high rates of birth, death, growth, infant mortality, maternal mortality and low life expectation.
- Socio-economic picture—joint family system with agriculture as occupation, low rates of per capita income, literacy rate, standard of living and medical care.

Changes in Indian Rural Life

Panchayat Raj System has come into effect to uplift villages and for democratic decentralisation. Three tier system of local self government is as under:

Gram Panchayat	-	at village level
Mandal Panchayat	-	at block level
Zilla Panchayat	-	at district level

Gram panchayat is responsible for village improvement.

Cooperative movement has brought cooperatives in agriculture, bank, marketing to facilitate village upliftment.

Following G.O.I. programmes are approved from time to time for rural development and for social and economic growth:

1. Indira Awas Yojana (IAY)—Shelter to shelterless
2. Jawahar Rozgar Yojana (JRY)—Sustained employment
3. Employment Assurance Scheme (EAS)—Assured employment
4. Million Wells Scheme (MWS)—open irrigation wells
5. Integrated Rural Development Programme (IRDP)
6. Development of Women and Children in Rural Areas (DWACRA)
7. Training of Rural Youth for Self Employment (TRYSEM)
8. Supply of Toolkits to Rural Artisans
9. Land Reforms (Surplus land distribution)
10. Waste Land Development
11. Old age pension scheme
12. Rural women delivery allowance.

Social Change

It is an alteration in basic structure of a social group. Social change is a continuously occurring social phenomenon in life. They are now intense in modern era. There has been a tremendous shift from traditional system to modern social system.

Determinants

Following are the determinants of social change:

i. Demographic – Age, sex, occupation, education

ii.	Behaviour	– Suicide, homicide, delinquency, sexual offences
iii.	Culture	– Values, custom, etc.
iv.	Social structure	– Family pattern, social control.

Influencing factors of social change:

- Physical environment
- Political environment
- Cultural environment

Change in social system in modern period is mainly due to economic influence, political influence and cultural influence.

Social Change Indicators

- Development of Science and Technology
- Agriculture Development
- Modernisation of Industry
- Ecological changes.

Standards of Living

It refers to ways of living as shown by spending capacity and acquiring capacity. This depends on:

a. National income
b. Total production
c. Population growth
d. Educational level.

Standard of living is related to health and disease. High standard of living brings down diarrhoea, cholera, tuberculosis and improves health status in population. Standard of living determines birth rate, death rate, nutritional level and life expectancy.

CULTURE

Culture is defined as values, ceremonies and ways of life characteristic of a given social group. Culture is one of the most distinctive properties of human social association. Culture stands for mode of living, language, custom and belief. Hence it is socially acquired and learned behaviour.

Cultural pattern in India : (examples)

Health and disease	– It is by supernatural factor It is by sin of past life.
Personal hygiene	– Bathing everyday done Apply oil before bath Pan, supari, lime eaten as custom Hukka smoking is a custom Walking barefoot is common.
Environmental hygiene	– Open field defecation, using river water for ablution purposes, washing animals in the same source of water.
R.C.H.	– Certain foods are avoided in pregnancy, lactation, infancy. Delivery is conducted by untrained indigenous Dai. Newborn is not given colostrum Cow dung application to cut end of umbilical cord Skin branding for headache.
Nutrition	– Higher caste do not eat non-vegetarian food. – Some foods are hot – Some are cold – Eating garlic is a taboo.

Above illustration gives us the cultural pattern of people which has direct bearing on health activities.

Understanding of culture is important to bring about changes in habit, custom and belief of the community, with respect to health of the individual and community.

SOCIAL SECURITY

It is defined as "Security that society furnishes through appropriate organisation, against risk to which people are exposed." Common risks are:

Sickness, Invalidity, Maternity, Old age, Death.

They are classified under 3 categories:

a. *For industry workers*
   Indian Factory Act, 1948
   E.S.I.S., 1948
   Workmen Compensation Act, 1923
   Central Maternal Benefit Act, 1961
   Family Pension Scheme, 1971
b. *For Civil Servants*
   Pension
   Gratuity
   P.F.
   Family pension
c. *For public*
   Insurance schemes
   P.P.F.

Social Security Benefits are distributed through three channels. They are:

(i) Social Assistance

It covers old age pension, widow pension, assistance to leprosy patients, F.P. assistance, old age homes, stipend for unemployed graduates, maternity assistance to the poor and senior citizen facility.

(ii) Social Defence

In includes Punishment of criminals, Anti Dowry Act, Eradication of beggary, Welfare of prisoners, Alcohol prohibition, Gambling control, Prostitution control, Suicide counselling.

(iii) Social Insurance

Like ESI, Crop insurance, Accident insurance, Insurance for health.

Social Agencies

As part of social cultural tradition, there are many social welfare services as an integral part of community development. In the field of social welfare, it is estimated that there are about 60,000 voluntary organisations in India doing yeomanly services. Coordination of social welfare is by Ministry of Social Welfare and Central Social Welfare Board. They are categorised as:

a. All welfare activities
b. Women welfare
c. Child welfare
d. Specific disease control
e. Specific welfare activities.

PSYCHOLOGY

Psychology is concerned with human behaviours. Both physical factors and mental factors (Bodily action/function and mental action/function) interact with each other which are more complicated than a circuit and computer.

Man has set certain do's and don'ts in his setting. His behaviour is determined by these factors. Acceptance or a sanction for treatment also is determined by his behaviour.

In nursing care we come across following types of behaviour which directs the individual towards acceptance or rejection of care.

a. **Health Behaviour:**
   Oral hygiene, care of teeth, care of genital organs, periodic health check-up to identify risks at early phase, eating habit, sleeping habit, bowel habit etc., are examples of health behaviour. They help in prevention of many diseases. Monogamy and marital harmony is another example of health behaviour which prevents S.T.D. and AIDS.
b. **Illness Behaviour:**
   In early part of sickness home remedy from enquiry with friends, advices from elders are common. This is a natural reaction to subjec-

tive manifestations of a disease. On the contrary, health awareness helps in early diagnosis and prompt treatment.

c. **Treatment Behaviour:**
Acceptance or no acceptance of activities suggested for disease form treatment behaviour. Some like oral, others parenteral (injections) medicine at advice. Many are scared of surgery and go for medical treatment only. In nursing care, taking drugs or medicamentation as directed and return for follow-up and advice is regarded as good treatment behaviour.

Definition

Psychology is "the study of human behaviour, the study of how people behave, the study of why they behave and which are within accepted norm".

Scope

Psychology is glued with every aspect of human life. It is seen in all types of human interaction. Understanding of human mind helps us to analyse intricacies involved in mental disorders. There are various branches of psychology which deal with day-to-day occurrence in human behaviour. These branches are:

- Social psychology
- Educational psychology
- Child psychology
- Applied psychology
- Psycho analysis
- Medical psychology (psychiatry)
- Adult psychology
- Women psychology
- Elders psychology.

Application to Nursing

Psychology helps a nurse in understanding the need of a patient. Nurse can motivate patient for required helpful activity useful for recovery. She can make patient think and reason out in medical emergencies. Understanding emotions and feelings of the sick will be the secret of success in effective nursing care. Psychotherapy may be required in cases of psychosomatic disorders like Asthma, Peptic ulcer, ulcerative colitis, hypertension etc.

Methods

Methods adopted in psychology, as a science of behaviour in abnormal behaviours and mental illnesses are:

- Psychoanalysis
- Psychodiagnosis
- Psychosocial counselling
- Psychotherapy.

Motivation

It is the driving force in human psychology. Man is driven to any social action by an inner force. Motivation thus, is the best determinant of behaviour. There are two sides of motivation. They are:

- Positive motivation (Right-doing-behaviour)
- Negative motivation (Wrong-doing-behaviour).

Occasionally manipulation is confused with motivation. MANIPULATION is acquiring phenomenon for a developed desire and urge.

Definition

Motivation is the desire, acquired to gratify the needs. It includes all activities and needs which are directed to acquire gratification.

Needs and Drives

Human needs are basic, additional and health needs. Some psychologists include luxury as a type of need.

To acquire and gratify above needs man has 2 major types of drives—One is innate and the other acquired.

Range and Classification of Needs and Drives

Needs are classified as under:

a. **Social need:** They are mainly desired needs like love, affection, recognition, education etc., which pertains to social nature of man.
b. **Economic need:** To fulfil the want of economic security is topmost need of the day.
c. **Ego need:** Self respect, power, position and status are present updated items under needs.
d. **Biological need:** They are mainly survival needs like water, food, shelter etc.
e. **Psychological need:** Sympathy, concern, attachment, influence are under psychological needs.

DRIVES which are called motive are classified as under:

a. **Innate drive:** They are desires to gratify the biological needs.
    i. **Primitive innate drive:** Has come from ancestors and are reflex oriented. To charge a man who beats you is similar to animal instinct.
    ii. **Reflex innate drive:** Hunger contraction motivates to acquire food. Typical example is seen with dog experiment by Pavlov.
    iii. **Universal innate drive:** Some innate drives are common in human beings like acquiring a house, to become a good singer, like to have a baby boy, like to have an auto mobile vehicle and so on.
b. **Acquired drive:** During the process of socialisation, child or adult acquires certain drives which are learned during social acts. A boy who wants to show off is acquired by observing others, dresses up most fashionably to meet a girl. This is an acquired drive to meet a psychological need.

EMOTIONS

They are strong feelings of human beings. Emotions always motivate men which are often irreversible. Visible changes of emotion are happiness, depression, anger, morose, hilarious etc. Invisible changes of emotion are rise in pulse, respiration, blood pressure, pain and tension. Both visible and invisible emotions usually return to normal with rest and relaxation (Fig. 2.2).

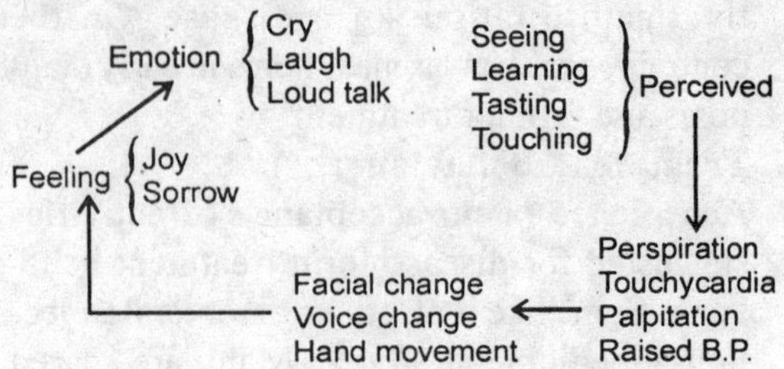

Fig. 2.2: General theory of emotion

Types of Emotions

Specific Emotions

Anger, Fear, Hate, Love.

Nonspecific Emotions

Grief, Joy, Jealousy, Lust, Moodiness, Pity, Sorrow, Sympathy.

Emotions are major barriers of communication. Only after "Pass-off" period of emotion, patient can talk freely and there is chance of effective nurse-patient interaction for nursing procedures.

Definition

Emotion is defined as "Sudden force surfacing in the mind in response to a situation."

States of Emotion

There are two states of emotion:

i. Positive state—Pleased, Joyous, Loved, Satiated etc.
ii.. Negative state—Sad, Sorrowful, Angry, Hateful, Fearful etc.

Emotion as a Motive

Emotion expressed becomes a motive to gratify the needs. A nurse falling unconscious at work attracts attention. Her friends get emotional to see her state of affair. It is a motive for quick interaction. Duty nurse is motivated to attend to her at her best out of emotional attachment to her professional colleague.

Both positive and negative emotions are found useful as motives in Health Care services.

- *Example of positive emotion as a motive:* Very low birth interval with low birth weight, repeated infection of newborn emotionally makes a mother to get motivated. She accepts "Spacing" as contraceptive method for the sake of health of newborn.
- *Example of negative emotion as a motive:* Showing a clinical case of tetanus to a mother who used to resist TT for her children, explaining her that TT as the only weapon to prevent tetanus. Emotions of fear and concern in the mother allow her child to get TT by negative motivation.

Emotion and Health

Various disorders are seen associated with emotions. These vary with age, sex and other demographic variables.

Adults – Loss of concentration
– Loss of appetite
– Increased accidents
– Loss of sleep
– Palpitation

Women – Anorexia nervosa
– Amenorrhoea
– Pseudo pregnancy

Children – Tantrums
– Abdominal pain
– Spasms
– Tics
– Aggressiveness

Control of Emotions:

Children – Love
– Affection
– Appreciation

Adults – Happy family life
– Reassurance
– Cultivating hobbies
– Habit of reading
– Recreation
– Adaptation of philosophy in life
– Understanding one's own limitations
– Development of sense of humour.

PERSONALITY

Since personality determines human behaviour and human behaviour is moulded by personality, they are inter-related. Personality of health professional influence prognosis of sick and hospitalized (Fig. 2.3).

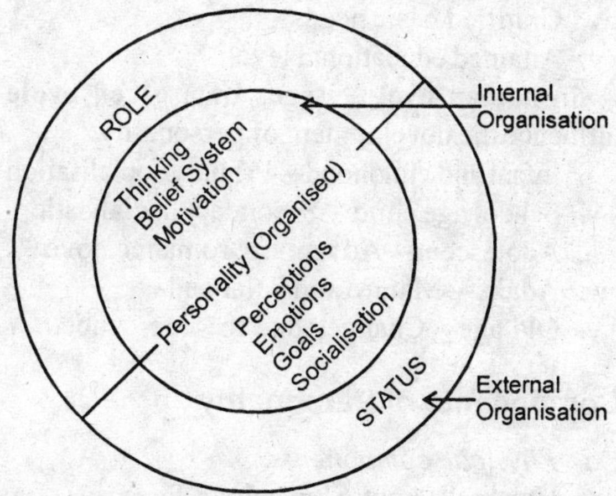

Fig. 2.3: Organisation of personality

Definition

Personality is defined as body pattern which are influenced by status role etc., externally and by thinking, desire, goals and motivation etc., internally and all these lead to an aspect of selfhood.

Types

According to Swiss psychiatrist Carl Jung (1875-1961), there are three types of human personalities:

i. *Extrovert:* A person always exhibits his feelings, easily mixes and active, deemed practical and daredevil in action.
ii. *Introvert:* A person always shy, keeps himself aloof, reserved.
iii. *Mixed:* A combination of extrovert and introvert.

Development of Personality

Following factors help in development of personality. They are:

i. Heredity (Parent's reflection)
ii. Physical environment
iii. Social environment
iv. Gratified basic needs
v. Attained educational level.

In human cycle, stages of a given cycle influence the development of personality.

i. Infant and childhood—Primary socialisation
ii. School age child—Secondary socialisation
iii. Adolescent—Adventure, romance, love
iv. Adults—Mature and balanced
v. Old age—Changes due to senescence.

Components of Personality

i. *Physical components:*
Height, Weight, Skin colour, Face.
ii. *Emotional components:*
Anger, Fear, Guilt, Jealousy, Love, Worries.
iii. *Intelligence components:*
I.Q.
iv. *Behaviour component:*
Kindness, Affection, Aggressiveness, Submissiveness, Balanced nature.

Personality Trait

It is defined as the stable personality manner and the tendency to behave in such a manner for a given social interaction. By 5 years 10 months, the child develops basic personality trait. In adulthood some traits are cultivated and some are concealed. Some of the examples of personality traits are:

- Kindness
- Reliability
- Sense of humour
- Loyalty
- Tactfulness
- Willingness to help
- Good manners
- Cheerfulness.

LEARNING

Learning is a psychosocial process that is required for survival and human progress. It is not equivalent to education but implies acquiring knowledge, skills and habit formation and perception development. Human intelligence has led to lot of change in learning. Age old observation and service at Gurukula for a learning which used to take years of exposure, has been reduced to a shorter spell of time where learning is processed even independently. Conscious learning is an adopted behaviour, whereas unconscious learning is a conditional behaviour.

Definition

Learning is an active and continuous process which results in relatively permanent behavioural change in man. This is reflected through thinking, feeling, doing and attitude of a learner. It is also an outcome of one's interactive experience with his surrounding.

Law of Learning

Learning has come up through all stages of human development—Birth, Marriage, Family-formation,

Service, Health, Sickness, Disability and even Death. Learning is appropriated for survival and progress. It is for habit formation and perception development. Law of learning helps an individual to face any psychosocial interaction by reflex and not allow him to succumb to injury or death.

Principles of Learning

Various theories of learning have evolved certain principles which are applied in learning activities to enhance learning.

The *Principles* of learning are:

a. Human learning is guided by many set goals to be achieved either at a short time or on a long-term.
b. Human needs in terms of physiological, safety, social, esteem, self actualization and aesthetic needs are strong reasons for learning.
c. Life oriented education through observation and participation form the basis of learning.
d. It is a voluntary process involving thinking, feeling and doing. Hence it involves the learner actively.
e. Basic styles of learning in man have been surface learning, deep learning and strategic learning.
f. There should be learning with an understanding which is called meaning orientation in learning.
g. Learning leads to knowledge and in turn should lead to application of mind.
h. Learning should be for a real life situation and real life problem solving.
i. Learning should begin from known and should proceed to unknown.
j. Reinforcement of learning is possible by feedback process.

Types of Learning

Present concept of classification in learning is called as "Taxonomy in Education".

There are three main types of learning. They are:

Bloom's "Cognitive Domain"

This is the area of intellectual skills. Learning is by acquiring, recalling and recognising a thing or an item.

Bloom and Krathwohl's "Affective Domain"

This is the area of learning communication skills. It deals with interpersonal relationships. Learning is considered by interest, attitude, values, appreciations and adjustment.

Krathwohl's "Psychomotor Domain"

This is the area of practical skill learning. It involves mind and perception. Further, human neuromuscular coordination determines this behaviour of learning.

Examples of above types of learning:

a. Knowledge Gain (Cognitive Domain):
- Nurse defines hypertension
- She enumerates APGAR scoring
- She understands normal menses to decide ideal contraceptive.

b. Communication skill (Affective domain):
- Nurse understands anxiety of patient going to O.T. room for operation.
- She gives reassurance to patient on the issue of scheduled operation.
- She helps to overcome emotion of the patient to cooperate in O.T.

c. Practical Skill (Psychomotor domain):
- Nurse learns and does cardiopulmonary resuscitation.
- Nurse learns and gives enema to a patient as preoperative procedure.

Methods of Memory

i. Recitation or learning by heart.
ii. Practical doing and undoing (Trial and Error).

iii. Observation and recording.
iv. Using mnemonic, phrases, anecdotes and proverb or life situations.
v. Personal exposure to experience.
vi. Group interactions.

THINKING AND REASONING

In man's perception, memory and imagination have given way to thinking. As a higher order of mental process there is a psychosocial analysis in brain called Reasoning.

Routine, skill use, performance of an activity create an opportunity for thinking.

Thinking may produce pleasant or violent aspect of thoughts. Outwardly expression of thinking is called extrovert and expressionless thinking is called introvert. Bizarre thinking produces psychopaths in the society.

Types of Thinking

i. **Objective thinking:** Here there is logical association between events and symbols. It is a disciplined imagination. Objective thinking leads to many scientific innovations and discoveries.
ii. **Wishful thinking:** Evading tendency of man leads to wishful thinking. It is also called Fantasies. This represents future anticipation of an individual. Very common wishful thinking area are Health and Wealth. Among adolescents it is romance that makes wishful thinking.
iii. **Imaginative thinking:** Day dreaming and thinking of impossibilities like magic world or wonder world is imaginative thinking. These do not serve any purpose in life except spending time in an unfruitful way.
iv. **Creative thinking:** It refers to thoughts brought out by an effective learning where there is scope for new ideas, new discoveries and new inventions. Creative thinking is a common word used in dress making, art, painting etc.

Development of Thinking

Education and commitment leads to development of objective thinking and creative thinking. Psychosocial norms should facilitate the process of required thinking and avoiding unrequired thinking. Unrequired thinking leads to worrying which is not a health process. Hence required thinking should be encouraged in an atmosphere of good psychosocial environment.

Camp lives, attending religious discourses, well developed hobbies regulate a covert activity of objective thinking. "Best thinking is to forget everything" makes you and allows you to effectively regulate ways of your thinking.

Reasoning

It is the highest stage of human thinking where he tries to solve problems in life which may be simple or complicated. Thinking and allowing the use of intelligence brings about reasoning. Careful reasoning disallows fallacies.

Types of Reasoning

i. Primitive reasoning comes from conventional outline. Problem solving in daily routine is from primitive reasoning where individual's experience, family experience and society experience play a vital role.
ii. Psychosocial reasoning comes from understanding of behaviour, personality and interpersonal relationships.
iii. Scientific reasoning is based on demonstrable scientific reasons in reasoning.

Problem Solving Methods

Thinking and reasoning are used in solving both simple and complicated issues in life situations. Collection and arrangement of information on a subject, drawing conclusions and testing conclusions are methods used in practical problem solving methods.

Examples of Problem Solving by Reasoning and Thinking

a. You are on a call to conduct normal home delivery in a house situated nearer the sub centre. When you visit the house, woman is in first stage of labour and there is rupture of amniotic fluid. Discuss your nursing line of management.
b. An elderly woman at home has fallen and has sustained fracture of neck of femur (Right side). Reason out your first line of management of this elderly woman at home.
c. In labour room, you have conducted a normal delivery and the mother with newborn is to be shifted to postnatal ward. You are expected to assess the mother before shifting. Describe your nursing procedure.

Here the nurse is expected to explain post partum techniques to be performed; viz., Assessing the mother by (a) Palpating the fundus and bladder (b) Evaluate the lochia (c) Inspect the perineum (d) Inspect and palpate the breasts to confirm normalcy before shifting.

INTELLIGENCE

Intelligence is an aspect of personality. It is defined as "an ability to see meaningful relationships between interrelated matters".

General Intelligence in Nursing

Taking over charge, handing over charge, morning assessment before clinical round, attending to duty doctor's instructions, drug administration, sample dispatch for investigation, getting report collected, recording 4th hourly pulse, respiration recording 6th hourly, body temperature recording 12th hourly, blood pressure recording etc., are commonly done routine nursing which is managed with general intelligence.

Special Intelligence in Nursing

Assisting in heart transplant operation, performing kidney dialysis, case management in ICU, ICCU, IPCU and emergency nursing care require special intelligence.

Concept of Mental Age in Intelligence

According to Benet and Simen (1896) who developed the concept, Mental age is determined by yearwise acquired and adopted tests which measures aptitude. Accordingly the outcome of test describes the mental age or intelligence by skill. It does not include details of the lowered or altered mental acumen to group the child under normal for age or not normal for the age. A 7 years child passing intelligence skill test of child aged 6 years does not mean that the child is dull. Thus mental age determination serves as a relative expression in psychoanalysis.

Intelligence Tests

Individual Performance Test

Understanding of language, general understanding, reasoning are used to measure psychological process of individual performance. Here time fixation is not a factor. There are specifications in test set to formulate evaluation of (a) Young children (b) Illiterates (c) Feeble mindedness (d) Monolinguist.

I.Q. Tests are applied which are concepts of mental age, improved upon to obtain a quotient by chronological age.

$$\text{I.Q.} = \frac{\text{Mental age}}{\text{Chronological age}} \times 100$$

Normal I.Q. ranges from 90 to 100 in our set up. When mental age and chronological age is same it comes to 100 which is an average.

According to level of I.Q. grouping of individual is done which is as follows:

Level of Intelligence	*I.Q.*
Genius	140 and above
Very superior	120–139
Superior	110–119
Normal	90–109
Low normal	80–89
Border line	70–79
Moron	50–69
Imbecile	25–49
Idiot	0–24

I.Q. measures the quality and potential intelligence. Higher performance is closely related to higher I.Q.

Adult intelligence is analysed based on item analysis. According to Thurstone, adult intelligence includes 8 components and item analysis of these 8 components proves efficient method of intelligence analysis.

They are:

i. Memory of words and ideas
ii. Ability of finding out principles
iii. Ability of using principles in solving problems
iv. Ability of expression with appropriate words
v. Ability of verbal comprehension
vi. Familiarity of elementary arithmetic
vii. Ability to perceive objects
viii. Flexibility and quickness of thought.

Uses of I.Q. Test in Psychology

- Arrangement of special education to low I.Q. individuals
- Selection of able individuals for a given task performance
- To test the eligibility of individual for an entry to a formal or informal education
- Help in work allotment according to ability of individual
- Common entrance tests for the selection to professional colleges
- Help in educational guidance
- Help in therapeutic prognosis.

EDUCATIONAL PSYCHOLOGY

Proper education of child starts from birth and the child is ready for formal education by 5 completed years. At this stage he is ready for learning only elementary things.

Meaning

Imparting sound education at different age levels is an arduous task because intelligence development and level of ability is found to vary from age to age. Children of same age are not alike in their mental capacity. The scientific study on individual differences has revealed that there are significant differences in the rate of mental growth and that different functions in the same child will grow at different rates. Vijay aged 9 years is found able to solve arithmetic problems whereas his elder sister Asha aged 12 years cannot solve arithmetic problem though she is more intelligent than Vijay. These variations in capacity render the problem of teaching even more difficult than it would otherwise be.

Scope and Aims

According to Kelly, purposes of educational psychology are as under:

- To give knowledge on the nature of the child.
- To give an understanding of the nature, aims and purpose of education.
- To give an understanding of the scientific methods and procedures which have been used in arriving at the facts and principles of educational psychology.
- To present the principles and techniques of learning and teaching.
- To give training in methods of measuring abilities and achievements in school subjects.
- To give knowledge on the growth and development of children.
- To assist in the better adjustment of children and help to prevent their maladjustment.

- To study the educational significance and control of emotions.
- To give an understanding of the principles and techniques of character training.

Individual Differences

It is obvious that people are physically different. Motor and sensory functions also differ greatly in individuals. Based on individual difference in intelligence men are classified into genius, normal, idiot etc.

But scientific observation has made it clear that all are qualitatively alike mentally, but differ in the degree of efficiency with which different functions work. Mind of a genius is similar to that of an idiot. But genius learns more easily, remembers easily and solves difficult problems.

Attitude

Meaning and Nature

Attitude is an expected response towards a stimulus. This describes the readiness to react. There are two types of attitude. They are:

Positive attitude: e.g., Person thinks that pneumonia is curable and penicillin is a weapon for it.

Negative attitude: e.g. Leprosy is not curable.

Attitude signifies individual preferences. They are acquired by social interactions and observed experiences. Attitude survey and attitude measurements are included in recent epidemiological approaches.

Development

Attitude is developed by experience and it is the effect of environmental stimuli. Attitudes are conditioned by the growth of intelligence.

Following are examples of attitude development:

- Young child has limited capacity for understanding world and so incapable of forming attitude.
- 7 years child can observe a picture and make out what is taking place in the picture. But it cannot interpret the reason for happening in the picture.
- 12 years child can interpret the reason for what happening in a picture.
- Adolescence is marked especially by the maturation of sexual emotions.

Factors Influencing the Development of Attitude Age

- Home influences
- The social environment
- School environment
- Movie, TV serial
- Teacher
- The curriculum
- Teaching methods
- Group memberships
- Associations.

Measurement of Attitude

Suitable scales are available to measure attitude.

Characteristics of an Effective Teacher

According to Robbins, following are characteristics of an effective teacher:

i. Makes the course interesting.
ii. Knows subject matter of the course.
iii. Shows enthusiasm.
iv. Has the material well organised.
v. Encourage student participation.
vi. Uses practical illustration.
vii. Has real sense of humour.
viii. Has friendly personality.
ix. Shows interest in the students.
x. Has pleasant voice.
xi. Neatly dressed.
xii. Has a poised and business like attitude.

Teacher-Learner Relationship

In educational psychology teacher-student relation is built up by abovementioned characteristics of an effective teacher. This is also an important element for a positive attitude in education.

HABIT

Habits are defined as accustomed way of doing things. They are acquired through repetitive act and are automatically executed. Habits are executed only under similar circumstances. They can become customs in due course to influence human behaviour. They may be grouped as under:

i. Good habits
ii. Bad habits
iii. Healthy habits.

Principles involved in habit formation are:

- It starts from early childhood.
- Frequently repeated.
- Occurs in due course of time.
- Emotions create habits.
- They are under human control.

Conflicts

It is a powerful repulsive action between two courses of actions. They are configured with emotions. Correct decision always keeps us away from conflicts. Conflicts cause emotional disturbances and leads to neurological disorders.

Frustrations

When man is unable to meet his needs and desires he ends up with frustrations. External causes are failure, defeat, unemployment and internal causes are poor health, low I.Q. etc.

Frustration can lead to nervous breakdown. Initially anger, dejection, hostility, suicidal tendencies are met with.

Frustration leads to drug abuse and alcoholism.

Defence Mechanisms

Problems, failures, difficulties make a man to employ certain defence mechanisms which help him to get a way to achieve happiness and success. Mentally healthy person uses them to achieve success or happiness. These defence mechanisms are:

a. Justification of behaviour: (Rationalisation) e.g., declaring grapes as sour.
b. Blaming others for fault: (Projection) e.g., Teachers are blamed for exam failure.
c. Enhancing self esteem by compensation: e.g., Poor in study shows up as good sportsman.
d. Escapism: e.g., Pretend ill at examination.
e. Displacing the situation: e.g., Office problem reflected at home.
f. Follow childhood practice: e.g., Crying.

SOCIAL PSYCHOLOGY

It is a branch of psychology and deals with behaviour of an individual in society. It studies attitude of individual towards culture and social values.

Group Behaviour

Interaction and social behaviour of individual in a group is called group behaviour. Man's activities are regulated by custom, law and social obligations. Group is led by a leader. It is responsible for solidarity of the group behaviour which is called "Group morale".

Group activity, group discussion, group opinion and group reaction are common psychosocial events in a society.

Group behaviour can lead to progressive reformation of society or can lead to civil unrest.

Social group is responsible for primary, secondary and re-socialisation of an individual. Social attitudes are shared by others in the community.

CHAPTER THREE

Health Statistics

INTRODUCTION

Statistics are of following types:

i. Health statistics which mainly deals with normal health aspect.
ii. Medical statistics which deals with data of case management.
iii. Vital statistics which deals with data pertaining to vital events like births, deaths etc.
iv. Biostatistics which deals with data of Biological and Biosciences.

These data are presently called "Health information" and the system or organisation which works for it is called "Health Information System".

Definition

WHO has defined health statistics as:

"A mechanism for the collection, processing, analysis and transmission of information required for organising and operating health science and also for research and training."

Mainly, statistics has a major role and is of great importance in National Health System. It has become a basic tool of management in public health.

Following terminologies are commonly used in elementary statistics:

Data : They are discrete observations and do not carry any meaning.

Information : They are tabulated data which give meaning.

Intelligence : They are transformed information based on social and political value.

Characteristics

Each individual is characterized by certain physical characters like age, sex, weight, Hb%, B.P., WBC count etc. Similarly there are some socio-economic characters like occupation, literacy, income. These qualities are called characteristics. These characteristics are grouped under two categories.

i. *Attributes:* Characters that are not measurable are called attributes. E.g., sex, death, survival etc. The person having attribute is countable and attribute as such is not countable.
ii. *Variable:* Characteristics that are measurable are called variables. E.g., Height, Hb%, etc.

Importance

Importance of statistics are enumerated as under:

a. It is a guide for nursing care services.
b. It is a tool for research.
c. It is a measure of health status of a community.
d. It identifies health problems.
e. It identifies health needs.
f. It helps in providing a scientific basis for recording, collection, compilation, presentation and analysis.

g. For comparing health status between individual to individual:
   - Society to society
   - Hospital to hospital
   - Community to community
   - District to district
   - State to state
   - Country to country.

h. For planning and health administration

i. It helps in finding out:
   - Impact of a health programme and health management.
   - Success or failure of an operation.

j. It helps in health programme evaluation.

k. It is a key to all health administration.

Statistics and Health Science

Application of statistical principles and methods are necessary, not only for understanding of biological and medical sciences but also for effective practice in health professions. Biological, clinical and laboratory data are variable and hence need statistics for understanding and interpretation.

In health science a course on statistics is necessary because:

- Decisions on diagnosis, prognosis and therapy are based on concepts of probability.
- Interpretation of tests, observations and measurements require knowledge of variations of physiological, observer and information.
- Epidemiological facts are necessary for controlling or preventing disease.
- Health workers who are primary data generators should know about statistics.
- Describing health level, health trend and health resources are possible through interpretations and inferences.
- Statistics in health sciences foster critical and analytical mind which are required during the course and later in professional practice.

Parameters

Parameter is a characteristic which describe population. When we say average size of family in India is 5.3, IMR in India is 71 per thousand LB, they indicate parameters.

When a sample is described by a unit it is called statistic. In a sample study of a village in Agra showed average family size as 6.0 and IMR of the same village as 74 per thousand LB, then characteristic describing this sample is statistic. Parameter is always single for a universe when compared to statistic which are many (for many samples).

Descriptive Statistics

Descriptive statistics are used to describe or characterise data by summarising them into more understandable terms without loosing or disturbing much of the information. *Examples:*

- Pie diagram
- Bar chart
- Frequency polygon.

DATA PRESENTATION

Raw Data, the Array, Frequency Distribution

Mass of raw data is available when they are collected. They do not mean anything for a profession to infer. No useful information is immediately evident from a mass of raw data. They are the array of number, words and response. These collected data need to be organised in such a way that the information they contain clearly reveals the pattern of variation.

Demographic Data

Before we can assess the magnitude of the health problem posed by a disease or impact of intervention we must have an idea of the size of the community we are dealing with, its composition with respect to various demographic characteristics and the magnitude of changes in relation to vital events.

Demographic data relates to health and illness of population for a community diagnosis.

They include:

- Population characteristics—size, age, sex etc.
- Health profile—risk factors.
- Environmental factors—Socio-economic aspect.
- Morbidity, mortality, fertility.
- Birth, death, migration.
- Reticulation—Boundary of census, unit etc.

Tabulation of Mortality

Crude and specific deaths, disease and cause specific deaths, age and sex specific deaths are considered for mortality data tabulation.

Tabulation of Morbidity

Disability, handicap, impairment, incidence, prevalence, population at risk, rate, ratio and population are considered for morbidity data tabulation.

Tabulation of Other Data

Fertility, current users, transition, relevance, health measures are considered for other data tabulation.

Diagrams

In addition to table and graph, diagrams are used which furnish a good impression of numbers and about idea. Real grasp of overall picture is possible by diagram. They are of course drawn based on set principles.

Bar Diagram

They are common and easiest diagrams for data presentation. They indicate the frequency of a character. Spacing between bars should be equal or more than half of the width of the bar. These are 3 types:

- Simple bar
- Multiple bar
- Component bar.

Line Diagram

When we present the data on a line it forms line (presenting variation by line) diagram. Since it produces many angles it is popularly called frequency polygon. In a line diagram the two ends need not be made to touch the X-axis. In frequency polygon the two ends of the graph is allowed to touch X-axis.

Frequency Curve

When numbers of observations are large and groups are more, the frequency polygon tends to loose its angulations and it forms a smooth curve called "Frequency curve".

When a frequency curve form bell shape and symmetrical around the mean of the distribution, it is called normal curve. We can define symmetry as frequencies at equal distances from the mean on either side are the same.

Pie Diagram

It is called a *sector diagram* where frequencies of the groups are shown in circle. Degrees of angle are denoted by frequencies and area of sector.

Total area of Pie diagram should be 100 percent and each angle is calculated as under:

$$\text{Angle} = \frac{\text{Class frequency}}{\text{Total observation}} \times 360$$

Dot Diagram

It is called *scattered diagram* where data show the nature of correlation between 2 characters (e.g., Age and weight).

This can also be called correlation diagram.

Picture Diagram

It is a method of illustration through picture (Figurative presentation).

Histogram

When data is represented in the form of column or rectangle it is called Histogram.

When midpoint of column or rectangle is joined it gives rise to a frequency polygon.

MEASURES OF CENTRAL TENDENCY

Computation of Mean, Median and Mode

For Ungrouped Data

10 nurses have I.Q. as follows:
158, 139, 120, 146, 111, 99, 114, 156, 111, 94.

Arithmetic mean = 158 + 139 + 120 + 146 + 111 + 99 + 114 + 156 + 111 + 94.

$$\textbf{Mean} = \frac{1248}{10} = 124.8$$

Median = We get mid value when they are arranged in an ascending order.

94, 99, 111, 111, 114, 120, 139, 146, 156, 158

$$\text{Median} = \frac{234}{2} = 117$$

Mode = Most fashionable number or the number which repeats most is taken which is 111, is mode.

Comparison and Uses of Mean, Median and Mode

Mean is best known and most widely used average. The median is not sensitive to extreme scores and is useful when the data are skewed. The mode is most frequently occurring value that has the largest frequency of scores.

Table 3.1: Comparative table of central values

Mean	*Median*	*Mode*
• Easy to calculate	• Easy to calculate	• Easy to calculate
• Easy to understand	• Not easy to understand	• Not easy to understand because not clearly defined
• Gets influenced by an abnormal value	• Not influenced by an abnormal value	• Not effected by abnormal value • We get more than one mode

MEASURES OF VARIABILITY (DISPERSION)

They include Range, Mean Deviation, Standard Deviation, Coefficient of Variation, Quartile Deviation and Variance.

Measures

Range: It is the value between minimum and maximum.

Mean Deviation: This is an average deviation from the mean.

Standard Deviation (S.D.)

For ungrouped data: Let us compute S.D. for I.Q. of 10 nurses which are as under:
158, 139, 120, 146, 111, 99, 114, 156, 111, 94.

x	$(\bar{x}-\bar{x})$	$(\bar{x}-\bar{x})^2$
158	33.2	1102.34
139	14.2	201.64
120	– 4.8	23.04
146	21.2	449.44
111	– 13.8	190.44
99	– 25.8	665.64
114	– 10.8	116.64
156	31.2	973.44
111	– 13.8	190.44
94	– 30.8	948.64

$$\bar{x} = \frac{1248}{10} = 124.8 \qquad \sqrt{\frac{\Sigma(x-\bar{x})^2}{n-1}} = \sqrt{\frac{4881.8}{8}}$$

$$\Sigma (x - \bar{x})^2 = 4881.8 \qquad S.D. = 23.24$$

Steps to Calculate S.D. of Ungrouped Data

- Find A.M. of I.Q.
- Find mean deviation of each
- Find square of each
- Find i.e. sum of squares
- Find the square root of above with D.F.= n or n-1 as denominator.

HEALTH INDICATORS

Concept, Importance

In order to evaluate the effectiveness and efficiency of a health treatment, health programme or health service, the extent of achievement of targets and objectives etc., we need the yardsticks called Health Indicators.

Health indicators measure health change, compare different stages of health and demarcate effective treatment. Inter-state and international comparison is possible through health indicators.

Examples of health indicators that are found appropriate in nursing health care services.

I. *Health status indicators:*
- Percentage of L.B.W.
- I.M.R., child mortality rate, under five mortality rate.
- Life expectation in years for a given age.
- MMR.
- Disease specific mortality rates.
- Disease specific morbidity rates.
- Disability rates.

II. *Indicator on the provision of nursing care:*
- Availability.
- Physical accessibility.
- Economic and cultural accessibility.
- Quality of care
- Level of health awareness.
- Availability of safe water within walkable distance.
- Conducting delivery by trained Dais.
- Availability of essential drugs.

III. *Socio-economic indicators:*
- Rate of population growth.
- Gross National and gross domestic product (GNP and GDP).
- Income distribution.
- Work availability.
- Adult literacy rate.
- Overcrowding (floor space per person).

IV. *Health policy indicators:*
- Level of political commitment.
- Allocation of adequate resources.
- Level of community involvement.

Rate, Ratio, Proportion

Magnitude of a disease, problem and event are expressed by rate, ratio and proportions. They are the basic tools in measurements of health and form common health indicators.

a. Rate = $\frac{\text{Numerator}}{\text{Denominator}}$ per 100, 1000, or 10,000 etc.

An event is measured in a population over a period of time and expressed per 1000 constitute rate.

Example:

$$\text{Birth rate} = \frac{\text{No. of Births in 1 year}}{\text{Mid year population}} \times 1000$$

Types of Rates are:

i. Crude Rates: e.g.: Death rate, Birth rate.
ii. Specific Rates: e.g.: Age specific Death by TB.
iii. Standardised Rates: e.g. : Standardised Death Rate.

b. *Ratio:* Ratio is an expression of relation in size between 2 random quantities. It is the result of dividing one quantity by another quantity.

Example:
Sex Ratio (986 females for 1000 males).
Nurse Population Ratio (1:21000).

c. *Proportion:* It is a ratio which indicates the relation in magnitude of a part to the whole, and is in percentage.

Examples:
Scabies in children is

$$\frac{\text{263 scabies children}}{\text{10000 children population}} \times 100 = 2.6\%$$

i.e., 2.6% children are scabies children.

Common Health Indicators

1. *Birth rate:* It is the number of live births during a year per 1000 mid year population.

$$\text{B.R.} = \frac{\text{No. of live births in 1 year}}{\text{MYP}} \times 1000$$

It is 25 at present (2003 estimate).

2. *Death rate:* It is the number of deaths per 1000 mid year population in 1 year.

$$\text{D.R.} = \frac{\text{No. of Deaths in 1 year}}{\text{MYP}} \times 1000$$

It is 8 at present (2003 estimate).

3. *Growth rate:* It is the difference between B.R and D.R and is expressed in percentage. It is now 1.7% at present (2003 estimate).
4. *Sex ratio:* It is the number of females per 1000 males. It is now 986.
5. *Dependency ratio:* This is proportion of persons above 65 years and below 15 years who are dependent on adult earning members.
   It is 55.5 in India at present (2005 estimate).
6. *Family size:* It is the total number of members in a family. It is 3.1 as per estimate in the year 2003.
7. *Literacy rate:* It is the number of literates (who can read and sign) (in his/her mother tongue) per 1000. It is now 65.38 as per 2001 census.
8. *Life expectancy:* It is expectation of life at birth i.e average number of years which a person of that age may be expected to live. It is now 62.10 for men and 64.00 for women at 2003 estimate.
9. *Age at marriage:* It is average age at which female marries and enters reproductive period of life. It is 19.5 years as per 1991 census data. Every 1 year increase in age at marriage brings down births by 4 to 5%.
10. *General Fertility Rate:* It is the number of live births per 1000 women in the age group of 15 to 49 years.

$$\text{G.F.R.} = \frac{\text{No. of Live Births in a year}}{\text{Mid year female population of 15-49 years}} \times 1000$$

It is 118.2 as per 1994 estimate.

11. *Total Fertility rate:* It is the average number of children a woman would have if she were to pass through her reproductive age group.
    It is 3.2 at present.
12. *Gross reproduction rate:* It is the average number of girls that would be born to a woman if she experiences the current fertility in her 15-49 age, assuring no deaths.
    It is 1.7 in India as per 1994 estimate.
13. *Net reproduction rate:* It is the number of daughters who deliver girl child during her 15-49 age assuming no deaths.
    It is 1.5 as per previous census data. NRR is a demographic indicator. Government of India has adopted a N R R of 1 by the year 2006 which is possible if couple protection rate is 60%.
14. *Pregnancy rate:* It is the number of pregnancies which include live birth, still birth, and not delivered by married women of 15-49 age.
15. *Maternal mortality rate:* It is death of women while pregnant or within 42 days of delivery per 1000 live births.

$$\text{MMR} = \frac{\text{No. of mothers dying due to pregnancy, Child birth within 42 days of delivery}}{\text{No. of live births}} \times 1000$$

It is 3.6 at present estimate.

16. *Perinatal mortality rate:* It is calculated by:

$$\text{PMR} = \frac{\text{Later foetal deaths (<28 wk gestation)} + \text{early neonatal death (1 wk) in 1 year}}{\text{No. of live births in 1 year}} \times 1000$$

It is 35 as per 2000 estimate

17. *Neonatal mortality rate:* It is calculated by:

$$\frac{\text{No. of deaths} < 28 \text{ days}}{\text{Live births}} \times 1000$$

It is 50 as per 1995 estimate.

18. *Post Neonatal mortality rate:* It is calculated by:

$$\frac{\text{No. of deaths from 28 days to 1 year age}}{\text{Live births}} \times 1000$$

It is estimated to be 26 at present.

19. *Infant mortality rate*: It is the ratio of infant deaths registered in one year to the live births of the same year.

$$\text{I.M.R.} = \frac{\text{No. of deaths below 1 year in 1 year}}{\text{Live births}} \times 1000$$

In India it is 66 as per 2003 estimate.

20. *1-4 year mortality rate:* It is calculated by:

$$\frac{\text{No. of deaths of 1-4 aged in 1 year}}{\text{1-4 age population}} \times 1000$$

It is estimated to be 112 as per previous census.

21. *Child mortality rate (under five mortality):* It is calculated by:

$$\frac{\text{No. of deaths of} < 5 \text{ years child in 1 year}}{\text{Live births}} \times 1000$$

It is estimated to be 96 as per 2000 estimate.

22. *Child survival index:* It is calculated by:

$$\frac{1000\text{—Under five mortality rate}}{10} \times 1000$$

Child survival rate is 90.4 as per 2000 estimate.

23. *Incidence*: It is number of new cases occurring in a defined population during 1 year.

$$= \frac{\text{No. of new cases in 1 year}}{\text{Population at risk}} \times 1000$$

24. *Prevalence:* It refers to the prevailing status at a point of time which include old and new cases.

Point prevalence is calculated by:

$$= \frac{\text{No. of old and new cases in a point of time}}{\text{Population at that time}} \times 100$$

Period prevalence is calculated by:

$$= \frac{\text{No. of old and new cases at 1 year}}{\text{Population at risk (MYP)}} \times 100$$

25. *Sullivan's index:* This is expectation of life free of disability. At life expectation of 58 years and disability or sickness period of 7.5 years, Sullivan index is 50.5. It is an advanced indicator available.
26. *Health adjusted life expectancy (HALE):* It measures healthy life expectancy. It includes time spent in poor health.
27. *Disability adjusted life expectancy (DALE):* It measures healthy life excluding time spent in poor health.
28. *Disability adjusted life year (DALY):* It measures burden of disease of a population. One year healthy life lost is equal to 1 DALY.
29. *Bed occupancy rate and bed turnover ratio:* Are utilisation rates which explain the extent of use of health services.
30. *Per capita income:* It is an index of standard of living. According to 1999 estimate it is Rs. 14712.

SOURCE OF STATISTICS

a. **Census:**
It is a major source of vital events. It is done once in 10 years. First census was in 1881 and latest 13th census was in 2001. Entire population is covered at one time for information on age, sex, marital status, birthplace, religion, literacy, occupation etc. The compiled data is published by census commissioner and Registrar General of India. It is a baseline data, helpful for research and Government activity including policy decision.

b. **Birth and death registration:**
It is a reliable source of information but is still in infancy because of following reasons:
- Lack of completeness.
- Lack of accuracy.
- Illiterate Primary Reporters.
- Revenue and police department transmits the data.
- People are not aware of its importance (ignorant).
- Lack of uniformity.
GOI Birth and Death Registration Act for registration of vital events came into effect in 1970.

c. **Notification of diseases:**
This is applicable to a list of diseases which help in proper recording, reporting and surveillance.

d. **Hospital records:**
This has been a major source over centuries. Since it is not community based it lacks in *power of data.*

e. **Health centres:**
After district health system, health centres are providing all information which is a good source of health statistics.

f. **Health surveys:**
It includes general survey and special surveys and sample surveys. They give good data for development of health indicators.

Uses of Statistics

i. It measures the state of health of a community
ii. It identifies health problems
iii. It identifies the health need
iv. Helps in comparison between:
   a. Past and present
   b. State to state
   c. Country to country
v. Helps in planning and administration of health
vi. Helps in evaluation of:
   a. Success of nursing care
   b. Failure of health programme
   c. Progress in professional care.

Survey

It is a basic tool of research in Health Sciences. There are many types like Impact survey, Utilisation survey, Gallup survey, Social survey, Morbidity survey, Mortality survey etc. Survey provides the denominator and hence enables comparison. Major uses of survey are:
- To assess magnitude of health problem.
- To guide planning.
- To evaluate national health activities
- Knowledge, attitude and practice can be studied.
- To know the extent of service utilisation
- Helps to test hypothesis on health related events.

Meticulous planning is needed for a survey. Survey instruments can be Interview, Observation, Questionnaire, Schedules, Techniques, Investigations.

Field Study

A designed research undertaken at community level constitutes field study. This can be Rural, Urban, Industrial or Nutritional in nature. It is an active process by a researcher to visit, observe and collect data at family level or at social unit level. This involves understanding of local customs, culture and traditional value. Field study requires local dialect for information collection.

Case Study

This is extensively used in nursing science and behavioural science. It involves in-depth study of one or a few cases as representative of a larger number of cases. The subject of investigations may be a few selected characteristics in individual or family. Case study do not generate information which can be adopted on a wider scale. However "case study" method can be used as an area for testing hypothesis.

SAMPLING

Meaning and Definition

In research it is not possible to study the whole universe which is called population. So we restrict to a sample from that population which is representative of whole population.

Sample is minimum number of objects or individuals for a study which is statistically determined and which represent the population in their characteristics.

What is a Good Sample

It is a sample size which is sufficient to answer the problem in research. It depends on the problem to be investigated, precision and resource available.

Types of Sampling

Random

Random sampling includes:

- Simple random sampling (by Lottery or random numbers).
- Stratified random sampling (sample from each strata).
- Systematic sampling (every 10th case).
- Cluster sampling (selecting natural groups).
- Multi-stage sampling (For HIV study 4 stages) is selected (primary), 4 districts in 4 states, (secondary), 4 villages in these 4 districts (final).

Non Random

- Area sampling (a non-probability sampling).
- Quota sampling (a non-probability sampling).
- Incidental sampling (a non-probability sampling).
- Purposive sampling (a non-probability sampling).

TOOLS FOR DATA COLLECTION

Data collection is a decisive step in research methodology. Hence, proper training of personnel who collect the data is mandatory. Pilot study conducted would have set right the deficiencies in proforma prepared.

There are many methods of data collection in a research design. Following are common and noteworthy as tools for data collection:

(i) Observation

Personal visit and observation by investigator help in observing many details who can detect the salient features of data collection. Qualitative evaluation is better done by the investigator. When more than one observer is involved there is a need for standardisation of evaluation technique.

(ii) Interview

Contact is done with individual or case by investigator. He elicits the response from the individual (a respondent). For a sustained prolonged interview, one has to maintain interest. The reaction and attitude of individual can be recorded.

(iii) Check List

This is a response sheet where questionnaires are recorded. Schedule or a questionnaire becomes useless if it is inadequately answered. The defect in check list cannot be compensated by any statistical means. Checklist should contain clear and unambiguous questions. As far as possible questions must be self-explanatory. Even answers like "not known", others etc., need entry in the check list.

As far as possible the reply is recorded by "a cross" or a "tick" or ringing a category which makes the tabulation also easier.

An assurance to the effect that information collected will be kept confidential makes the respondent free to express his opinion.

(iv) Survey

The coverage of survey may include few individuals to whole community. Survey provides denominator which enables comparison. Health, morbidity and utilisation survey are common types of surveys.

(v) Case Study

It is an in-depth analysis of a few cases or subjects. The method entails a comprehensive work up. The data collected will be enormous, when compared to surveys. But case study does not give a denominator and hence cannot be compared.

(vi) Sociometry and Sociogram

Sociometry is a technique of determining and identifying good respondents. It also identifies the non-cooperative. When such preference or rejection is seen in a society by prior visit, advanced briefing and motivating for interrogation is advisable.

Sociogram is a map or description which allows the investigator to know the cooperative and non-cooperative group. It is a description of social reaction, either by active group or by shy group. Sociogram developed at pilot study needs attention by frequent visits and motivation.

Scaling Methods

There are four types of scales that are used by the investigator for data collection. They are:

- Nominal scale (Category or quality described)
- Ordinal scale (Category where distance between category not known).
- Interval scale (accepted physical measurement)
- Ratio scale.

Pilot Study

This is pre-survey check of planning done. After preparation of proforma and questionnaire, they are subjected for a test in the field, by administration of proforma. Reliability of questions and response is checked and necessary alteration can be made for the future reliability of the study. Unclear and ambiguous areas are removed replacing clear and standardised ones for a high yield study.

CHAPTER FOUR

Demography and Family Planning (F.W.P.)

DEMOGRAPHY

Importance

Community health nursing or public health nursing is directly connected with people. Public health is related to population change, size of family, type of family, composition of family, morbidity and mortality of the family and hence public health nursing serves population to meet the health needs which might have been met or unmet. Moreover population is influenced by marriages, migrations and social mobility which are occurring as a natural process.

Terminologies

Demography

Demography is the study of human population with respect to size, type, composition, pattern and distribution.

Population Dynamics

Population dynamics is the study of mode of change of population and the factors responsible for such changes.

Social Mobility

Social mobility is movement of people with the purpose of family settlement, occupational placement and temporary stay on account of religious, philanthropic and national purpose.

Marriage

The term marriage can well be defined as the socially acceptable bondage in the process of family formation.

Fertility

Fertility is the child-bearing process in the reproductive age group.

Demographic Gap

Demographic gap is the difference between births and deaths. It helps to know the rapid growth of population.

Malthusian Theory of Population Explosion

This theory postulates that overpopulation is controlled by natural calamities like volcano, earthquake, floods, epidemics, etc. Though it is not a scientific version it can only be an antithesis of population.

Improvident Maternity

Improvident maternity is said to occur to a mother giving birth to a child who has already given birth to three children of whom one is alive. It is 42.8% in India.

Population Education

Population education is a health education programme which provides for a study of population

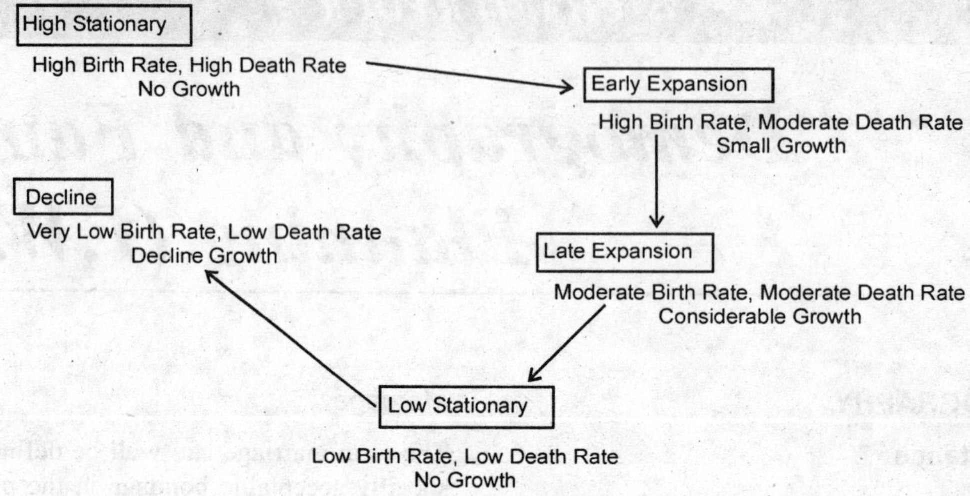

Fig 4.1: Demographic cycle

situation in the community, country and world with the purpose of developing rational and responsible attitude among present generation towards family planning behaviour.

Demographic Cycle

With change of time, population change occurs which are noted is 5 cycles (Fig. 4.1).

Major Sources of Demographic Data

There are many sources of data for demography and they are ongoing over many centuries. But, of late, importance is given through legislation (like Registration of Birth and Death Act) and a national commitment towards population census. Four major sources are to be noted. They are:

- Registration of births, deaths, marriages and migration.
- Census.
- Hospital records, health centre records.
- Notification of diseases.

Effects of Overpopulation

Impact of overpopulation on the society is many. Major effects noticeable are hindrance to national development, unemployment, illiteracy, poor housing, non-availability of health care facility, poor environmental sanitation and fast development of slums and shanty towns with its consequences.

Fertility

Fertility is child bearing among women of 15-45 age group. Uninterrupted marriage life, without protection that can allow 8-10 children is the fertility status. Factors which influence fertility are :

i. Age at marriage—On an average age at marriage in India is 19.5 years among girls.
ii. Married life—Longer married life has high fertility rates.
iii. Spacing—Postponement of pregnancies.
iv. Literacy—Illiteracy is associated with high fertility.
v. Income—Higher income (per capita income) show low fertility.
vi. Religion and caste—Studies from International Institute for population science, Mumbai has shown its observation.
vii. Nutrition—It indirectly influences fertility.
viii. Acceptance of family planning—This has determined the fertility rate.

Fertility Indicators (Table 4.1)

Table 4.1: Fertility indicators

Birth rate = 22		
General fertility rate = 118.0		
General marital fertility rate = 153.0		
Age specific fertility rate =		
15-19 years -	0.054	
20-24 years -	0.226	
25-29 years -	0.188	
30-34 years -	0.109	
35-39 years -	0.055	
40-44 years -	0.026	
45-49 years -	0.008	
Total fertility rate (15-44 age)		3.29
Total fertility rate (15-49 age)		3.32
Total marital fertility rate		4.9
Gross reproduction rate		1.7
Net reproduction rate		1.46

World Demography

In the year 1800 world reached 1 billion population. Later we noticed population explosion and doubling of population as under:

In 1930—two Billion recorded (130 years)
In 1960—three Billion recorded (30 years)
In 1974—four Billion recorded (15 years)
In 1987—five Billion recorded (12 years)
In 1999—six Billion recorded (12 years)

Now, annual growth rate of the world is 14 percent. China and India are among the most populous countries. Present demographic picture of the *world* are:

Population	– 6054,000,000
Annual Growth Rate	– 1.4%
Birth Rate	– 22 per 1000 MYP
Death Rate	– 9 per 1000 MYP
Current Growth	– 176 per minute (92,543,000 per year)

India—Demography

India reached 1 billion population on 11-05-2000. India thus has 2.4% of land area and 16.87% of world population. As per census report, post independent India population is as under: (First census was in 1881):

Year		Population
1951	-	361,088,080
1961	-	439,234,771
1971	-	548,159,652
1981	-	683,329,097
1991	-	846,302,688
2001	-	1027,051,247 (Total 35 states/UT[5])

The total population of India as at 0.00 hours on 1.3.2001 stood at 1,027,015,247 persons. With this India become only the second country in the world after China to cross 1 billion mark. The population of India rose by 21.34% between 1991-2001. The sex ratio (female to male) in 2001 is 933 and 986 as per 2003 estimate. The literacy rate is reckoned at 65.38%.

Rural urban proportion of India is as under:

	Population	*Percentage*
Rural	741,660,293	72.2
Urban	285,354,954	27.8
Total	1,027,015,247	(100.0)

Male and female proportion of India is as follows:

	Population	*Percentage*
Male	531,277,078	51.7
Female	495,738,169	48.3
Total	1,027,015,247	(100.0)

Dependency ratio (above 65 years and below 15 years) is 55.5% (8.3% and 47.2% for 65 + and below 15 respectively).

Density of population in India as per 2001 is 324 persons per square kilometre area.

Average family size is 3.1 members per family. Literate is 65.38% and life expectancy is 62.10 for males and 64.00 for females. India has 3 mega cities (10 million population) viz., Mumbai, Kolkota and Delhi.

Proportion of population by age and sex are as follows:

Age	Male	Female
0-4	11.2	11.1
5-14	24.9	24.2
15-44	45.2	46.4
45-64	13.4	13.5
65 +	5.3	4.8
	(100.0)	(100.0)

The age structure of a population is best represented as age pyramid. The age pyramid of India has broad base and a tapering top. In developed countries it (pyramid) shows bulge in the middle and a narrow base.

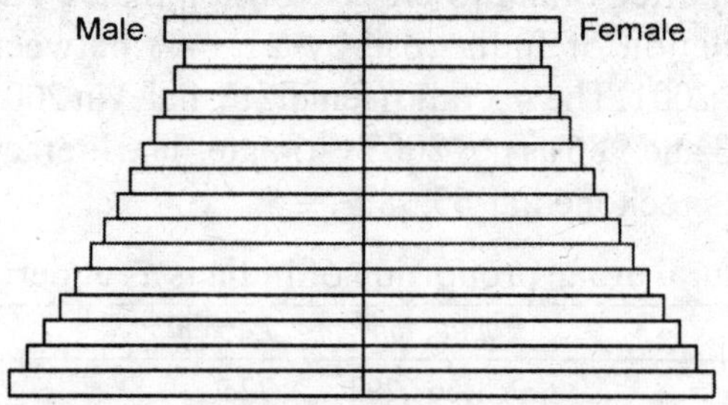

Fig. 4.2: Age pyramid of developing countries

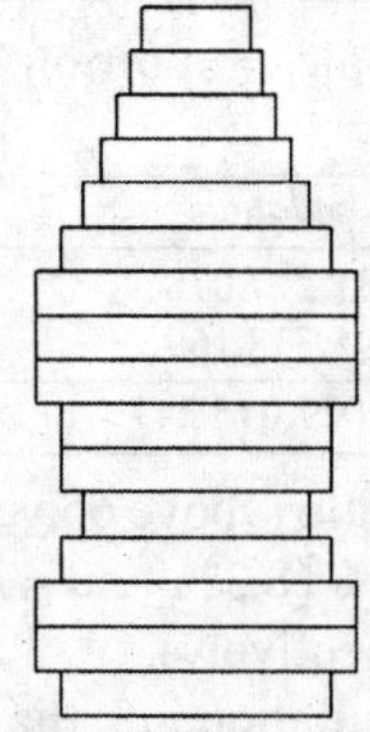
Fig. 4.3: Age pyramid of developed country

NATIONAL POPULATION POLICY

To achieve National Demographic goals India developed National Population Policy in 1976, modified in 1977 and restructured in 2000. The National Population Policy of 2000 has laid emphasis on women's education, child survival and unmet needs of family planning, coverage of under-served population, adolescent health and education and participation of men in Planned Parenthood. Following are the demographic goals of NPP by 2010:

1. Service, supply and infrastructure for unmet needs of RCH.
2. Free and compulsory education upto 14 years of age and school drop-out reduced to below 20%.
3. IMR to 30 per 1000 live births.
4. MMR to 1 per 1000 live births.
5. 100% coverage of UIP.
6. Age at marriage for girls 18 years.
7. 100% deliveries by trained persons.
8. Cafeteria approach of family planning methods.
9. Registration of vital events 100%.
10. Integrated approach for RTI and STD.
11. Control of communicable disease by priority.
12. Integration and availability of Indian system of medicine for RCH care and home visiting.
13. Total fertility rate is brought to replacement level by 2010 by promoting small family norm.
14. F.P. is made as family welfare and as a people centred programme.

Population Dynamics in Nursing

Population statistics has made the task possible in population size determination. The increase in population may be any of the following ways:

1. Natural increase
2. Arithmetic progression
3. Geometric progression.

FAMILY PLANNING

Importance

Reproductive and sexual health care including family planning is a key intervention for improving the health of women and children along with considering human right. Beijing platform for action has aptly said:

"Reproductive rights embrace certain human rights that are already recognised in national laws, international human rights documents and other relevant consensus documents. These rights rest on the recognition of the basic right of all couples and individuals to decide freely and responsibly the number and spacing and timing of their children and to have the information and means to do so, and the right to attain the highest standard of sexual and reproductive health."

The benefits of family planning can be tabulated as under (Table 4.2):

Terminology Used

Family planning: Family planning refers to practice that help individuals or couples to attain certain objectives like:

a. To avoid unwanted births
b. To bring about wanted births
c. To regulate the interval between pregnancies
d. To control the time at which births occur in relation to the age of the parents
e. To determine the number of children in the family.

Small Family Norm: "A concept to stabilise the country with 2 children per family which help to achieve NRR 1 and made acceptable into the lifestyle of people."

Spacing: "Postponing succeeding pregnancy to maintain 3 to 4 years difference between 2 children."

Eligible couple and target couple: The eligible couple rate is 150 per 1000 population in India. Eligible couple register is basic document in public health nursing. The priority group in target couple is eligible couple which can be differentiated by Table 4.3:

Table 4.3: Difference between target couple and eligible couple

Target couple	*Eligible couple*
Age group of 15-45 years	Following are deducted from target couple – Primary sterility – Secondary sterility – Early menopause

Unmet Need for FP: There is a gap between women's reproductive intention and their contraceptive behaviour. And it is a KAP gap (Knowledge attitude and practice). When married women prefer to avoid pregnancy but nevertheless not using method are attended on priority basis. This unmet need is estimated to be 25 percent among eligible women.

Couple Protection Rate: It is an indicator of the prevalence of contraceptive practice in the community. It is the percentage of eligible couples effectively protected against childbirth by approved methods of family planning. By 60% of CPR we can achieve N.R.R. of 1.0.

Incentives and Disincentives in Family Planning

These are measures to encourage couples to practice family planning as a strategy (Fig. 4.4).

Table 4.2: Benefits of family planning

Women	*Children*	*Men*	*Families*	*Nation*
• Protect from unwanted pregnancies • Saved from unsafe abortions • Are health benefits	• Save life of children	• Better life in family	• Family well being	• National Development • Economic improvement

Table 4.4: Incentive and disincentive in family planning

Incentive	*Disincentive*
• Tubectomy 200.00	Improvident maternity
• Laparoscopy 145.00	No housing loan
• Vasectomy 180.00	No subsidised medical treatment
• Motivation of tubectomy 10.00	
• Motivation of vasectomy 40.00	
• One special increment	
• 14 days leave (women)	
• 7 days leave (men)	
• Green card to individual acceptances (for special attention)	

Health Aspect of F.P.

a. *Women health:* By not allowing unwanted pregnancy, limiting the number of children to two, and timing of pregnancy for above 20 years to 35 years we can bring down maternal mortality and morbidity.

b. *Foetal health:* Timing of pregnancy can avoid congenital anomalies. The quality of health of foetus is better if proper planning of the family is done.

c. *Infant and child health:* Family size and spacing of pregnancy has an impact on infant and child health. Growth and development is good with small family norm.

Organization of F.P. Services

Health and family welfare are essential component and is primary responsibility of Government for its delivery to the community. There is an organised set up for the F.W. programme in India.

Family planning organisation in India is sideline of health services and it is accounted from central government to village (Fig. 4.4 and Table 4.5).

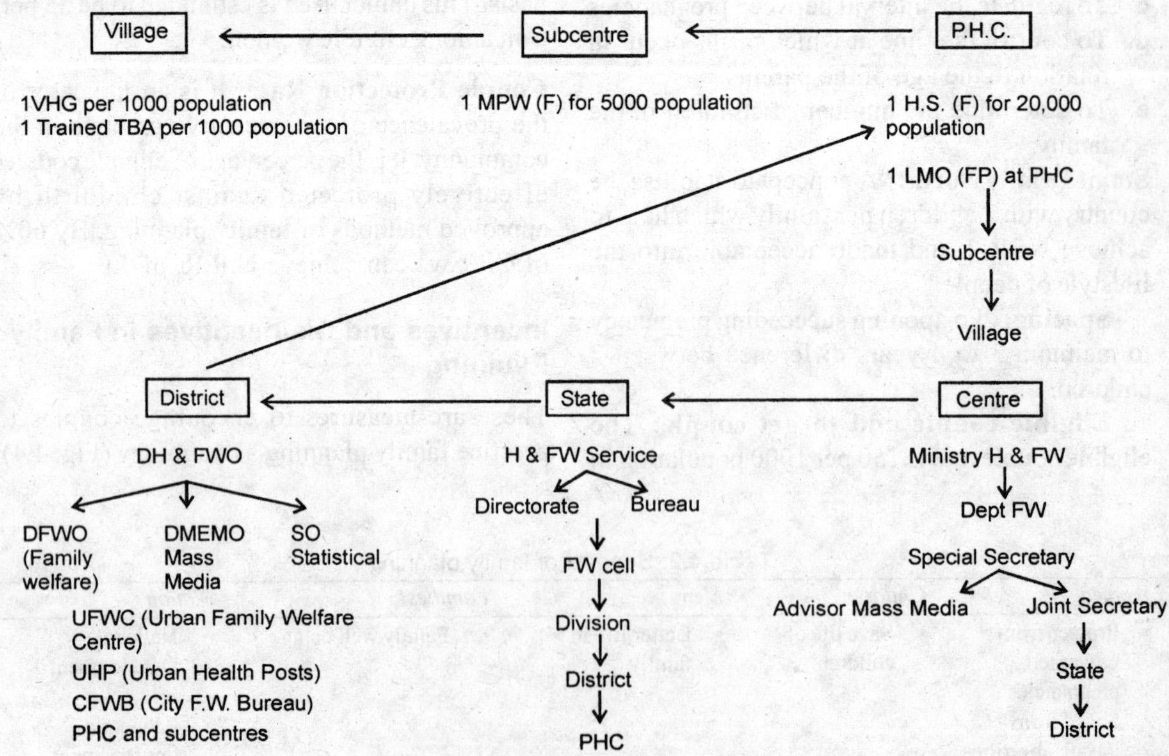

Fig. 4.4 : Organization of F.P. in India

Table 4.5: Voluntary F.P. organisations

National level	*International level*
1. Family Planning Association of India	1. International Planned Parenthood Association
2. Family Planning Foundation	2. UNFPA
3. Population Council of India	3. USAID
4. Indian Red Cross	4. The Population Council
5. I.M.A.	5. Ford Foundation
6. Rotary Club	6. Pathfinder Fund
7. Lions Club	7. World Bank
8. Citizen's Forum	8. WHO
	9. UNICEF

Abortion

Abortion is termination of pregnancy before 28 weeks of pregnancy. They can be induced abortion or spontaneous abortion. Spontaneous abortion is natural method of family planning. Induced abortion can be either legal or illegal, which carry health hazards resulting in maternal mortality and morbidity. Early complications like haemorrhage, shock, sepsis, performing injury are well-known. Late complications can be infertility and ectopic pregnancy. As per IPC 1860 and CCP 1898 abortion is a crime except under life saving process. Hence Government of India brought out a legal abortion called MTP Act, 1971.

The MTP Act, 1971 (Medical Termination of Pregnancy)

This lays down the conditions, persons to perform and place to perform for MTP.

Indications

Medical—When pregnancy cause injury or death to mother.

Eugenic—When abnormal growth is established.

Humanitarian—When rape has caused pregnancy.

Socio-economic—When socioeconomic cause can lead to death or injury to mother.

Failure of contraceptive—Failed F.P. methods causing pregnancy.

Written consent of guardian when pregnant woman is lunatic or minor is a requirement.

Person to Perform MTP

- By RMP if below 12 weeks, who has experience in OBG.
- By 2 RMP opinion if above 12 weeks who have experience in OBG.

Place to Perform MTP

It must be in a hospital, health centre or any approved place.

Following Amendments are done in 1975 in MTP:

i. DH and FWO can certify a doctor to conduct MTP.

ii. An RMP who conducts 25 MTP in a hospital is permitted to conduct MTP.

iii. Experience in OBG means.
   - 6 months experience as house surgeon in OBG.
   - PG in OBG.
   - RMP of before 1971 needs 3 year OBG practice.
   - RMP of after 1971 needs 1 year OBG practice.

iv. DH and FWO can certify place of conducting MTP.

Thus MTP is a safe, legal abortion made universally available for family planning in the country.

Family Planning Methods

Fertility Awareness Based Methods (FABM):

Fertility awareness means that a woman learns how to tell 'when the fertile time of her menstruation starts and ends'. This helps a woman to know when she could become pregnant. The couple avoids pregnancy by changing their sexual behaviour during fertile days.

i. *Abstain from vaginal intercourse:* Avoiding vaginal sex completely during fertile time. This is called periodic abstinence and natural F.P. method.
ii. *Use of withdrawal (coitus interruptus)*: The male withdraws before ejaculation and avoids semen deposit into vagina. There are other sexual contacts without vaginal intercourse as per studies conducted in sex behaviour in communities.
iii. *Calendar calculation:* A woman can count calendar days to identify the start and end of the fertile time. The number of days depends on the length of previous menses (Fig. 4.5).

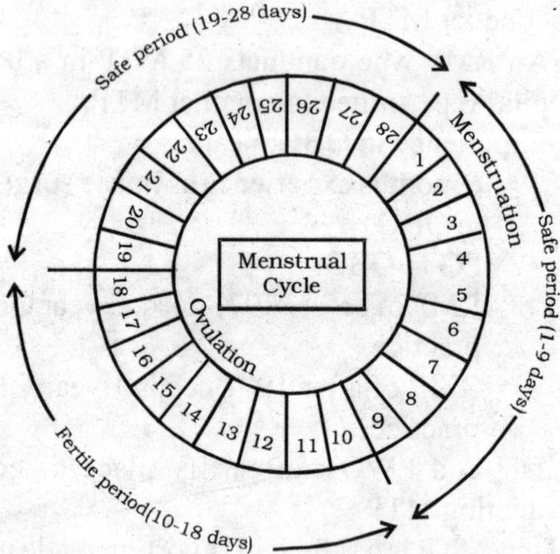

Fig. 4.5: Fertile period in menstrual cycle

iv. *Cervical secretions:* When a woman sees or feels cervical secretions, she may be fertile. This is to be differentiated with just a sense of vaginal wetness.

During lactation, circulating hormones, particularly progesterone gives hypo-thalamus a signal that there is no need of L.H. (Leutinising Hormone) and F.S.H. (Follicle Stimulating Hormone) and thus ovulation is prevented. As long as continuous breast feeding is there, the cycle is expected, but not 100 % sure. Once menstruation occurs LAM cannot be considered as a contraceptive device.

Vaginal Methods

Vaginal methods are contraceptives that a woman places in her vagina shortly before sex. Common vaginal methods are:

Spermicides

They include foaming tablets or suppositories, melting suppositories, foam, melting film, jelly and cream. The active ingredient is a surface acting agent which attaches to sperm and inhabit their oxygen intake.

Diaphragm

It is a soft rubber cup that covers the cervix. It should be used with spermicidal jelly or cream. Checking proper placement of a diaphragm is very important (Fig. 4.6).

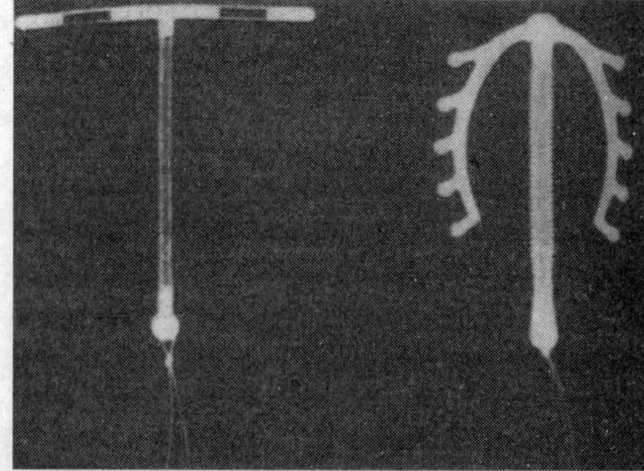

Fig 4.6: Commonly used copper T and multiload MLcu 375

Cervical Cap

It is similar to diaphragm but smaller, but not widely available in developing countries.

Vaginal Sponge

It is available by trade mark 'Today', made of polyurethane foam sponge with nonoxynol-9 as spermicide. But failure rate is high with vaginal sponge.

Intra Uterine Device (IUD)

An I.U.D. is usually a small, flexible plastic frame. It has copper wire or copper sleeves on it. (Exception—Lippy's Loop). It is inserted into women's uterus through her vagina. All brands have strings or threads tied to them. The strings hang through the opening of the cervix into the vagina. The user can check that the IUD is still in place by touching the strings. A nurse can remove the IUD by pulling gently on the strings with forceps. Earlier it was called IUCD (contraceptive device). Specific IUD's are:

- Copper T
- T Cu—380 A
- M L Cu 375 (multiload)
- Nova T
- Progestasert
- LNG—20.

Lippes loop is no longer used in India.

Most commonly used I.U.D.'s are T Cu 380 A and MLcu—375.

Types of IUD are:

i. First generation IUD (nonmedicated IUD)
ii. Second generation IUD (copper containing)
iii. Third generation IUD (Hormone releasing).

There are many advantages of copper-T. They are:

a. Low expulsion rate
b. Low side effects
c. Easy to insert
d. Better tolerated
e. High protection rate, and
f. Useful as post coital contraceptive.

Contraindications

1. Acute pelvic infection
2. Chronic pelvic infection
3. Menorrhagia

Before putting IUD, one has to exclude the following:

Pregnancy
Anaemia due to iron deficiency
Anaemia due to hook worm
Large fibroid

Side effects of IUD and their management (Table 4.6):

Table 4.6: Management of IUD side effects

Side Effects	*Management*
Increase in menstruation	Watch for anaemia
Uterine cramp	Exclude other causes
Extrusion	Check threads frequently
Pregnancy	Always remove IUD
Anxiety	Support and reassure

Most ideal time for IUD insertion is during menstruation or within 10 days of the beginning of a menstrual period. Post puerperal insertion has several advantages. Follow up of IUD cases are required and nursing staff should encourage this.

Condom

A condom is a sheath or covering made fit over man's penis. They are known by many trade names. Most condoms are made of thin latex rubber. Some are coated with a dry lubricant or with spermicides. Different sizes, shapes, colour and texture are made available in some places.

Nirodh is available in 3 brands

a. Dry nirodh
b. Delux nirodh (lubricated)

c. Super delux nirodh (thin and lubricated).

Its use has shown pregnancy rate 2-3 per 100 women year. It is a common barrier method of contraceptive used in F.P. programme.

Sterilisation

Tubectomy

Female sterilisation provides permanent contraception for women who will not want more children. It is a safe and simple surgical procedure. It can usually be done with just local anaesthesia and light sedation. Proper infection prevention procedures are required. The common approaches are mini-laparotomy and laparoscopy. They are also called V.S.C. (Voluntary Surgical Contraception), T.L. (Tubal Ligation), Minilap, etc.

Laparoscopy

Sterilisation is done by using laparoscope. Abdomen is inflated with nitrous oxide tubes. When tubes are accessible, clips are put and tubes are occluded. It has to be done only in 2nd month after delivery. Post operative observation is for 48 hours. Multi-purpose worker (female) and health supervisor will pay home visiting on 10th day and 12th month after operation. Least complications are recorded in the hospital practice.

Minilap Operation

With a small incision under local anaesthesia, tube is identified, ligated and sterilised. This is also called as Pomeroy technique. Because of safety, efficiency and ease, it is used in tubectomy camps. It is suitable for postpartum tubal sterilisation.

Vasectomy

Vasectomy provide permanent contraception for men who decide they will not want more children. It is safe, simple, quick surgical procedure. It can be done in a clinic, a camp with proper infection prevention procedures. Guidance and counselling at nursing care require telling that it is not castration and it does not affect testicles or it does not affect sexual ability.

New, No-scalpel Vasectomy

The difference noticed from conventional procedure are:

a. Use of a small puncture (instead of 2" incision) in the scrotum.
b. Special anaesthesia technique needs only 1 needle puncture instead of 2 or more.

Advantages are:

a. Less pain
b. Less bruising
c. Short recovery time
d. Less operating time.

Main advice given after vasectomy is that usually until 30 ejaculations, the persons will have the chance of impregnating his partner. Vasectomy does not alter sperm production or hormone output. It is simpler, faster and less expensive sterilisation method.

Side effects noticed after vasectomy are:

a. Sperm granules
b. Spontaneous recanalisation
c. Rise in circulating antibodies against ones own sperm as an auto-immune response is seen
d. Anxiety and psychological depression.

Implants

They are subdermal implants for long-term contraception. Commonly used Norplant is a set of 6 small plastic capsules.

Each is about the size of a small matchstick. The capsules are placed under the skin of a women's upper arm. They contain progestin similar to a natural hormone that woman's body makes. It is released slowly from all 6 capsules. Thus the capsules supply a steady, very low dose. It does not contain oestrogen.

Injectable Hormones

Women who use this method receive injections to prevent pregnancy. Common preparations are:

DMPA (Depot Medroxy Progesterone acetate).

NET—EN (Norethisterone enantate).

Common type of injectable is RMPA given every three months. It contains a progesterone similar to the natural hormone that a woman's body makes. The hormone is released slowly into the blood stream. (Trade names : Depo provera, Depo Megestron) NET–EN is given every 2 months.

Mode of Action: The suppression of ovulation through feedback mechanism.

Injectables do not affect breast milk:

Contraindications:

- Hypertension
- Diabetes
- Large Fibroid

Side Effects:

- Irregular bleeding
- Amenorrhoea
- Delayed return of ovulation
- Hypertension
- Changes in carbohydrate metabolism.

Injectables are given during first 5 days of menstrual cycle deep IM to gluteus maximus. Post injection massage is disallowed.

Oral Contraceptives

They are effective contraceptives when properly used, which have nearing to 100% effectiveness. Oestrogen and progesterone by gonads are called physiological steroids. Synthetic oestrogens are ethyl oestradiol and mestraol. Synthetic progesterone are norethisterone lynestrenol and levonorgestrel. They are grouped under 5 heads:

1. Combined (oestrogen progesterone pill)
2. Progesterone only pill (POP)
3. Post coital pill
4. Long acting pill
5. Male pill.

Combined Pill

Women who use oral contraceptives swallow a pill each day to prevent pregnancy. Combined O.C. contain 2 hormones similar to the natural hormones in a woman's body:

a. Oestrogen
b. Progesterone.

Present day combined O.C. contains very low dose hormones. Hence they are called L.D.C. O.C. (Low dose combined oral contraceptives). There are 2 types of pill pockets. Some contain 28. These contain 21 *active* pills which contain hormones, followed by 7 *reminder* pills of a different colour that do not contain hormones. Other type contain only 21 *active* pills.

Reaction and Effects of Combined Pill

Medically not Significant

- Decreased menstrual loss
- Amenorrhoea
- Mid cycle spotting
- Weight change
- Breast tenderness
- Breast milk reduced
- Facial pigmentation
- Nausea in first month.

Medically Significant which Require Attention

- Jaundice
- Hypertension
- Thromboembolism
- Glycosuria
- Severe headache
- Chronic cervical erosion
- Monilial vaginitis
- Fibroid enlargement.

Contraindications for Combined Pill (Fig. 4.7)

Table 4.7: Contraindications of combined pill

Absolute contraindication	*Careful supervision*
Acute liver disease	Renal or cardiac disease
History of Thromboembolism	Diabetes
Cancer breast	Hypertension
Lactation	Sickle cell anaemia
Prediabetes	Major surgery

Government of India has commercialised two types of combined oral contraceptives. They are:

1. Mala N (Free supply through health and nursing care)
   Norgestrol 0.3 mg
   Ethyl oestradiol 0.03 mg
2. Mala D (21 active 7 brown placebo) (Under social marketing at low cost)
   Norgestrol 0.3 mg
   Ethyl oestradiol 0.03 mg

Progestogen Only Pill (POP)

Women who use progestogen only pill, swallow a pill everyday to prevent pregnancy. Progestogen—only pill contain very small amounts of only progestin (one tenth of dose of combined pill). They are best for breastfeeding women. They do not reduce milk production.

Contraindications

There are no contraindications to POP:

Side effect of POP:

Irregular bleeding at first
Amenorrhoea later
Increased pregnancy risk

It is suitable for women who are:

Lactating
Sub-fertile
Spacing of children

POP to be taken everyday. It is best to take at the same time each day. Taking pill more than a few hours late increase the risk of pregnancy and missing two or more greatly increases the risk.

After 1 pack, one should take first pill from next pack on the very next day. All pills are active, hormonal and there is no wait between packs.

Post Coital Contraceptive

They are recommended within 48 hours of unprotected intercourse.

a. IUD Copper-T is inserted if acceptable.
b. Double the dose of standard combined pill. i.e., 2 oral contraceptive tablets immediately followed by another 2 pills 12 hours later.
c. As emergency contraception 4 tablets of pills containing 30 mg oestrogen, at one time itself.

Long Acting Once a Month Pill

Quinestrol + progestogen is advocated but is associated with high failure rate.

Male Pill

A derivative of cotton seed oil "gossypol" for 6 months orally has produced azoospermia in men. It is not in routine clinical use.

Vaccines for Birth Control

Only known vaccine known by clinical trail is "hcG vaccine" i.e., beta sub-unit of human chorionic gonadotrophin, which blocks continuation of implanted ovum. Booster dose at 12th month is recommended. Birth control vaccine is only an academic interest and not in clinical practice.

National Family Planning Programme (NFPP)

In 1952 India launched FP programme. The approach is "Extension education approach" for motivating people to accept small family norm. Since 1965 to 1970 IUD (Lippes loop) made a mark in F.P. programme. Later Copper-T has been used under National F.P. programme. In 1966 Ministry of Health got bifurcated to Health and F.P. wings. The infrastructure of F.P. was strengthened. In every 5 years plan, top priority is being given to F.P.

PPC in 1970 and MTP in 1971 were added as additional forces in Family Planning. National population policy gave vivid picture for action in 1976.

In 1977 F.P. was renamed as FWP since it involved family welfare activities.

Primary health care approach, HFA approach, long-term demographic goal of NRR 1 by 2007 which imply two-child family norm, goal of BR 21, goal of DR 9 and CPR of 60% are strategic phenomena under NFPP in India.

Seventh Five Year Plan incorporated UIP, ORT (under CSSM) under F.W. planning.

Since 1997 we have unified R.C.H. integrated with Eighth Five Year Plan for need based, client oriented service.

In the year 2000, Government of India reinforced the comprehensive National Population Policy.

Financial allocation to FWP is better reviewed by following table (Table 4.8):

Table 4.8: Financial allocation to FWP

Year	*Expenditure*
First 5-year plan	0.65 crore
Fifth 5-year plan	285.6 crore
Ninth 5-year plan	14170 crore

National F.P. programme is evaluated from time to time through evaluation of :

- Need
- Plan
- Performance
- Effects
- Impact.

RCH programme integrates all the related programmes of National Five Year plans. This need based, client oriented, demand driven and high quality integrated service has taken up CSSM programme at various levels. Following Drug and equipment kits were supplied in the said programme.

MATERNITY CARE KIT

Item	*Nos.*
1. Umbilical cotton (0.3 cm × 25 cm)	2
2. Blade with holder	1
3. Cotton swab 7.5cm × 7.5 cm (2.5 gm)	3 pieces
4. Surgical gauze pieces 5 cm × 7.5cm- 12 ply	2 pieces
5. Sanitary pad no. 4	1
6. Drape—polyethylene sheet 75 cm × 100 cm	1
7. Trolley cover	1

DAIS KIT

Item	*Nos.*
1. Aluminium kit box	1
2. Stainless steel straight scissors (blunt–pointed)	1
3. Stainless steel teaspoon	1
4. Enamel irrigator with rubber tubing and ebonite nozzle	1
5. Enamel bowl (large)	1
6. Aluminium bowl	2
7. Mackintosh sheeting (90 cm square)	1
8. Hand towel	2
9. Soap dish with soap	1
10. Nail brush	1
11. Absorbent cotton wool (sterilized)	1 packet
12. Gauze (sterilized)	1 packet of 12 pieces
13. Umbilical cord tape (sterilized)	6 pieces
14. Dusting powder in a plastic container	1
15. Antiseptic lotion	1 bottle

KIT FOR HEALTH GUIDES

S.No	Item	Quantity
*1.	Foetoscope	1
2.	Stainless steel straight scissors (blunt- pointed)	1
3.	Sterile cotton wool	1 packet
4.	Sterile gauze	1 packet
5.	Roller bandage	1
6.	Triangular bandage	1
7.	Adhesive plaster	1
8.	Soap dish and soap	1
9.	Towels	2
10.	Clinical oral thermometer	1
11.	Slide box containing 10 glass slides	1
12.	Cloth for cleaning slides	1
13.	Hagedorn needle	1
14.	Graduated medicine glass	1
15.	Suitable containers for drugs	18
16.	Stainless steel teaspoon (9 ml)	1
17.	Spring scale (hanging)	1
18.	Mid-upper arm circumference strip	1
19.	Measuring tape	1
20.	Exercise book (200 pages)	1
21.	Pencil	1
22.	Forms for reporting blood smears	
23.	Health education materials	
24.	Kit bag	

* Not to be included in the kits meant for Male Health Guides.

KIT FOR COMMUNITY HEALTH WORKER

1. Slides (5) in slide Hagedorn box
2. Cloth for cleaning slides
3. Hagedorn needle
4. Pencil
5. Clinical oral thermometer
6. Graduated medicine glass
7. Scissors
8. Razor blade
9. Cotton wool
10. Gauze
11. Roller bandage
12. Triangular bandage
13. Adhesive plaster
14. Soap dish and soap
15. Towels (2)
16. Nirodh packets (50)
17. Suitable containers for drugs (17)
18. Forms for reporting of blood smears
19. Franked envelopes addressed to the Primary Health Centre
20. Exercise book (200 pages)
21. Diary
22. Health Education Materials (flip chart on family welfare, set of contraceptives)
23. Manual for Community Health Worker
24. Kit-bag.

Medicines to be Carried by Community Health Worker

For Internal Use

1. Aspirin, Phenacetin and Caffeine (APC) tablets
2. Chloroquine tablets
3. Cough mixture
4. Kaolin powder
5. Magnesium hydroxide tablets
6. Rehydration powder (chorosol).

For External Use

7. Antiseptic lotion
8. Benzyl benzoate emulsion
9. Menthol and eucalyptus oil ointment
10. Mercurochrome 2 per cent
11. Methylated spirit
12. Methyl salicylate ointment
13. Potassium permanganate crystals
14. Sulphacetamide eye and ear drops 10 per cent
15. Sulphanilamide skin ointment
16. Sulphonamide dusting powder
17. Whitfield ointment.

Additional material to be kept with selected members of the community

1. Bleaching powder in pots.

Medicines for Inclusion in Health Worker's Kit

For Internal Use

1. Acetyl salicyclic acid tablets
2. Belladonna and phenobarbitone tablets
3. Chloroquine phosphate tablets
4. Cough mixture
5. Dried aluminium hydroxide tablets
6. Ergometrine maleate tablets
7. Iron and folic acid tablets
8. Kaolin pectin suspension
9. Magnesium hydroxide tablets
10. Magnesium sulphate
11. Mepyramine (antihistamine) tablets
12. Mebendazole tablets (Pantelmin)
13. Oral rehydration powder
14. Paracetamol tablets
15. Phthalyl sulphathiazole tablets
16. Piperazine citrate/ Piperazine adipate tablets
17. Sulphadimidine tablets
18. Vitamin A solution.

For External Use

19. Acriflavine ointment
20. Antiseptic lotion
21. Benzoic salicyclic ointment
22. Benzyl benzoate emulsion
23. Chloromycetin eye ointment (Applicaps)
24. Gentian violet 2%
25. Menthol and eucalyptus oil ointment
26. Mercurochrome 2%
27. Methyl salicylate liniment
28. Sulphacetamide eye and ear drops 10%
29. Tetracycline eye ointment
30. White vaseline.

Reagents

31. Chemistrips (Miles India Ltd.)
32. Litmus paper (blue and red).

Medicines to be kept at Sub Centre

For Internal Use

1. Bephenium hydroxy naphthoate granules
2. Calcium gluconate tablets
3. Liquid paraffin
4. Mist alkaline
5. Mist carminative
6. Mist chloral hydrate
7. Mist sedative expectorant
8. Multivitamin tablets (A,B,C,D)
9. Prochlorperazine tablets (Stemetil)
10. Syrup ferric citrate
11. Vitamin C tablets
12. Injection methyl ergometrine maleate (Methergen).

For External Use

13. Boric acid powder
14. Calamine lotion
15. Methylated spirit
16. Tincture benzoin co.
17. Tincture iodine
18. Zinc boric dusting powder.

List of Drugs to be Supplied to Sub Centre

Essential drugs

For Internal use:

1. Acetyl salicylic acid tablets
2. Belladonna and phenobarbitone tablets (Antispasmodic tablets)
3. Chloroquine phosphate tablets
4. Ergometrine maleate tablets (Methergen tablets)
5. Iron and folic acid tablets
6. Liquid paraffin
7. Mebendazole tablets (Panhelmin)
8. Mepyramine (Antihistamine) tablets
9. Oral Rehydration Salt packets
10. Paracetamol tablets

11. Prochlorperazine tablets (Stemetil)
12. Sulphadimidine tablets
13. Syrup ferric ammonium citrate
14. Vitamin A solution
15. Injection methyl ergometrine maleate (Methergen injection).

For External use

16. Acriflavine ointment
17. Antiseptic lotion (Savlon/Dettol)
18. Benzyl benzoate emulsion
19. Boroglycerine
20. Gentian violet 2%
21. Sulphacetamide eye and ear drops 10%
22. Tetracycline eye ointment
23. Zinc boric dusting powder
24. Absorbent cotton wool
25. Absorbent gauze
26. Roller bandage (98 × 61 cm)
27. Reagent strips (URISTIX).

Optional Drugs

For Internal Use

1. Bephenium hydroxyl naphthoate granules
2. Calcium gluconate tablets
3. Cough mixture
4. Dried aluminium hydroxide tablets
5. Kaolin pectin suspension
6. Magnesium hydroxide tablets
7. Magnesium sulphate
8. Mist alkaline
9. Mist carminative
10. Mist chloral hydrate
11. Mist sedative expectorant
12. Multivitamin tablets (ABCD)
13. Phthalyl sulphathiazole tablets
14. Piperazine citrate/Piperazine adipate tablets
15. Vitamin C tablets.

For External use

16. Benzoic salicylic ointment
17. Boric acid powder
18. Calamine lotion
19. Chloromycetin eye ointment(Applicaps)
20. Menthol and eucalyptus oil ointment
21. Mercurochrome 2%
22. Methyl salicylate ointment
23. Methylated spirit
24. Tincture benzoin co
25. Tincture iodine
26. White vaseline.

KIT FOR HEALTH WORKER FEMALE

General Kit:

Sr.No.	Item	Quantity
1.	Kit bag (brown) with nylon tray, rectangular aluminium tray, side pocket, rear pocket, cover flap and shoulder strap	1
Cover flap		
2.	Spring type dressing forceps stainless steel (150 mm)	1
3.	Surgical straight scissors (blunt-stainless steel) (140 mm)	1
4.	Pencil with eraser	1
5.	Teaspoon—stainless steel	1
Side pocket		
6.	Nail brush	1
7.	Soap dish	1
8.	Soap	1
9.	Nail clipper	1
Rear pocket		
10.	Clear vinyl plastic sheeting (910 mm wide)	1 metre
11.	Huck towel (430 × 500 mm)	2
12.	Folding aluminium shield (BCG)	1
13.	Polythene self-sealing bag (125 × 200 mm)	12
14.	Sterile gauze pads (12 ply) (76 × 76 mm square)	6

No.	Item	Quantity
15.	Arm circumference scale	1
16.	Nylon tray	1
17.	Absorbent non-sterile cotton wool	1 roll (113 gm)
18.	Vinyl-coated fibreglass tape measure (1.5 metre/60")	1
19.	Safety pins (medium/40 mm)	1 bag of 12
20.	Adhesive zinc oxide tape (25 mm × 0.9 metre)	1 roll
21.	Alcohol lamp with screw cap-metal (60 ml)	1
22.	Safety razor blades (double edge)	1pkt of 5
23.	Clinical oral thermometer (35 to 42°C)	1
24.	Clinical rectal thermometer (35 to 42°C)	1
25.	Gauze bandage (non-sterile) (25 mm × 9 metres)	1 roll
26.	Triangular cloth bandage (910 mm slides)	1
27.	Microscope slide box	1
28.	Microscope slides (plain) (75 mm × 25 mm)	1 pkt of 10
29.	Cloth for cleaning micro slides	1
30.	Stick swabs	1 bag
31.	Rubber solid stopper (bottom 16 mm top 20 mm)	1
32.	Specimen tube-glass (1900 × 75 mm)	1
33.	Keith abdominal suture needle (44 mm)	1
34.	Anaemia recognition card (English/Hindi)	1
35.	Nelaton solid-tip one eye urethral catheter (12 Fr)	1
36.	Urinalysis outfit (test tubes/ bottle/clamp)	1 set
37.	Mayo Ochsner haemostat straight forceps—stainless steel (160 mm)	1
38.	Umbilical tape (non-sterile)	1
39.	DeLee tracheal catheter with glass mucus trap	1
40.	Rectangular aluminium tray	1
41.	Medicine cup—polypropylene (30 ml)	1
42.	Lubricant jar—plastic	14
43.	Amber dropping bottle—glass (10 ml)	3
44.	Wide–mouth screw cap square bottle (60 ml)—polyethylene	9
45.	Screw cap sputum container	4

Immunization kit (one for each Sub centre)

No.	Item	Quantity
46.	Rubber ring	2
47.	File for BCG ampoules (6 mm × 50 mm)	1
48.	Wooden block for ampoules	1
49.	Sharpening stone (50 mm × 19 mm × 6.3 mm)	1
50.	Bifurcated needles- stainless steel (65 mm)	12
51.	Luer hypodermic needles (0.90 mm × 25 mm/20 G × 1")	1 box of 12
52.	Luer hypodermic needles (0.60 mm × 25 mm/23 G × 1")	2 boxes of 12 each
53.	Luer hypodermic needles (0.45mm × 10 mm/ 26 G × 3/8")	1 box of 12
54.	Luer nylon hypodermic syringe (2 ml × 0.1 ml)	2
55.	Luer glass hypodermic tuberculin syringe (1ml × 0.01ml)	2
56.	Test tube holder—two piece plastic	1
57.	Vacuum insulated thermocontainer (300 ml)	1
58.	Aluminium box (180 mm × 100 mm × 40 mm)	1

CHAPTER FIVE

Environmental Health Including Medical Entomology

IMPORTANCE

Physical development, health and survival are influenced by physical, chemical, social, spiritual and biological environments. Man lives in this group of environment where he adjusts and readjusts to the surroundings. Control of these environments which exercise or may exercise a deleterious effect on his health, constitute environmental health.

Sanitation is equally a forceful word in environmental health which is defined as the *Science of Safeguarding Health.* According to the National Sanitation Foundation of USA "Sanitation is way of life". It is the quality of living that is expressed in the clean home, the clean farm, the clean business, the clean neighbourhood and the clean community. It comes from people, it is nourished by knowledge, grows as an obligation and an ideal in human relations."

Types of Environment

i. *Physical environment* includes housing, human congregation, meteorology, air, ventilation, noise, lighting, radiation, water, solid waste and liquid waste.
ii. *Chemical environment* include organic and inorganic chemicals that exist in human placement and human occupations.
iii. *Social environment* includes ways of living, religion, caste, customs, culture, attitude, beliefs, mores, education, occupation and standard of living.
iv. *Spiritual environment* include integrity, principles, ethics, purpose of life and commitment to some higher being.
v. *Biological environment* include bacteria, virus, rickettsiae, fungi, helminths, protozoa, insects, rodents and other animals.

Biological environment is detailed under communicable diseases, social and spiritual environment is detailed under sociology and psychology and chemical environment is detailed under human occupations. In the present chapter all physical and materialistic surroundings are highlighted.

PHYSICAL ENVIRONMENT

HOUSING

House refers to a physical structure where unit of society the *family* lives, but the concept is slowly changing to "Human settlement" which allows the extended outlook of a house, where people live, interact and pursue their goals, W.H.O. has coined the word residential environment which is used by man for his activity and desired devices for his family well-being.

Healthful Housing

American Public Health Association has given basic principles of healthful housing. On similar lines W.H.O. has given following Healthful Housing Criteria:

- It gives physical protection and shelter.

- Adequate provision for cooking, eating, washing and excretory functions.
- It prevents spread of infections and communicable diseases.
- Protects from noise.
- Protects from atmospheric pollutions.
- Housing material is free from toxic and harmful chemicals.
- Encourages personality development.
- Promotes mental health.
- To attain social goals like:
  - Family life
  - Access to community facility
  - Social participation
  - Economic stability.

Need of Housing

i. *Physical needs* like air, temperature, lighting, rest, recreation.
ii. *Physiological needs* like privacy, family life.
iii. *Health needs* like water, sanitary latrine, balanced diet, protection from insects and animals.
iv. *Protective needs* like accidents, fire, electricity etc.

Housing Standards

Environmental Hygiene Committee of Government of India has given some minimum housing standards that are to be maintained by building regulations through Municipality, Corporation, Town Planning and Urban Development authorities (Fig. 5.1).

Bathing facility: House should have adequate bathing facility.

Cubic space: It should be 500 cubic feet per person.

Floor: Pucca floor, no crack and damp proof.

Floor area: 100 square foot per person.

Garbage disposal: Daily removal by sanitary method for proper disposal.

Kitchen: Adequate provision for separate and sanitary area for food preparation.

Lighting: It is expected to have a D.F. (day light factor) of 1.0 or above 1.0.

Privy: Sanitary RCA latrine and water carriage system is a must under criteria of healthful housing.

Roof: It should be more than 10 feet.

Rooms: According to family size and needed privacy, number of rooms are suggested.

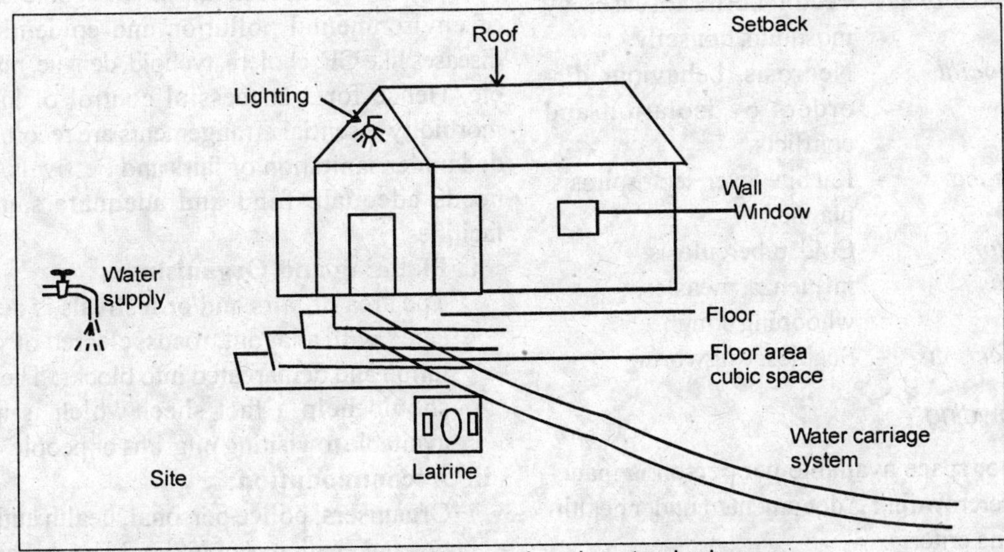

Fig. 5.1: Minimum housing standards

Refuse disposal: Daily disposal and transport for sanitary disposal is advocated.

Site of the house: In an elevated place, in a residential area of a town and subsoil water must be below 10 feet.

Setback: The built up area is restricted to 2/3rd of site. Wind direction and ventilation are considered.

Walls: Strong and weather resistant.

Windows: Window area shall be 1/5th of floor area.

Water supply: Safe and wholesome water supply is guaranteed.

Washing: Should have provision for washing facility.

In case of rural housing criteria, additional considerations are suggested and recommended. They are:

- Cattle shed 25 feet away.
- Manure pit at the backyard or side yard.

Housing Related Diseases

Accidents – Home accidents like fire, electrocution, fall and fracture.

Arthropod Borne – Vector borne diseases by mosquito, housefly.

Psychosocial – Neurosis, behaviour disorders by isolation and conflicts.

Rat Menace – Rat bite fever, leptospirosis, plague.

Respiratory Infections – Cold, tuberculosis, influenza, measles, whooping cough.

Skin Infections – Scabies, ringworm.

Overcrowding

If the floor space available per person is inadequate, overcrowding is documented under healthful housing criteria.

Accepted standards are:

- 70-90 sq.ft.—for 1 person
- Infant is not counted
- Child 1-10 years is ½ person.
- 2 persons above 9 years, not husband wife, of opposite sex, are not obliged to sleep in the same room.

Current Status

Absolute homeless families are in lakhs in India. Urban housing crisis is increasing due to hiked inflation. Slum and shanty town has no healthful and housing conditions. N.B.O. (National Buildings Organisation), HUDCO (Housing and Urban Development Corporation) and HHF (Hindustan Housing Factory) are functioning to achieve goals of healthful housing to the community, under IAY (Indira Awas Yojana) house with 1 room, 1 kitchen and RCA latrine, a bath and a smokeless chullah are being constructed which also give employment opportunity to rural youth.

FAIRS AND FESTIVALS–SANITATION

Fairs and religious festivals have become source of environmental pollution and epidemics of diseases like GE, cholera, typhoid, dengue, malaria etc. Hence for a successful control of human morbidity essential arrangements are recommended under sanitation of fairs and Festivals. This needs adequate fund and adequate sanitary facilities.

i. **Planning and Organising:**
   The area of fairs and/or festivals is demarcated with a layout, roads, cleared of vegetation and demarcated into blocks. The plan should help a fact sheet which is made available to visiting pilgrims or people.

ii. **Accommodation:**
   Organisers, police personal, health authorities and visiting people should have required

accommodation. It should have sanitary conveniences. Room accommodation should be 10 feet height and 10% of floor area with window. Pits, pools etc. are smoothened to avoid future breeding places.

iii. **Health Facility:**
The area should be under supervision of a health officer and assisted by required health assistants. Facility for routine treatment, first aid and an ambulance are prime requisites. Treatment facilities for burns, accidents are facilitated.

iv. **Water Supply:**
Adequate, safe and wholesome water supply arrangement is looked into through feasible methods like:
- Filtered, chlorinated water from water works.
- Deep tubewells.
- Piped water connection.

v. **Conservancy:**
Sweeping of roads, residential blocks are got done by whole time conservancy staff. They are also delegated the duties of cleaning of latrines, urinals.
One sanitary worker for 2000 expected pilgrims or people is the standards aimed at.
Dustbins at reachable to collect dust, their removal by trucks are to be arranged.
Latrine for males and females are to be planned separately. Trench latrine is ideal which is to cater as under:
- 1 day fair—2 seats per 1000 people.
- More than 1 day—1 seat per 100 people.

Adequate urinals are to be provided in fairs.
A pit 4 feet square, 5 feet depth is filled with broken bricks. At corner of pit kerosene tin filled with saw dust and bottom perforated is placed.
Satisfactory arrangement for refuse disposal is expected.

vi. **Food Hygiene:**
Supervision of food sale is exercised. Glass cover to cut fruits, sweets and eatables is enforced to avoid fly nuisance, care of food handlers and hygiene of food catering area are also enforced.

vii. **Immunisation:**
This depends on the place of fair or festival. Depending on its geographic location, vaccination for cholera, typhoid and meningitis are advocated. Pilgrims are expected to get vaccinated before specified days and before coming to Mela, as specified by corporation health authorities. In some of the international congregation, certification of vaccination is mandatory.

viii. **Health Inspection Check Post:**
Health staff is posted in check post to keep surveillance on patients with infectious disease, who are not allowed to fairs and festivals, to avoid spread of diseases.

ix. **Vigilance on Social Problems:**
Personnel from police and volunteers are drawn to check goondaism, theft, public unrest, prostitution, alcoholism and drug abuse.

METEOROLOGICAL ENVIRONMENT

These are physical surroundings that comprise: (a) Temperature (b) Humidity (c) Atmospheric pressure (d) Rainfall (e) Wind (f) Clouds; these are summated to represent meteorology or weather forecasting for the given geographical area.

Temperature

Atmospheric temperature is variable during the day, during the season and at given latitude. It is higher at ground level and goes on reducing as we move up to higher attitude. To measure atmospheric temperature, thermometers are used.

Mercury thermometers are used to record maximum temperature, because of its great expansible character. Ether is used to record lower temperature because of its great condensation power.

Dry Bulb Thermometer: Commonly used to record air temperature.

Wet Bulb Thermometer: When bulb of thermometer is kept wet by a muslin cloth, it shows air temperature depending on the dryness of air.

Maximum Thermometer: It is a mercury thermometer.

Minimum Thermometer: It is an alcohol thermometer.

Six's Maximum and Minimum Thermometer: It is a combination of maximum and minimum thermometers which are used in Indian Meteorological observations.

Globe Thermometer: Bulb of thermometer is painted with matt-black paint which absorbs radiant heat and air temperature.

Kata Thermometer: It is used to find out cooling power of the air.

Cooling power of the air is expressed as milli calories per square cm per second.

Indices of Comfort in Kata Thermometer

Dry kata 6 and above Wet kata 20 and above	Indicate thermal comfort

Types of kata are:

a. Standard kata—range 100-95°F (Red).
b. High temperature kata—130-125°F (Dark blue).
c. Extra high temperature—150-145°F (Magenta).

Common heat stress indices are available like: (a) Equatorial comfort index (b) Heat stress index (c) Predicted four-hour sweat rate.

Heat stress index upto 10 is tolerable and heat strain starts with 10 and 40 HSI, is severe heat strain.

Health Effects

- Heat stroke.
- Heat hyperpyrexia.
- Heat exhaustion.
- Heat cramps.
- Heat syncope.

Prevention of Heat Stress is by:

- Water replacement.
- Salt replacement.
- Regulation of work.
- Light loose clothing.
- Protection by goggle, shield.
- Air and ventilation of working area.

Effect of lower temperature:

- Numbness.
- Loss of sensation.
- Muscular weakness.
- Immersion foot (Trench foot).
- Frostbite.

Above cold stress can be prevented by protection and using warm water.

Global Warming

Emission of green house gases to atmosphere mainly CO_2 can bring about rise in global surface temperature, rise in sea level and extreme climatic events like cyclone, heat wave and draught. This affects global ecosystem.

Humidity

Humidity is expressed in terms of the water content in air (Aqueous Tension). Air temperature determines humidity. We notice dew collection when air temperature is very low. If it is measured in percentage it is called *Relative humidity*. If humidity is expressed in actual by weight for a given value it is absolute humidity. Below 30% of relative humidity and above 65% of relative humidity is not comfortable. Low humidity cause dryness of nasal mucosa and cause ENT problems.

To measure humidity following instruments are used:

i. Hygrometer (Dry and wet bulb thermometer).
ii. Sling psychrometer (Dry and wet bulb with rotation facility).
iii. Assmann psychrometer.

Rainfall

Water precipitated from atmosphere is rain water. Depending on level of precipitation the water may be in the form of snow, hail, dew or frost. Rainfall is measured by "Rain gauge". Rainfall of 8 mm in a day or 41 mm in a month is unit of expression with the measure by Symons Rain Gauge.

Wind Velocity

Air velocity is measured by anemometer, gives the unit metre per second. Accordingly we have the following meteorological terminologies.

0.5 meter per second – Calm wind
3.3 meter per second – Slight breeze
10.0 meter per second – Strong wind
15-20 meter per second – Storm
25-30 meter per second – Gale
30-50 meter per second – Hurricane

Direction of wind is measured by wind vane.

Clouds and Weather

It gives sequence of weather in a geographical locality. Common man uses the word bad weather, good weather by these observations. Satellite installation by Government of India has given highly sensitive and accurate idea of weather and values for weather forecasting.

AIR AND VENTILATION

Air

Biosphere has life only by the presence of air which supplies oxygen, cools the body, gives stimulus to special sense. Polluted air can cause high morbidity and mortality.

Composition of Air

1. Nitrogen 78.1 %
2. Oxygen 20.93 %
3. CO_2 0.03 %
4. Other gases
5. Water vapour
6. Ammonia traces
7. Suspended matter:

   Air gets polluted very easily by:

   a. Traffic, trade
   b. Organic matter decomposition
   c. Combustion of oil, gas, coal
   d. Human and animal respiration.

   Nature simultaneously disallows air pollution through:

   a. Wind
   b. Sunlight
   c. Rainfall and
   d. Green plant life.

Effect of Overcrowding

Both physical changes and chemical changes are noticed due to overcrowding. Physical changes include rise in temperature, increase in humidity, reduced air movement, emission of body odours and microorganisms from patients if they are suffering from diseases. Chemical changes include raised CO_2 level and reduced O_2 content.

Overcrowding causes headache, drowsiness and inability to concentrate. Discomfort in overcrowding is due to physical changes and not because of chemical changes.

Measurement of Thermal Comfort

i. Cooling power of the air by kata thermometer.
ii. Corrected effective temperature (CET) which combines air temperature, humidity, air movement and radiant heat. Globe

thermometer is used in recording air temperature.

iii. Predicted four hours sweat rate (P_4SR).

It is called McArdle's maximum allowable sweat rate which is 3 for an upper limit of comfort zone (Table 5.1).

Table 5.1: Comfort zone

	CET	*P_4SR*
Comfortable	77-80°F	—
Comfort zone	—	1-3 litres
Hot, uncomfortable	81-82°F	—
Just tolerable	—	3-4.5 litres
Intolerable	86°F	4.5 + litres

Air Pollution: Air is said to be polluted if substance of human and animal activity is raised and that can cause human ill health. Air can get polluted by:

a. Motor vehicles which emit hydrocarbons, CO, lead, nitrogen oxide and particulate matter.
b. Industry emit smoke, SO_2, Nitrogen Oxide and fly ash.
c. Domestic combustions of coal, wood etc.
d. Others like nuclear energy, pesticide spray etc.

Man is in direct effect of 10 kms of atmosphere and not above that from the earth's surface. Rise in atmospheric temperature make pollutions to diffuse vertically. If cooling of lower layer has occurred then vertical air diffusion is not possible allowing pollutants to get trapped at lower level as *smog.* This is called *temperature inversion.* Important pollutants are CO, CO_2, H_2S, SO_2, SO_3, NO_2, organic compounds, metals, radio active compounds and photo chemical oxidants (Table 5.2).

Table 5.2: Indoor air pollutants

Possible source	*Pollutant*
Smoking	Tobacco particle
Combustion	CO, CO_2
Coal	SO_2
Resin products	Benzene
Fire proofing	Asbestos
Appliances	Mineral fibre

Hazards of Air Pollution

i. Respiratory tract irritation
ii. Impaired lung function
iii. Lung cancer
iv. Cough, ARI
v. Asthma, Chronic bronchitis
vi. Hindrance in neuropsychological development.

Control of Air Pollution

a. By air monitoring for SO_2, smoke index and dust measurement
b. Follow up of criteria and guidelines for maximum permissible allowance for individual substances
c. Monitoring of air pollution through data base in selected cities.
d. Containment of harmful substances
e. Discarding and replacing old technology process with new safe process
f. Vegetation and development of green belt.
g. Acts and amendments to enforce clear air.
h. Development of network of Laboratories
i. Air disinfection by ventilation, ultraviolet radiation and allowing clean air by triethylene glucol vapour (Table 5.3).

Table 5.3: Maximum upper limit of chemicals in air

Substance	*Maximum limit*	*Averaging time*
CO	30 mg/m³	1 hour
H_2S	150 microgram/m³	24 hours
Lead	0.5-1.0 microgram/m³	1 year
NO_2	150 microgram/m³	24 hours
SO_2	350 microgram/m³	1 hour

Ventilation

Ventilation is a process of controlling air quality in terms of temperature, humidity and purity. Minimum fresh air supply to man is 300 to 3000 cubic feet per hour per person. Air is allowed to have recommended cooling power of the air.

Optimum floor space suggested is 50-100 square feet.

Natural Ventilation

A. Wind movement in a chamber is called perflation. When there is obstruction, it is aspirated. Windows or doors when facing each other cross ventilation occurs.
B. When a small space is provided air is diffused slowly.
C. Temperature difference outside and inside make air movement possible.

Mechanical Ventilation

A. Exhaust fan takes the air out and is called exhaust system.
B. Centrifugal fans blow air inside and is called plenum system.
C. A combination of exhaust and plenum system is used.
D. Air conditioning in O.T., hospital, ICU, ICCU, IPCU is very helpful. The air is filtered and saturated with water vapour. The excess moisture is removed and the air is heated to desired temperature. Care is taken to see that outside and inside temperature is maintained to below 20°F.

NOISE

Noise is defined as unwanted sound i.e. wrong sound, in wrong place at wrong time. Modern life is associated with noise pollution. Major source comes from automobile, factory, industry, airway, roadway, television and sound systems (Table 5.4 and 5.5).

Table 5.4: Acceptable noise level

Home	40 dBA
Office	45 dBA
Industry	60 dBA
Classroom	40 dBA
Hospital ward	20 dBA

Table 5.5: Noise level in decibels

Whispering	10 dB
Talking	60 dB
Speech	80 dB
Radio music	85 dB
Shouting	80 dB
Crying	80 dB
Road roller	120 dB
Plane take off	150 dB

Above 90 dB and 4000Hz, whistling and buzzing in ears occur. Temporary or permanent hearing loss is affected based on noise level and duration of exposure. Sleeplessness, psychosis, neurosis and fatigue are common due to noise pollution.

Suggested Measures to Control Noise Pollution

i. Town planning
ii. Vehicle and traffic control
iii. Noise proof constructions
iv. Source reduction in industry
v. Ear plug and ear muff use
vi. Legal regulations
vii. Public awareness on noise pollution.

LIGHTING

Lighting is an essential part for good vision, efficiency, physiological functions and vitamin D synthesis. Brightness of light is measured by candle power whereas amount of light reaching surface is measured by foot candle.

D.F. (Daylight Factor)

$$D.F. = \frac{\text{Indoor Illumination}}{\text{Outdoor Illumination}} = \times 100$$

Daylight Factor is a ratio between instantaneous illumination indoors and simultaneously occurring illumination outdoors. Living room should have 8% D.F. and kitchen 10%. Since artificial lighting is to be depended, systems of artificial lighting like direct, indirect, semi-direct, semi-indirect and direct-indirect have come up in daily life. Light from above and from left is ideal for reading and studying; lighting standards are laid down for each visual activity. Avoiding glare, an illumination of above 30 times the requirement is rule of thumb for visual task.

RADIATION

Men are continuously exposed to radiation through cosmic rays, U.V. rays, X-rays, α rays , β rays and γ rays, both natural way and man made exposures. Further over the past 25 years, therapeutic procedures have been developed in the field of Radiology, based on (mainly) angiographic techniques. Diagnostic procedures involving injection of contrast media comes under the heading of invasive diagnostic radiology. Interventional radiology on the other hand comprises procedures with a predominantly therapeutic objective. Here from nursing care point of view it takes care of informed consent and the level of acceptable risk for diagnosis.

Natural Radiation

From outer space cosmic rays are emitted. In soil and rock radioactive elements like thorium, Uranium are emitted.

Somatic effect: Acute (Radiation Sickness and Acute Radiation Syndrome).

Chronic (Blood cancer, Other cancers, Foetal abnormalities, Reduced lifespan).

Genetic effect: Chromosomal aberrations, point mutations.

Thorium, uranium, radium are present, even human body does contain minute quantity of isotopes of K_{40}, Sr_{90} and C_{14}.

Manmade Radiation

X-Ray is the greatest source used in hospital practice. Nuclear explosions release energy and ionising radiation. T.V., luminous watches etc., also contribute to our exposure. Ionising radiation is one where radiation penetrates the tissue and gets deposited in tissues.

Effects of Radiation

Since man is exposed to radiation during diagnosis and for intervention, the scope has widened to cover fluoroscopy, ultrasound, computerized tomography (CT scan) and magnetic resonance imaging (M.R. scan).

Radiation Protection

i. Pregnant women are not exposed to radiation unnecessarily.
ii. Leakage of X-ray machines and defective machines are avoided and discarded.
iii. All working in X-ray unit, isotope unit, cobalt therapy unit, luminous parts industry and atomic energy are subjected for periodic check-up.
iv. Dosimeter or Film badge is used by people working in Radiology department, which checks the dose of ionization.
v. Lead apron to prevent X-ray entry to workers' body.
vi. Adaptation of ICRP recommendations on radiation dose levels (International Commission on Radiological Protection).

WATER

Most of the developing countries are not getting required quantity of safe and wholesome water. Water is not easily accessible, not only in adequate quantity but also found invariably contaminated. Water is a necessity for survival. This is related with socio-economic development of human population. Safe drinking water is a basic need of primary health care which is the key to attain health for all. There is considerable improvement in urban water supply in late 2000, but rural India has not attained the requisite provision of protected water for the community. Now Government

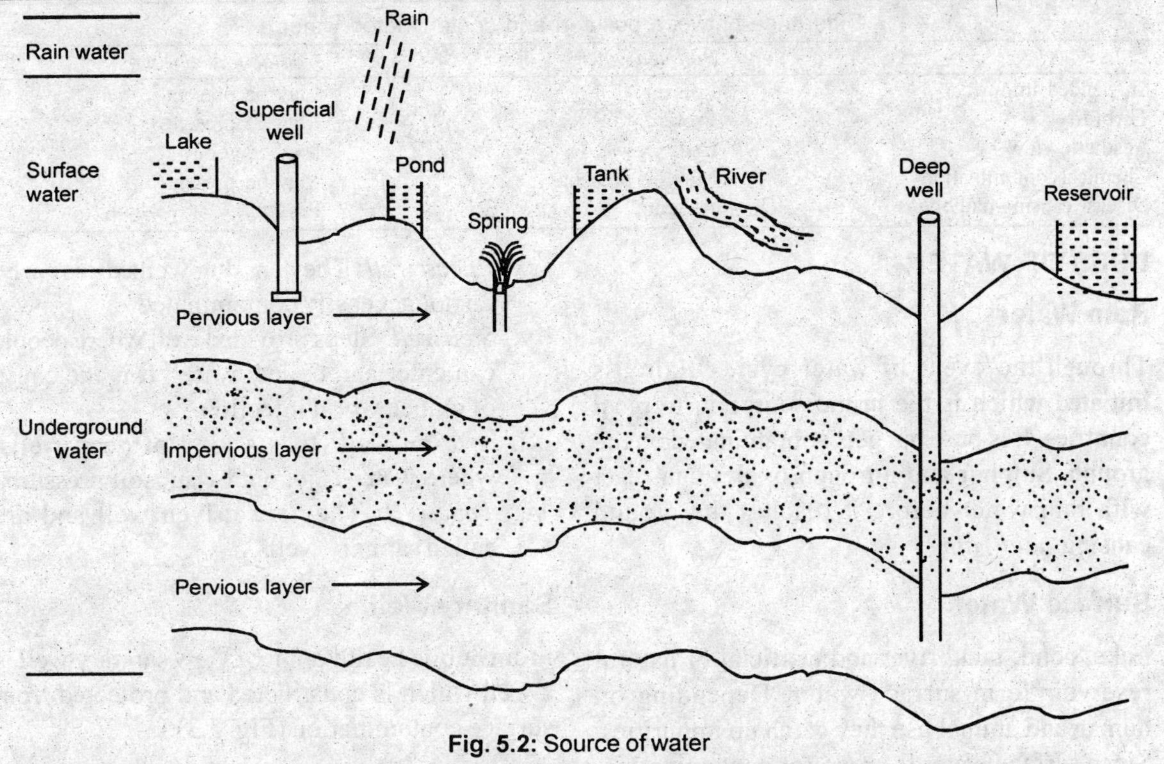

Fig. 5.2: Source of water

Table 5.6: Uses of water

Domestic	*Public*	*Industry*	*Agriculture*
Drinking Cooking Washing Bathing Ablution Gardening	Swimming pool Fountain Ponds Fire force Public park	Raw material Process material Cooling material	Irrigation Farming Plantation Cash crops Food crops
Power	*Carriage system*		
Hydropower Steam power Sullage	Solid waste Liquid waste Sewage		

of India has included water as a component in RCH, Nutrition programme and health awareness programme.

Safe and Wholesome Water

The criteria for safe and wholesome water are:

i. It should be potable.

ii. It should meet aesthetic value by colour, taste, turbidity.

iii. It should be free from harmful chemical substances.

iv. It should be free from pathogens (Fig. 5.2 and Table 5.6).

Difference between polluted and contaminated water

	Polluted water	*Contaminated water*
Suspended impurity	Present	May be present
Turbidity	Present	May be present
Aesthetic view	Bad	May be good
Chemical contamination	May be present	May be present
Disease causing pathogens	Absent	Present

USES OF WATER

Rain Water

Through the event of water cycle "Rain" is initiated which is the prime source in tropical countries. It is pure but gets contaminated on the ground. Sulphur and nitrogen oxides can react with rain water before it reaches the ground causing *acid rain.*

Surface Water

Lake, pond, tank, river and artificial or natural reservoir form surface water. Depending on human and animal use they catch up impurities. Since surface water is prone for contamination, it needs purification before use.

Underground Water

Wells, spring are typical source of underground water which is the major source of water in India. The water drawn from below the impervious layer is safe since it is not amenable for contamination. Hence deep well and deep springs are safe sources of water.

Types of Wells

i. *Shallow well:* It taps water from above the impervious layer, soft often grossly contaminated and not long lasting.
ii. *Deep well:* It taps water from below the impervious layer, hard, bacteriologically pure and provides constant supply.
iii. *Katcha well*: They are dug wells dries early, gets easily contaminated.
iv. *Pucca well:* They are dug wells dries early, do not get easily contaminated.
v. *Step well:* Steps provided well where people can enter and collect water. It is the cause of guinea worm infection.
vi. *Artesan well:* It is a kind of deep wells, where water is jet out by subsoil pressure.
vii. *Tubewell:* They are driven well and are called sanitary wells.

Sanitary Well

From public health point of view sanitary well is a well which is constructed and protected from surface contamination (Fig. 5.3).

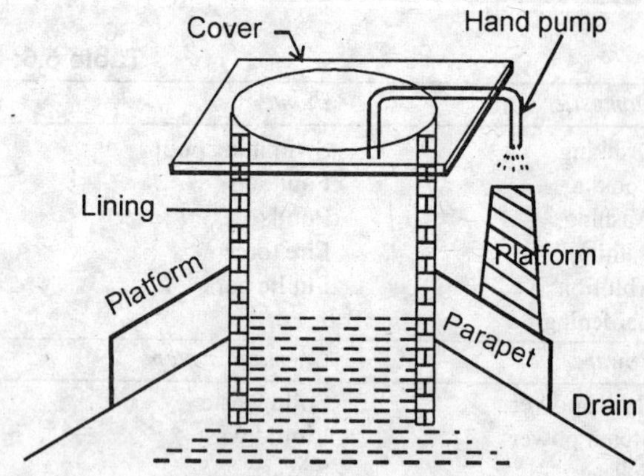

Fig. 5.3: A sanitary well

A sanitary well should be 50 feet away from likely source of contamination. Lining of the well wall must be of brick and cement. It should have a parapet wall and a platform round the well. Drain is provided which drains beyond the zone of influence. Well is covered and a pump set is fixed.

Water Pollution

The impurities derived from atmosphere, catchments area and soil, pollutes a given source of water. Industry and urbanization worsen the pollution. Sullage, sewage, industry waste and agricultural wastes dominate in water pollution. Cross connection and leakage also cause water pollution.

Water Pollution is indicated by:

i. Suspended solids
ii. B.O.D. (Biological Oxidation Demand)
iii. C.O.D. (Chemical Oxidation Demand)
iv. Nitrogen
v. Dissolved oxygen.

Water Borne Diseases

Bacterial	–	Typhoid, paratyphoid, dysentery, infantile diarrhoea, cholera
Viral	–	Hepatitis A, poliomyelitis, infantile rota virus infection
Protozoal	–	Amoebiasis, giardiasis
Helminthic	–	Roundworm, threadworm
Leptospiral	–	Weil's disease
Others	–	Schistosomiasis Guinea worm infection Fish tape worm

To control water pollution, Parliament has passed "Prevention and Control of Pollution Act", 1974.

Purification of Water

Domestic Scale

Boiling for 10 minutes and keeping in the same vessel.

Bleaching powder commercially available contains 33% of available chlorine. In case of stabilized bleaching powder it is about 70% of available chlorine.

Chlorine tablet—0.5 grams of one tablet is sufficient for 20 litres of water.

Iodine—It is only for emergency disinfection.

$KMnO_4$—Though it is good, not accepted from aesthetic point of view.

Filters

Candle filters are commercially produced. In this contaminated water is allowed to filter slowly through a porous ceramic material. This cannot filter virus. Types of filters available are Pasteur Chamberland Filter, Berkefeld Filter and Katadyn Filter.

Double Pot Method

Double pot is a product of NEERI, Nagpur. There are 2 pots one placed inside the other. Inner pot has hole in upper portion and in outer pot the hole is 4 cm above the bottom. Mixture of 1:2 Bleaching powder and coarse sand is kept in inside pot. When water enters there is slow release of chlorine for action. It is lowered and immersed in the well for well disinfection (Fig. 5.4).

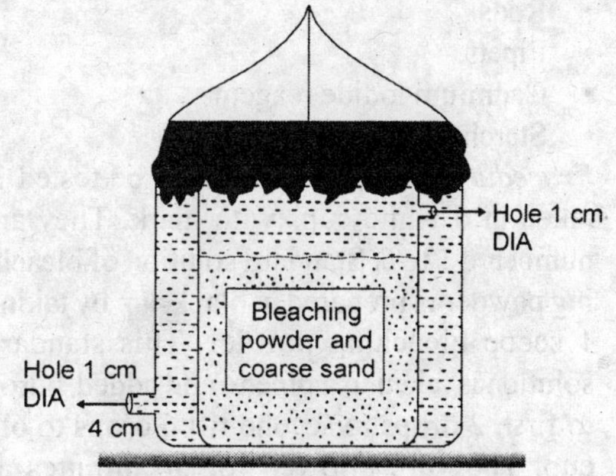

Fig 5.4: Double pot

Well Disinfection

Subsoil water through well is a major source of water and well disinfection is to be periodically done in rural India to prevent water borne disease.

Following steps are followed in well disinfection:

a. Volume of water in a well is determined by following formula:
   i. Circular well with metric values:

$$\text{Volume of water (Litres)} = \frac{3.14 \times d^2 \times h}{4} \times 1000$$

where d = Diameter of well
h = Depth of water

   ii. Rectangular well with British value:
   Vol (Gallon) = Length × Breadth × 6.25 × Depth of water
   iii. Circular well with British values:
   Vol (Gallons) = $D^2 \times W \times 5$ = gallons
   Where D = Diameter of well
   W = Depth of water

b. Bleaching powder demand is found out by Horrock's Test.
   Apparatus contains:
   - Six white cups
   - One black cup
   - Scoop (2 G)
   - Rods
   - Pipette
   - Cadmium iodide reagent
   - Starch solution.

   Procedure: Sample of water to be tested is taken in 6 white cups with mark. They are numbered 1 to 6. Standard solution of bleaching powder is prepared in black cup by taking 1 scoop bleaching powder. This standard solution is taken in a pipette and added 1 drop to first, 2 drops to second till 6 drops to 6th cup. They are allowed for 30 minutes as contact period by constant stirring. After 30 minutes 3 drops cadmium iodide and 1 ml starch solution are added and observed for colour change. From the inference, bleaching powder demand is calculated (e.g., if 3rd cup onwards blue colour appeared, then 3 × 2 = 6G. of bleaching powder is needed for 100 gallons of water. (Note: If there is no change, experiment is repeated with 6 to 12 drops of standard solution).

c. Required quantity of bleaching powder is taken in a bucket, prepared to paste in the beginning and later to a homogenous solution.
d. Supernatant solution of (c) is taken in a bucket and mixed to well water by constant jerky movement (in the evening times at village).
e. Allowed overnight for action.
f. Next morning well water is tested for residual chlorine which should be at least 0.5 PPM (1 PPM after 1 hour contact period is ideal) by ortho-toluidine test.

Large Scale

In a water reservoir, procedure followed are: (i) Storage (ii) Filtration and (iii) Chlorination.

Storage: 24 hours storage help in settling of suspended impurities, oxidation by aerobic bacteria can occur and sunlight may help in certain disinfection.

Filtration: It can be either slow sand filtration or rapid sand filtration. In case of more suspended solid content and high turbidity of source of water, prefiltration with gravel or other course material before sand filtration is an effective means of preventing the rapid blocking of the sand filters. Raw water is passed vertically or horizontally through different compartments and collected in outlet chamber. If vertical flow is chosen, either up-flow or down-flow is possible, but up-flow filters are easier to clean and thus more likely to operate effectively.

Slow Sand Filtration

Slow sand filtration improves physical, chemical and microbiological quality of water. It is reliable and less expensive and is therefore particularly useful in small community water supplies. The *Biological* layer (it is also called vital layer or Zoogleal layer or schmutzdecke) is made of algae, plankton, diatoms and bacteria which is responsible for removal of organic matter and oxidize ammoniacal nitrogen.

Essentials of Slow Sand Filtration are tabulated as under (Table 5.7 and Fig. 5.5):

Table 5.7: Essentials of slow sand filter

1. Occupies large area
2. Rate of filtration is 3 million gallons per acre per day
3. Effective sand size is 0.3 mm.
4. Prefiltration is plain sedimentation
5. Washing of bed is by scraping
6. Operation is not skilled work
7. Loss of head allowed 4 feet
8. Turbidity is removed
9. Colour is removed
10. 100 percent bacterial purity (99.9%)

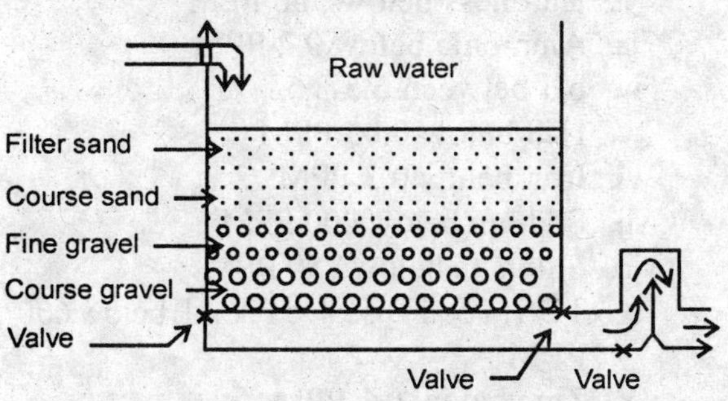

Fig. 5.5: Element of slow sand filter

Loss of head is, resistance offered by sand, in due course of time of filtration, which needs periodic cleaning (Fig. 5.6).

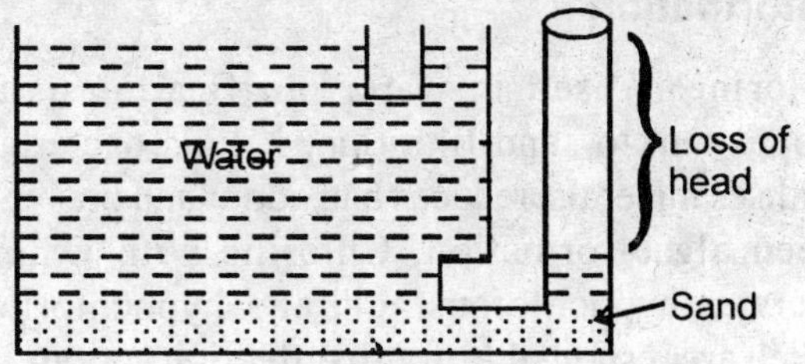

Fig. 5.6: Loss of head

Rapid Sand Filtration

There are two types of Rapid Filters, Paterson Filter acts on the gravity and Candy's Filter acts on the pressure. Before filtration or prefiltration, coagulation is allowed in rapid filtration which takes off suspended impurities.

Including prefiltration process, rapid sand filtration has following components (Fig. 5.7):

Essentials of rapid sand filter are tabulated as under:

1. Occupies small space.
2. Filters 200 million gallon per unit filter.
3. Sand size is 0.4 mm.
4. Prefiltration include coagulation, sedimentation.
5. Cleaning is done by back wash.
6. Operation is a skilled one.
7. Loss of head 6 feet.
8. Removes turbidity.
9. Removes colour.
10. Bacteriological purity 99%.

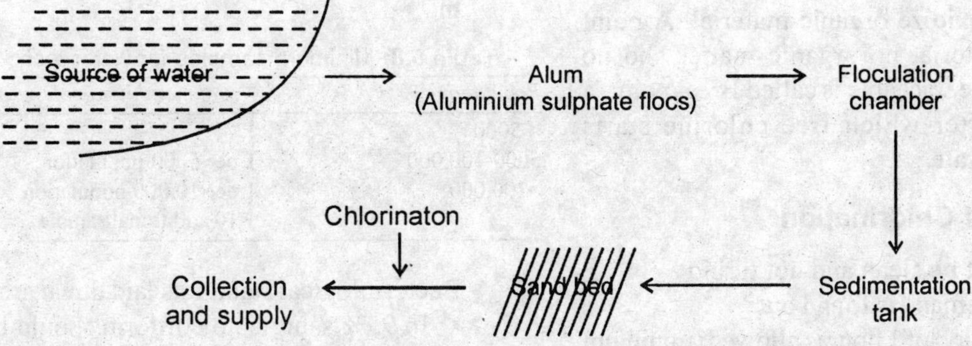

Fig . 5.7: Rapid Sand Filter Unit

Chlorination

Chlorine is used in water purification as a supplement to sand filtration. It kills bacteria, oxidises minerals, reduces bad odour and prevent green algae-formation. Chlorine with water liberates hypochlorous acid and hypochlorite which are responsible for disinfection action.

$H_2O + Cl_2 \rightarrow HCl + HOCl$

$HOCl \rightarrow H + OCl$

Types of chlorination are:

a. Pre chlorination
b. Post chlorination
c. Combined chlorination
d. Super chlorination
e. Break point chlorination (Fig. 5.8).

For chlorination chlorine used will be in the form of: (a) Gas (b) Chloramine or (c) Perchloron.

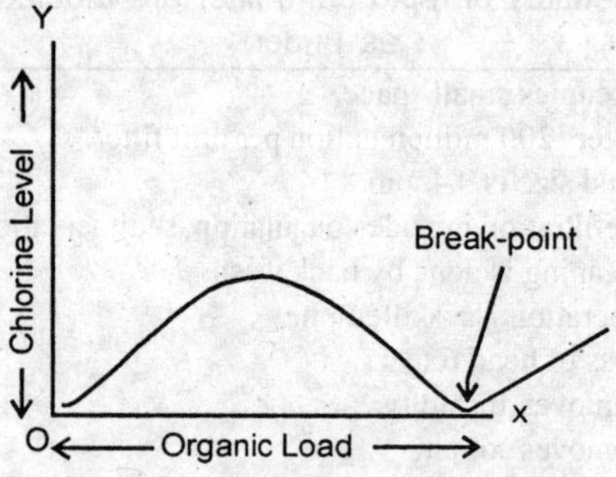

Fig. 5.8: Break point chlorination

Figure 5.8 illustrates that chlorine added kills bacteria and oxidize organic material. A point where no bacteria, no organic matter and no chlorination are traceable is called Breakpoint (a misnomer) after which free chlorine starts appearing in water.

Principles of Chlorination

1. Water must be clean and not turbid
2. Chlorine demand is found out
3. Contact period of 1 hour is allowed (minimum 30 minutes)
4. Residual chlorine of 0.5 mg/litre after 1 hour contact period is allowed.

Guidelines for Drinking Water Quality

I. Acceptability
 a. Physical
  i. Should not be turbid
  ii. Should not have colour
  iii. No bad smell or taste
  iv. Should be cool.
 b. Inorganic
  i. Chloride less than 600 PPM
  ii. Hardness below 500 PPM
  iii. Ammonia below 0.2 PPM
  iv. pH between 6.5-8.5
  v. H_2S below 0.05 PPM
  vi. Iron below 0.3 PPM
  vii. Sodium below 200 PPM
  viii. Sulphate below 250 PPM
  ix. TDS (Total Dissolved Solid) below 600 PPM
  x. Zinc below 0.1 PPM
  xi. Manganese below 0.1 PPM
  xii. Dissolved O_2 (level for not to cause bad odour)
  xiii. Copper below 1 PPM
  xiv. Aluminium below 0.2 PPM
II. Microbiological:
 a. Coliform organisms are tested by multiple tube method. They should be less than 10 MPN (Most Probable Number) per 100 ml.

Table 5.8: Minimum samples for water test

Population	*No. of monthly sample*
< 5000	1
5000-100,000	1 per 5000 population
>100,000	1 per 10,000 population + 10 additional sample

Bacteriological standards laid down are:

- In 95% sample no coliform should be seen

- No E.coil in any sample in 100 ml
- MPN (Coliform) should be below 10/ 100 ml
- Should not be positive in two consecutive samples.

b. Virologically it must be pure
c. Biologically no organism should be present.

III. *Chemical aspect:*
Following upper limit are fixed for criteria under potable water (all ppm):

Arsenic	0.005
Cadmium	0.003
Chromium	0.05
Cyanide	0.07
Fluoride	1.5
Lead	0.01
Mercury	0.001
Nitrate (NO_3)	50
Nitrite (NO_2)	Zero
Benzene	10

IV. *Radiological aspect:*
α Radioactivity below 0.1 Bq/L*
β Radioactivity below 1.0 Bq/L.*

Note:
* Unit of Radioactivity was called curie (Ci).
* Now it is called Becquerel (Bq).

Surveillance of water supply to the community should have following measures:

i. Check at new source of water
ii. Water source is protected
iii. Sanitary survey carried out
iv. Sampling done properly as per specifications
v. Bacteriological surveillance includes:
 a. PCT (Presumptive Coliform Test)
 b. Detection of faecal contamination
 c. Colony count
 d. Biological examination
vi. Chemical surveillance is done.

Hardness of Water

Temporary hardness is due to bicarbonates and permanent hardness is due to sulphates and chlorides. Soft water has less than 1 mEq/Litre of hardness whereas very hard water has over 6 mEq/Litre of hardness. Hardness causes: (a) More soap usage (b) Scaling of boilers (c) Fabrics do not last longer (d) Not suitable for industries.

Removal of hardness is as under:

i. Boiling (for temporary hardness):
 $Ca\ (HCO_3)_2 \rightarrow CaCO_3 + H_2O + CO_2$
ii. Addition of lime (for temporary hardness):
 $Ca\ (OH)_2\ +\ Ca(HCO_3) \rightarrow 2\ CACO_3\ +2\ H_2O$
iii. Addition of sodium carbonate (for both temporary and permanent hardness):
 $-Na_2Co_3\ +\ Ca(HCO_2)_2 \rightarrow 2\ NaHCO_2\ +\ CaCO_2$
 $-CaSO_4\ +\ Na_2CO_2\ CaCO_3\ +\ Na_2SO_4$
iv. Base exchange process:
 Sodium permutit, a complex compound of sodium, aluminium and silica is used ($Na_2\ Al_2\ Si_2O\ H_2O$). By change process it softens the water.

Hard water has a protective role in cardiovascular disease.

Fluorine Content: Normal level is 0.5 to 0.8 PPM. Low level is associated with caries. High level is associated with fluorosis.

SWIMMING POOL SANITATION

Health hazards associated with swimming pool are:

- Fungal infection of skin
- Warts
- Eye, Ear, Nose, Throat infection
- Respiratory infection
- Intestinal infection
- Accidents.

Preventive Measures

i. Rules and regulation for personal hygiene is advocated.
ii. Everyday 15% of water is replaced.
iii. Chlorination and maintenance of residual chlorine 1 PPM is advocated.

Health Education

It includes convincing felt need of protected water and for giving up unhygienic practices.

National Water Supply and Sanitation Programme

It was started in 1954. In 1972 it envisaged Accelerated Rural Water Supply Programme. Government identified problem villages (no water within distance of 1.6 km and at depth of 15 metres) for assistance. A norm of water supply of 40 litres per head per day and one hand pump for every 250 population was planned. Current status is that 85% of population are getting safe water supply.

Waste Disposal

Health hazards due to improper disposal of waste are known and its need is to be understood by nursing professionals. They are called upon to give advice on some occasion.

SOLID WASTE

This depends on lifestyle, living standard, urbanization and industrialisation. Per head solid waste produced on an average works out to be 1.0 to 2.0 kg per day. Vector borne diseases will increase with the accumulation of solid waste material. Sanitary disposal of waste is a must for positive health. Following sequence follows which can lead to diseases if dumping is done:

- Ferments and decomposes
- Fly breeding
- Vector borne diseases occur
- Water pollution
- Soil pollution
- Aesthetic point of view.

Terms used:

Garbage – Fruit and vegetable waste.

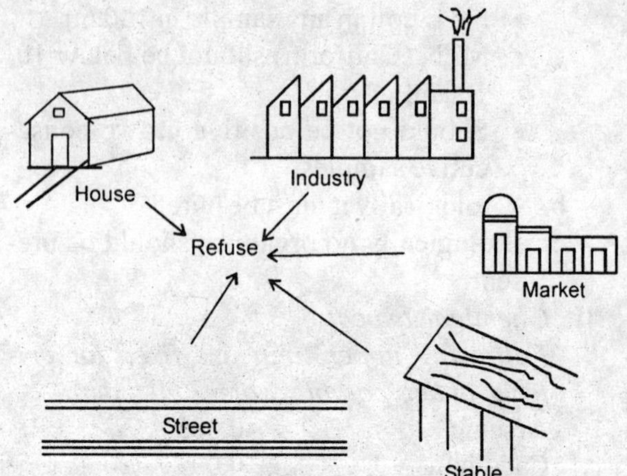

Fig 5.9: Sources of refuse

Rubbish – Paper, plastic, wood, metal, old container, glass pieces, bricks, pipes, sludge and solid of domestic waste.

Ash – Burnt material in powder form

Storage – By waste bin, plastic bin etc.

Collection – House to house collection by closed cart, closed truck, corporation van etc.

Sanitary Methods of Disposal

a. **Urban Area:**

i. *Controlled tipping on sanitary landfill* (Raised temperature at 60°C kills pathogens)

- Trench method (when land is available) 1 acre per 10,000 population is sufficient. Trench at 9 metre width and 3 metre height works out better.
- Ramp method (when slope is there)
- Area method (when depressions are there).

ii. *Incineration:*(Best suited for hospital waste)

Hospital waste which are contaminated, paper and waste that can be burnt are put to incinerator and destroyed by burning.

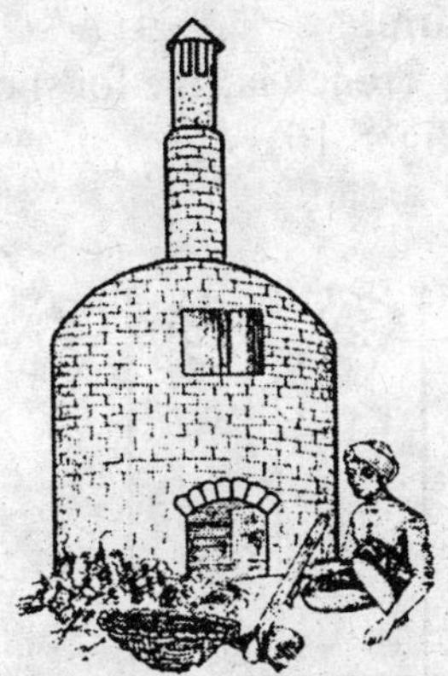

Fig. 5.10: Incinerator

The ash left out is called *clinkers,* is used for metal road. Parts of incinerator are:

- Furnace built fire proof
- Platform for tipping refuse
- Stoker for raking refuse to fire
- Baffle plate to drive fumes to chimney.

Common pattern of incinerators are:

- Double cell meldrum type.
- Single cell horsfall destructor type.

iii. Composting: Bangalore Method of composting)
Pattern of filling gives room for hot fermentation and decomposition. After 3 months harmless manure is made available:

b. **Rural area :**
- By manure pit
- By gobar gas plant.

c. **Camp life:**
- Burial into ground
- Burning to ashes.

LIQUID WASTE

Excreta Disposal

Faecal borne diseases like Typhoid, Paratyphoid, Diarrhoea, Dysentery, Cholera, Hookworm, Roundworm are common because of soil pollution, water pollution and food contamination by excreta.

Where open field defecation is common, pollution of environment occurs. Enteric fever and hookworm anaemia is highest in their prevalence in such areas (Fig. 5.11).

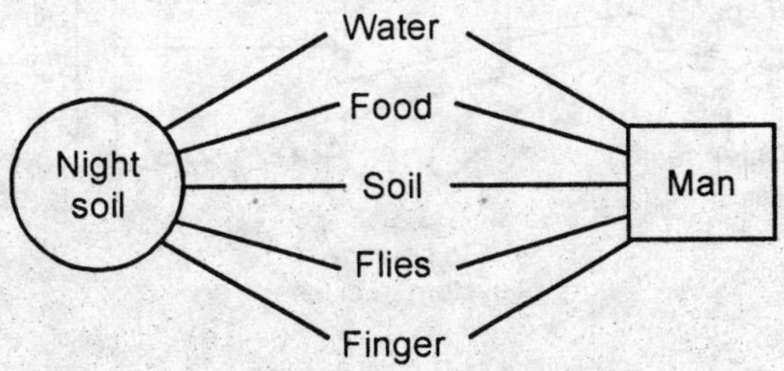

Fig. 5.11: Faecalborne disease transmission

i. *Bore hole latrine (Fig. 5.12):*

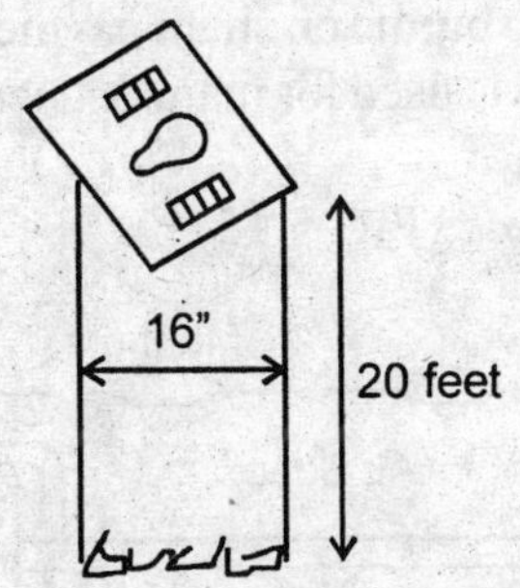

Fig. 5.12: Bore hole latrine

ii. *Dug well latrine (Fig. 5.13):*

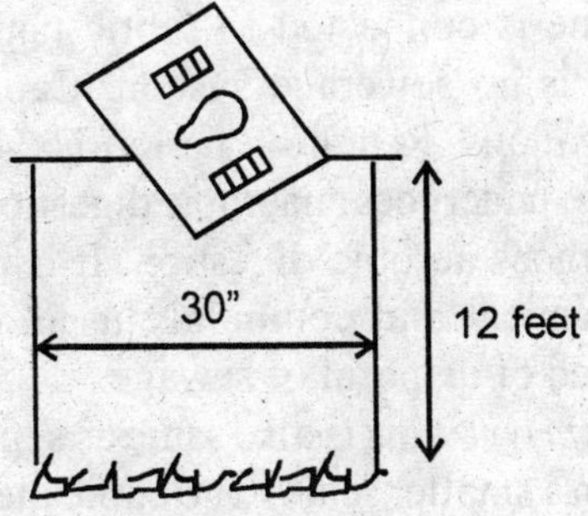

Fig. 5.13: Dug well latrine

iii. *R.C.A. Latrine (Research cum action):*

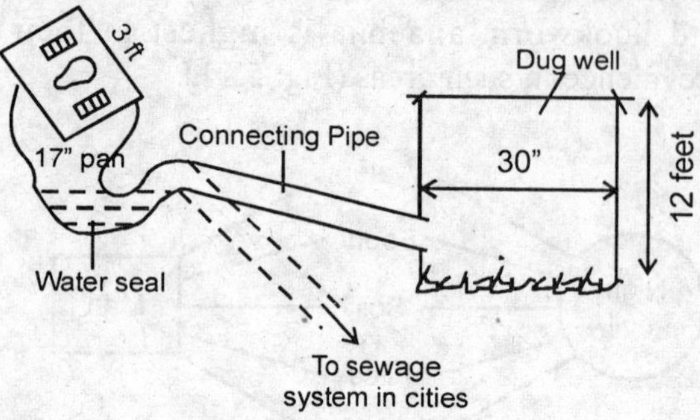

Fig. 5.14: R.C.A. latrine

iv. *Sulabh Shouchalaya:*
It is founded by Sulabh organisation of Dr. Bindeshwar Pathak to provide clean toilet facility to public on small payment. Amount collected is used for maintenance of sulabha souchalaya.

v. *Septic tank* (Fig. 5.15):

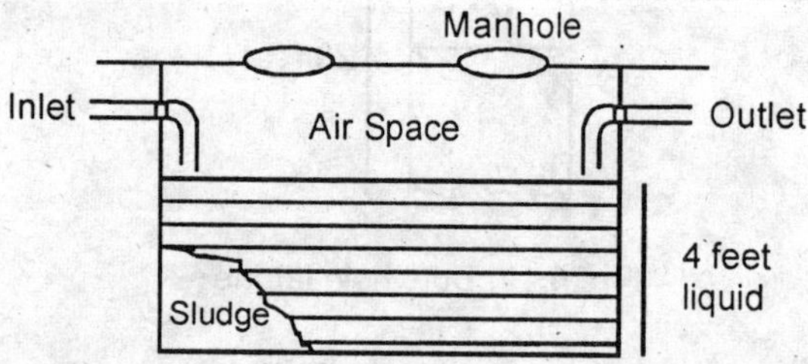

Fig. 5.15: Septic tank

Latrine is connected to septic tank when there is no sewerage system. Capacity is 500 gallons. Retention period is 24 hours. Sludge undergoes anaerobic digestion, scum undergoes aerobic digestion. It is the best economical and commonly used sanitary method of disposal of sewage.

vi. *Aqua privy:* This is also same as septic tank but on a smaller scale. One cubic metre size is sufficient for a family of 4 members for 5 years.

For camp life:

- Shallow Trench latrine for short duration camp (Fig. 5.16)

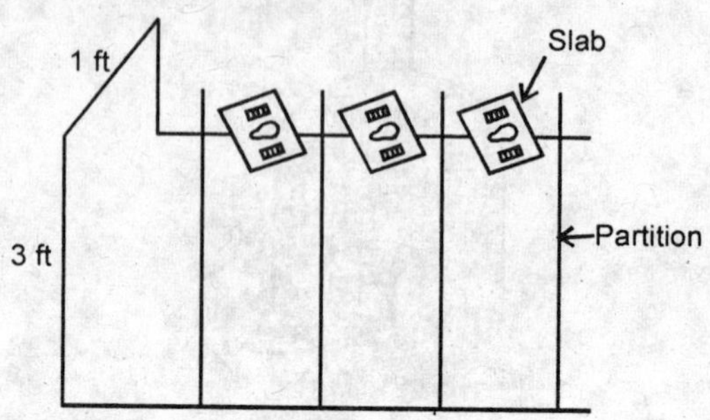

Fig. 5.16: Shallow trench latrine

- Deep trench latrine (Fig. 5.17)
  For long duration camp

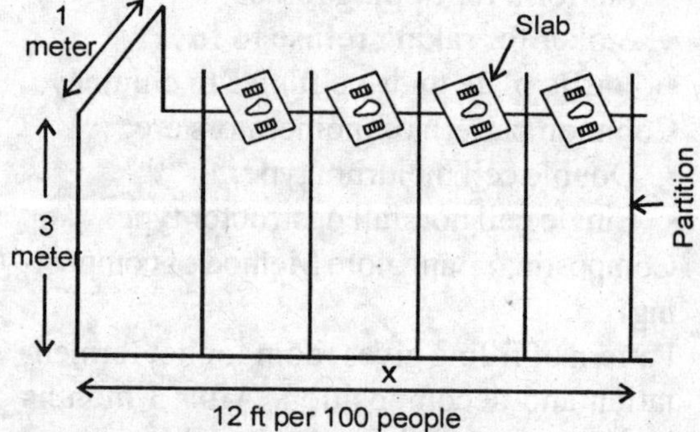

Fig. 5.17: Deep trench latrine

When Sewerage System is Available

i. **Water Carriage System (Fig. 5.18):**
Water carriage system is called sewerage system which collects and transports liquid waste and human excreta for sewage treatment away from residential area. Liquid waste is sullage which is not mixed with night soil. Sullage with excreta is sewage.
Sanitary indicators of sullage and sewage:

a. *B.O.D. (Biological Oxygen Demand):* It is O_2 absorbed in 5 days at 20°C. It is weak at 100mg/L and strong at 300 mg/L.

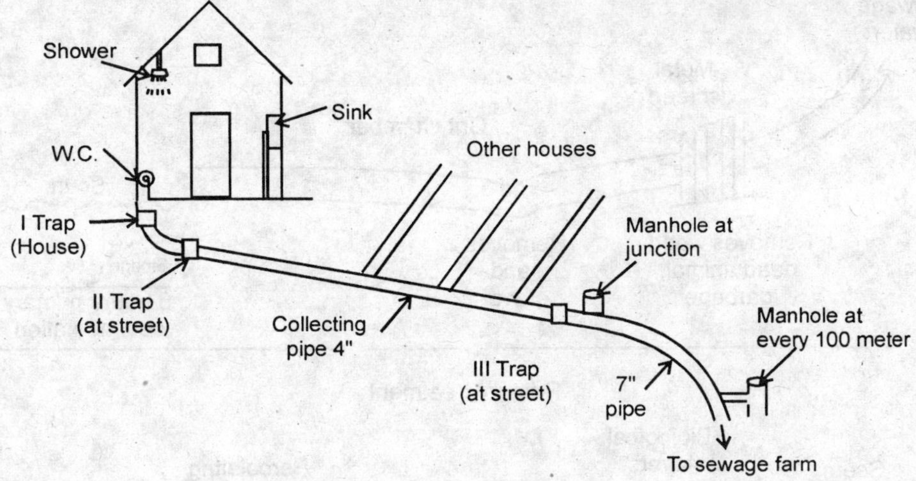

Fig. 5.18: Water Carriage System

b. *C.O.D. (Chemical Oxygen Demand):* It measures organic load.

c. *Suspended solids:* It is weak if s.s. is 100mg/L and is strong if s.s. is 500 mg/L.

ii. **Modern sewage treatment (Fig. 5.18):** Liquid waste from sewerage is screened and sedimented. Later it is subjected for aerobic oxidation either by Trickling Filter or by Activated sludge process. Later, secondary Sedimentation allows to treat sludge and to dispose effluent. The working of sewage treatment is depicted in Fig 5.19.

iii. **Oxidation pond:** This is an open pool containing liquid waste and sewage which undergo both aerobic digestion and anaerobic digestion which take place at the outskirt of a town. In Bhilai first experiment of oxidation pond by public engineers was successful for a population of 1 lakh.

DISPOSAL OF DEAD BODY

Dead body disposal is always associated with religious rituals and varies from country to country. However sanitary practice of throwing dead body to vultures, to river, to maintain God lead to health hazards.

Two sanitary proposals seen are:

a. Burning
b. Burial

In normal process both Burning (Cremation) and Burial are satisfactory methods for dead body disposal.

Recent introduction of (c) Electric Crematorium has solved urban problem of sanitary disposal of dead body.

Burial has to be done in the corporation allocated area only.

Municipally Act has given guidelines for the disposal of the body of those who died due to acute infections diseases. These guidelines are to be strictly followed. Handling of dead in this case needs use of gloves and personal protection. A cover sheet dipped in formalin is worn over the body and tied properly. In case of burial, it shall be deep burial (> 3ft.) and addition of lime crystals with mud covering.

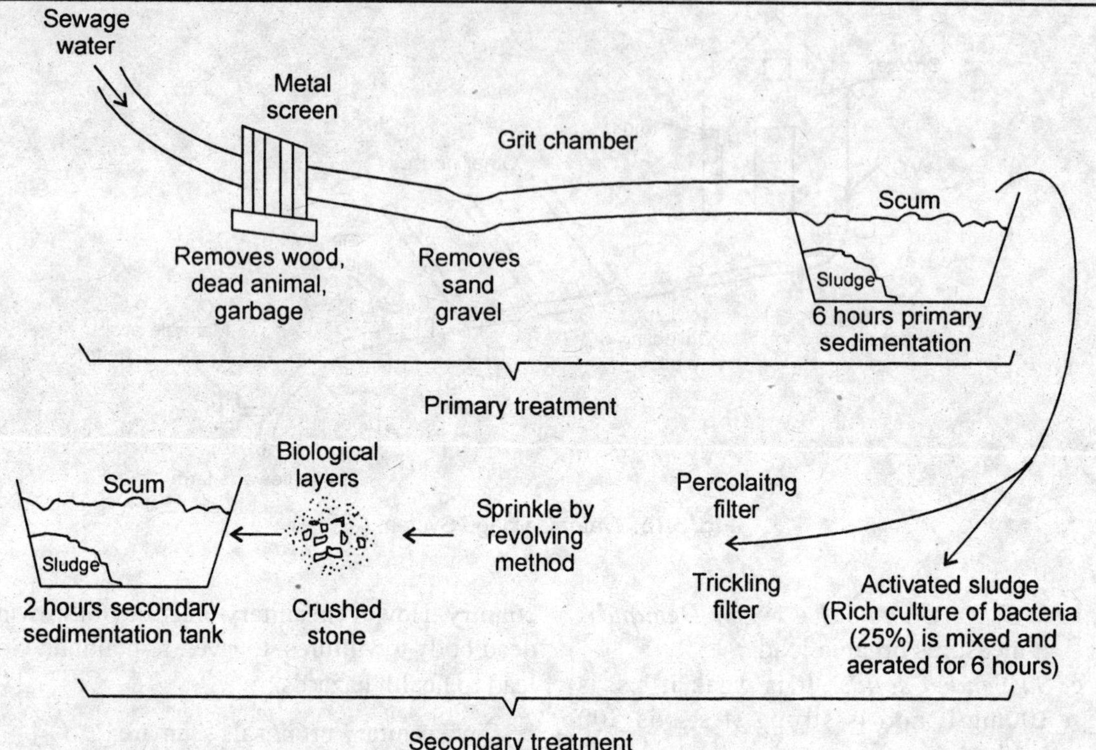

Fig. 5.19: Modern sewage treatment

MEDICAL ENTOMOLOGY

IMPORTANCE

Insects, arachnids, crustaceans and other arthropods cause pathological conditions in man, which are known from the time of Old Testament (Exodus 8:24) which described grievous swarm of flies and in sixth century when Shushruta recorded Filaria infection. The science is directly concerned with the biology and control of offending arthropods and with the recognition of the damage they cause. All of them are related to individual health as well as group health. The field of entomology made a good appearance after 1910. Greatest entomological discoveries on record are:

- Plague
- Malaria
- Yellow fever
- Typhus.

Experiencing disease, human death and search for survival gave great impetus to the subject and we started to know about vectors on these lines–How they live? How they carry disease ? How they are classified ? What is the biology ? and How they may be destroyed ?

In 1874 Othmar Zeidler synthesized DDT in Germany and its value was shown by Paul Muller in 1939 in Switzerland.

Scope

The subject helps us to understand morphology, life cycle, bionomics, disease transmitted and control measures. Both medical and public health importance are proved beyond doubt.

HEALTH PROBLEM

In day-to-day patient care and nursing care we come across umpteen number of vector borne (arthropod borne) diseases. Malaria, Filaria, Brain Fever, Dengue Fever, Typhoid, Diarrhoea, Typhus, Plague, Monkey Fever, Scabies and Guinea worm infection are very common diseases in nursing care services. All the vectors are (colloquially) called "Insects" whose population in 1 square mile is equal to human population in the world. This identifies the area of importance around us. Millions of people are getting diseases through the bite of insects. Severe malaria is causing deaths; filaria and brain fever is incapacitating people. Trachoma is causing preventable blindness.

Classification

Group	*Example*	*Characters*
1. Crustaceans	Cyclops	Head thorax joined, 5 pair legs 2 pair antennae, no wings, Live in water
2. Arachnida	Ticks Mites	No body division 4 pair legs, No antennae, No wings, Live on land
3. Insecta	Mosquito Flies Lice Flea	Head, Thorax, abdomen are seen, 3 pair legs, Antennae 1 pair, some have wings, live on land

MODE OF TRANSMISSION

Direct Contact

Transfer of arthropod from man to man occurs. For example in scabies and pediculosis disease occurs with 2 living factors. *Man* and *arthropod* (Either itch-mite or head louse) (Fig. 5.20).

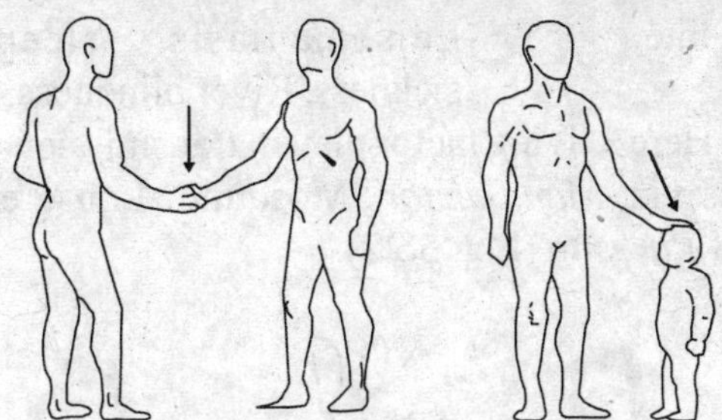

Fig. 5.20: Direct transmission

Mechanical

Mechanically disease agents is transferred by arthropod to a man. Examples are diarrhoea, dysentery, typhoid, food poisoning and trachoma. Here, disease occurs with 3 living factors viz. *Man, arthropod* (House Fly) and *parasite.*

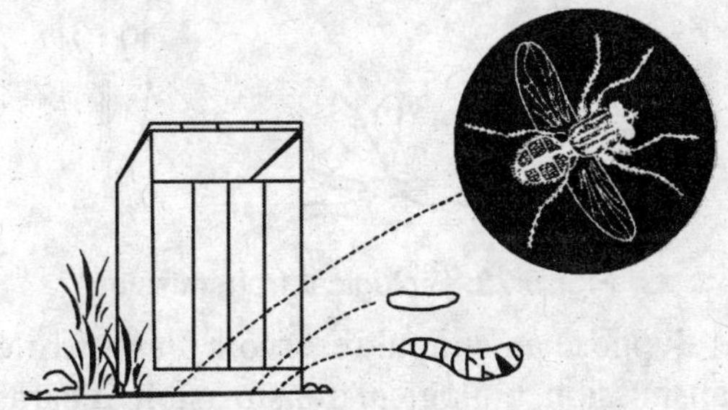

Fig. 5.21: Mechanical transmission

Biological Transmission

They are of 3 types:

i. Propagative—e.g., plague bacteria multiplies in Rat Flea.
ii. Cyclopropagative—e.g., malaria parasite multiplies and undergoes cyclical change in mosquito.
iii. Cyclodevelopment—e.g., filaria parasite undergoes cyclical changes in mosquito. E.g.Guinea worm undergoes cyclical changes in cyclops.

Parasite is transmitted from man to man by arthropod (Mosquito bite). Examples are :

Mosquito bite : Malaria, Yellow fever, Dengue Fever, Filaria

Louse bite : Epidemic typhus, Relapsing Fever

Fly bite : Leishmaniasis, sleeping sickness, River blindness.

Here 3 living factor play in transmission process viz, *Man, vector* (Mosquito, Louse etc.,) and *Parasite* (Fig. 5.22).

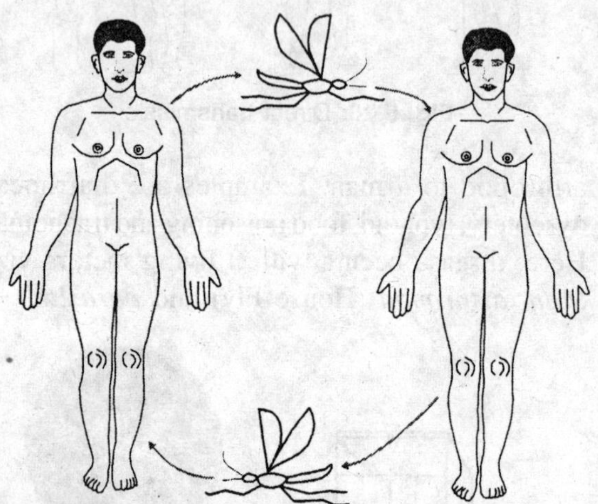

Fig. 5.22: Biological transmission

Suppose an animal reservoir play its role in transmission, biological transmission of parasite to man by arthropod (Flea etc.) from animal reservoir (rat) occurs. Here 4 living factors play their role viz. Man, Vector (Flea etc.), Parasite (plague bacilli etc.) and animal reservoir (rat etc.)

Examples: Plague – Rat flea – Rat – Man
K.F.D. – Tick – Monkey – Man

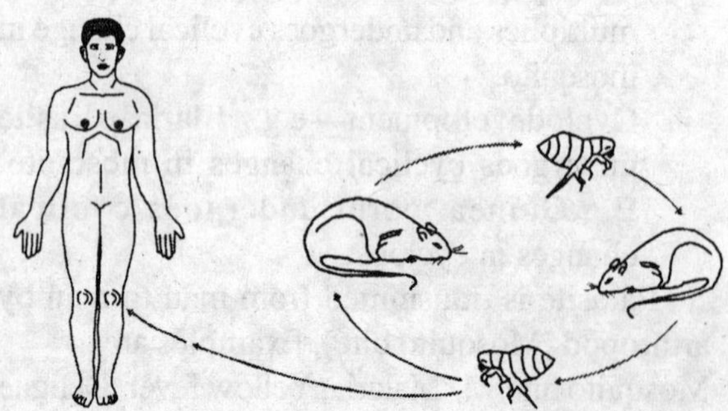

Fig. 5.23: Biological transmission where animal reservoir is seen

ARTHROPOD BORNE DISEASES (Table 5.9)

Table 5.9: Arthropod borne diseases

Vector	*Disease*
Cyclop	Guinea worm
Hard Tick	Typhus, Viral encephalitis, K.F.D.
Soft Tick	Relapsing fever
Mite	Typhus
Itchmite	Scabies
Mosquito	Malaria, Filaria, J.E., Dengue, Yellow fever
House fly	Typhoid, cholera, G.E., Trachoma
Sand fly	Kala-azar, sand fly fever
Tsetse fly	Sleeping sickness
Lice	Typhus, relapsing fever
Flea	Plague
Black fly	River blindness

Vectors of Public Health Importance

CYCLOPS (Fig. 5.24)

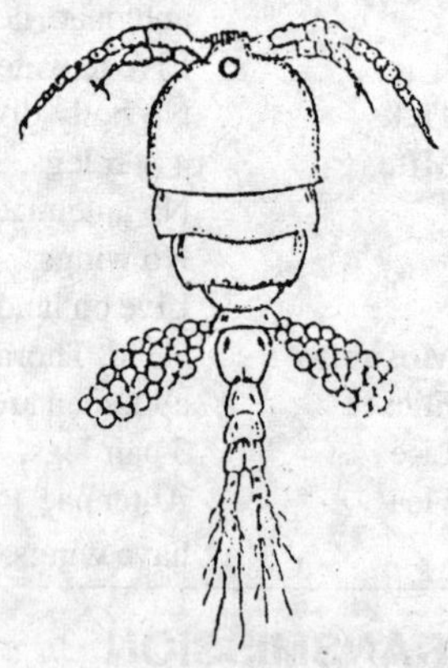

Fig. 5.24: Cyclops

Cyclops is a tiny vector of the size of a pin head. It is pear shape, body is semitransparent and the tail is forked; Pigmented eye, 5 pair legs and 2 pair antennae are present.

Diseases transmitted—Guinea worm infection (D. medinensis) and Fish tape worm (D. latum) infection.

Control Measures

Physical methods:

- Straining with muslin cloth
- Boiling the water

Chemical methods:

- Bleaching powder to water (5 PPM)
- Lime (4 grams per 5 litre)
- Abate (1 PPM)

Biological method:

- Barbel fish will eat cyclops
- Gambusia fish will eat cyclops.

Social method:

- Abolition of steep wells and introduce pipe water supply.

TICKS

They are of 2 kinds (a) Hard Tick (b) Soft Tick. They are oval shape, 4 pairs legs, no antennae. Males are smaller. Soft tick can withstand starvation. Life cycle passes through stages of egg, larva, nymph and adult (Fig. 5.25).

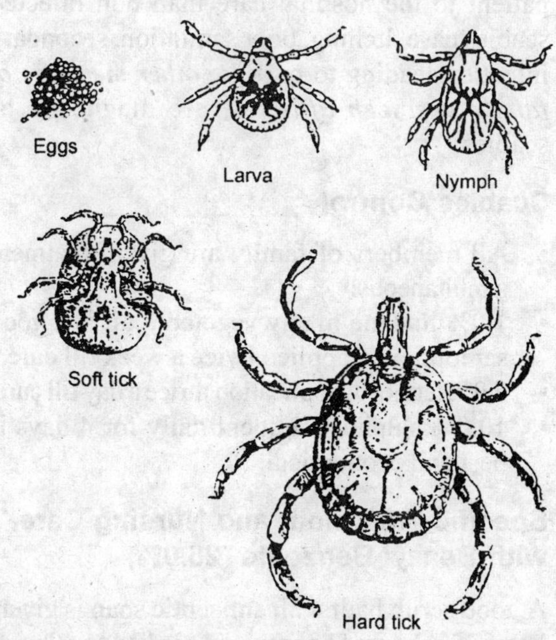

Fig. 5.25: Life cycle and morphology of ticks

Major identification points between hard and soft tick are (Table 5.10):

Table 5.10: Major points to differentiate hard and soft tick

Ticks	
Hard	*Soft*
Hard scutum cover back	No hard scutum
Head at anterior end	Head on underside
Feeds always	Can starve for 6-12 months

Diseases Transmitted

Hard Tick	*Soft Tick*
Tick Typhus K.F.D.	Relapsing Fever

Special Note on Transmission of Tick Borne Disease

Ticks suck blood and cause anaemia. They secrete a neurotoxin at bite causing local neurotoxic effect. Larva stage and nymph stage can also bite and transmit disease. Hence *transtagial* is used for disease transmission at other stages also. It is proved by entomological experiments that successive generation can transmit the disease in case of ticks. This type of transmission is specific to Tick borne diseases and is called *transovarian transmission.*

MITES

They resemble ticks but have different bionomics which differentiates them as different entity. Two forms are medically important. They are:

a. Trombiculid mite and
b. Itch mite (Fig. 5.26).

Mites are spider like in their appearance. They pass through stages of egg, larva, Nymph and adult. Life cycle takes about 6 weeks and Life span is observed to be 6 months.

Disease transmitted by Trombiculid mite is scrub typhus.

Control measures for ticks and mites are the same. They include:

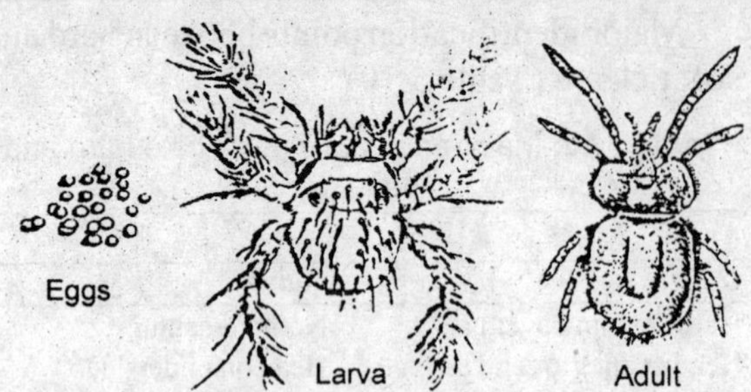

Fig. 5.26: Life cycle of mite

- DDT, Lindane or malathion at 1 pound per acre as insecticide.
- Insecticide dust on pet dogs which harbour ticks and mites.
- Abolition of crevices in residential area reduces the vector density.
- Repellents are used by workers who are exposed in areas where ticks and mites are prevailing.

Sarcoptes Scabiei (Itch Mite) (Scabies)

Scabies is one of the oldest known diseases of poor sanitation. Small globular arthropod is just visible to naked eye. Female mite burrows to epidermis, breeds in epidermis and cause intense itching; hence the name Itch mite (Figs 5.27 and 5.28).

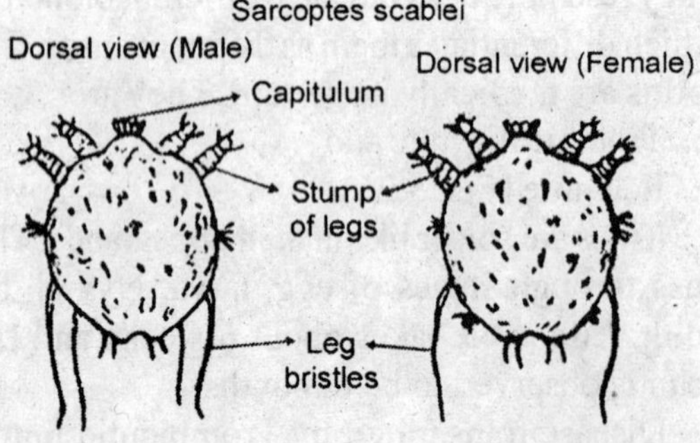

Fig. 5.27: Dorsal view of itch mite

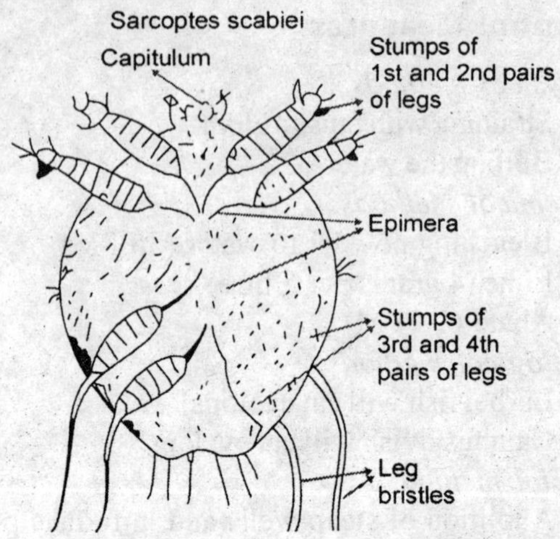

Fig. 5.28: Ventral view of itch mite

Female itch mite is differentiated when skin scrape of scabies patient is examined under microscope. It is bigger than male and has long tubular suckers in all 4 pairs of legs. Close contact and contaminated clothes spread scabies from person to person. Hands, Wrist, Elbow are common sites of scabies. Infected scabies draws patient to the hospital care than non infected scabies case. Itching, poor sanitation, secondary infection leading to pustule, *other members of family are seen afflicted,* are diagnostic of scabies.

Scabies Control

- All members of family are given treatment simultaneously.
- 1.0% lindane in any vegetable oil is a good sarcopticide, applied twice a week till cure.
- 5.0% tetmosol application thrice a day till cure.
- 10.0% sulphur ointment daily for 4 days is best and economical.

Specific Treatment and Nursing Care with Benzyl Benzoate (25.0%)

A good scrub bath with antiseptic soap is given. Later 25% benzyl benzoate is applied to all parts of body below chin and allowed to dry; later repeated after 12 hours. Further 12 hours later thorough bath is given; all clothings are immersed in boiling water and washed with detergent soap. Application as above is limited to 2 applications per week.

MOSQUITOES

Mosquitoes are ubiquitous in nature, disease transmitting groups are anopheles, culex, aedes and Mansonia. Characteristics are depicted in Fig. 5.30. The body is divisible into head, thorax and abdomen with a probosis (sucker), a pair of antennae (feelers), a pair of palpi (sensory), a pair of wings and 3 pair of legs.

Life cycle passes through the stages of egg, larva, pupa and adult. Life cycle takes about 1 week; life span is about 15 days (Fig. 5.29).

Main point to differentiate and disease transmitted in 4 different groups are tabulated in Table 5.11:

Mosquitoes Control

Integrated approach where more than one method is used for best result. Common measures are enumerated as under:

1. Protection from mosquito bites by mosquito net, screening to doors and windows and use of mosquito repellent.
2. For larva
   a. Source reduction by breeding control.
   b. Mineral oil once a week to suffocate and kill larvae.
   c. Paris green (stomach poison) as 2% dust.
   d. Abate 100 grams per hectare.
   e. Gambusia fish, lebister fish to eat larvae.
3. For adult
   a. Residual spray
      i. Lindane 0.5 gram per square meter; residual effect is 3 months (DDT is banned, and is resistant).
      ii. Malathion 2 gram per square meter; residual effect is 3 months.

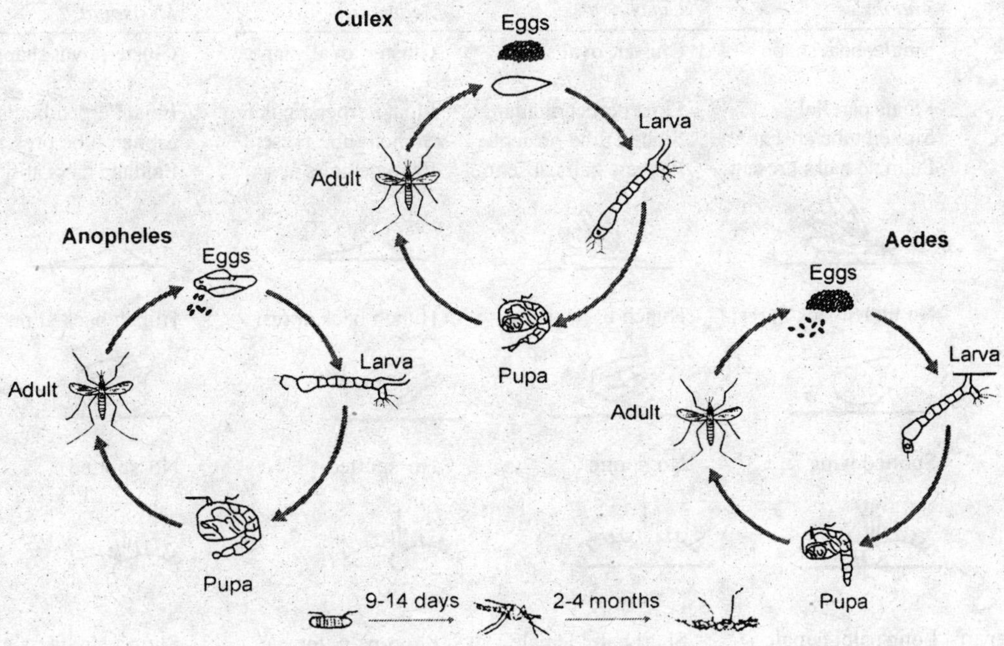

Fig. 5.29: Life cycle of mosquitoes

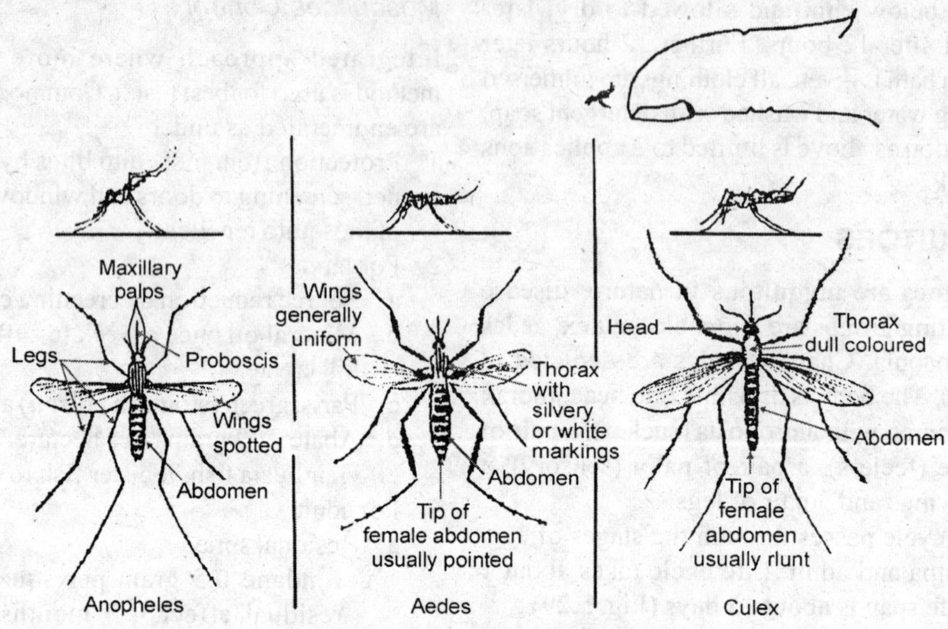

Fig. 5.30: Characteristics of different mosquitoes

Table 5.11: Differentiation and disease (mosquitoes)

	Anopheles	*Culex*	*Aedes*	*Mansonia*
Egg	Single, boat shape	Cluster, oval shape	Cluster, oval shape	Cluster, oval shape
Larva	Floats parellel Siphen tube absent Palmate hairs present	Float perpendicular Siphen tube present Palmate hairs absent	Float Perpendicular Siphen tube present Palmate hairs absent	Float Perpendicular Siphen tube present Palmate hairs absent
Adult Resting	No hunchback at rest	Hunch back at rest	Hunch back at rest	Hunch back at rest
Wing	Spotted wing	No spotted	No spotted	No spotted
Mouth part	Long palpi female	Short palpi female	Short palpi female	Short palpi female
Disease	Malaria	Urban filaria J.E.	Dengue	Rural filaria

b. Space spray
   Pyrethrum 1.02 gram per 1000 c.ft.
c. Fogging by fenitrothion.
d. Releasing sterile male to atmosphere is still at research phase and feasibility not sound.

FLIES

House Fly

They are non-biting common house fly called musca domestica. Their density is an index of poor sanitation.

It has head, thorax and abdomen, a pair of antennae, a pair of eyes, a probosis, a pair of wings and 3 pair of legs.

Life cycle passes through stages of egg, larva (maggot), pupa and adult. Life cycle is about a week to 10 days and life span is about 15 days (Fig. 5.31).

Larva infestation is common in wounds, lesions or post injury, post operative, Late cancer phases. The condition is called Myiasis. It is a nursing care problem.

Daily application of irritant to remove maggots and cleaning is a cumbersome process in regular nursing care. Fly control and good sanitation and not allowing their lying eggs on wounds is both cost benefit and effective.

They are vectors for Typhoid, diarrhoea, cholera, GE and trachoma by mechanical transmission.

Fly Control Measures

i. Elimination of breeding place.
ii. Proper disposal of garbage, refuse, night soil and animal dung.
iii. Lindane 0.5% sprays.
iv. Malathion 5% spray.
v. Liquid bait or crystal bait.
vi. Formalin in milk with sugar (50 ml formalin in 1 pint milk).
vii. Fly papers (2 Lb resin + 1 pint castor oil).
viii. Fly proof windows, doors.
ix. Health awareness by health education of community.

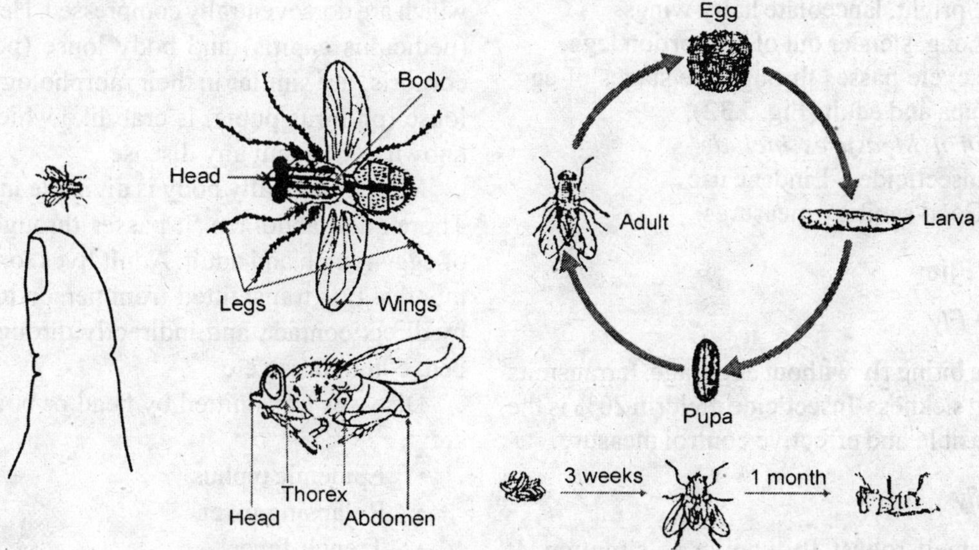

Fig. 5.31: Life cycle of house fly

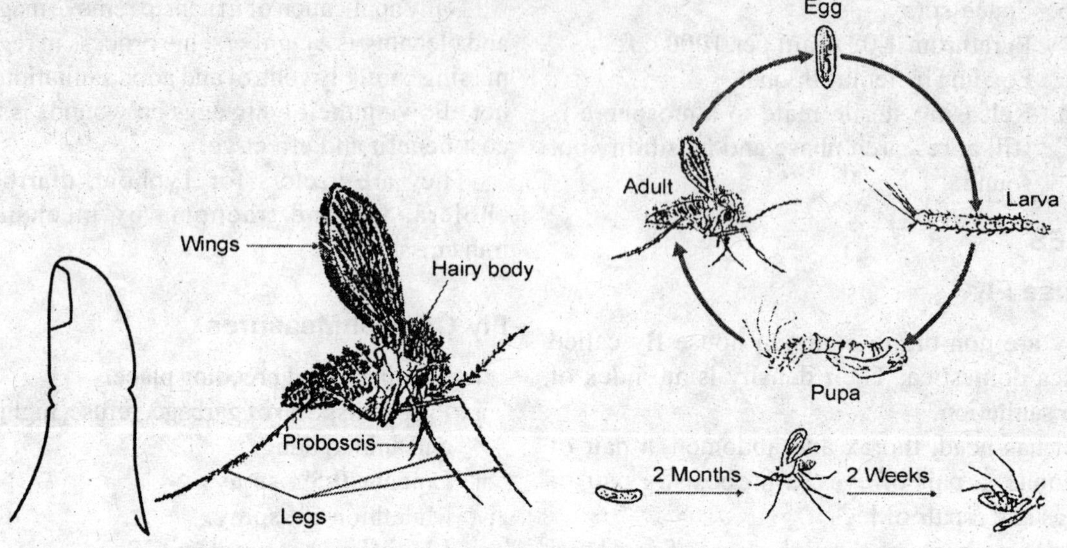

Fig. 5.32: Adult sand fly and life cycle

Sand Fly

They are smaller but visible by disproportionate legs. They are important vectors of kala-azar, oriental sore and sand fly fever.

They are differentiated from mosquitoes by:

- Smaller size than mosquito.
- Upright, lanceolate hairy wings.
- Long, slender out of proportion legs.

Life cycle passes through the stages of egg, larva, pupa and adult (Fig. 5.32).

Control Measures include:

- Insecticide—Lindane use.
- Good sanitary measures.

Other Flies

Tsetse Fly

This is a biting fly without egg stage. It transmits sleeping sickness. Insecticide dieldrin 20% is the only feasible and effective control measure.

Black fly

It is a small robust fly known as simulum. It transmits "river blindness" by onchocerciasis. Adult control is becoming very difficult. Abate 1 PPM for 10 minutes is found an effective control measure.

LICE

They are small wingless ectoparasite of man which are dorsoventrally compressed. Head louse (pediculus capitis) and body louse (pediculus corporis) are similar in their morphology. Pubic louse (phthirus pubis) is crab like which is not known to transmit any disease.

Morphologically body is divisible into head, Thorax and abdomen. It passes through stages of egg, nymph and adult. Adult lives for about 2 months. It is transmitted from person to person by direct contact, and indirectly through cloth, bed, comb, brush etc.

Diseases transmitted by head or body louse are:

- Epidemic typhus
- Relapsing fever
- Trench fever
- Dermatitis.

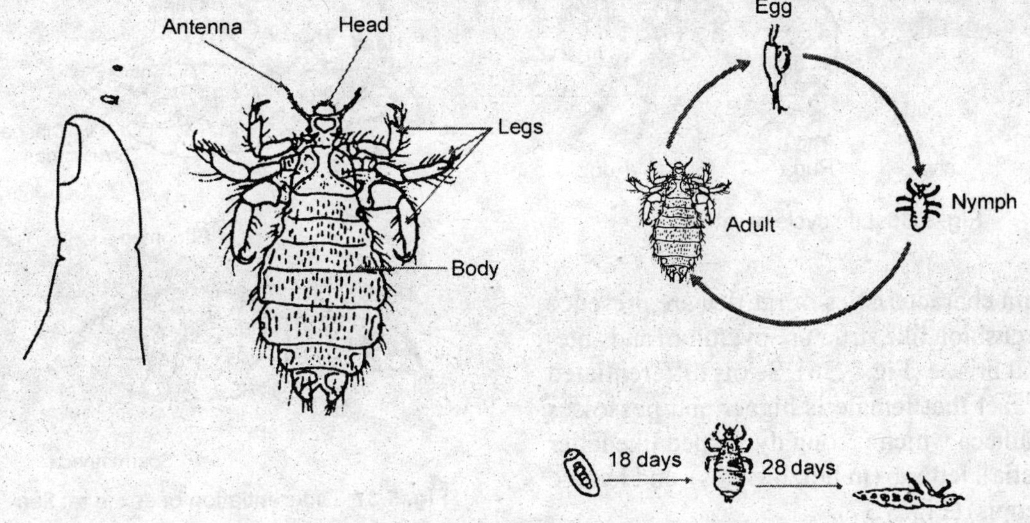

Fig. 5.33: Lice (Morphology and life cycle)

Pubic louse in pubic area and in perineal region is a nuisance. Their presence is suggestive of poor personal hygiene (Fig. 5.33).

Species

Pediculus humanus capitis (Head louse)
Pediculus humanus corporis (Body louse)
Phthirus pubis (Pubic louse)

Diseases transmitted by head and body louse:

- Epidemic typhus
- Relapsing fever
- Trench fever
- Vagabond's disease.

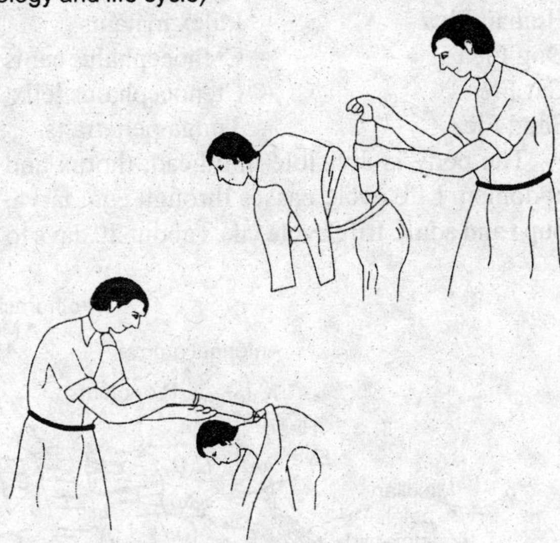

Fig. 5.34: Delousing method

Control Measures

Personal hygiene, mass delousing and use of insecticide are very effective (Fig. 5.34).

Body louse: 1% malathion with carbaryl as powder is sprayed on the body by a hand operated duster. Powder is brushed down the neck, up the sleeves, into trousers from several angles, both front and back. Two applications with 1 week apart, each time using 50 grams powder per person is found to eradicate pediculosis.

Head louse: 0.5% malathion lotion applied to head, allowed for 24 hours and later hair wash is given.

FLEA

They are wingless, bilaterally compressed ecto-parasites. Public Health importance is Rat Flea (Oriental Flea) (Fig. 5.35).

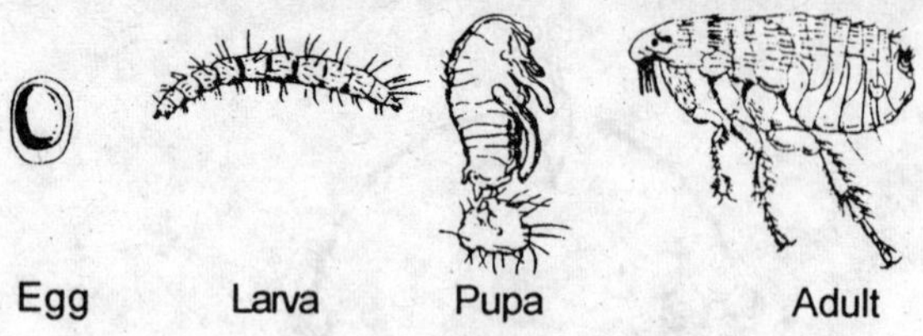

Fig. 5.35: Life cycle of rat flea

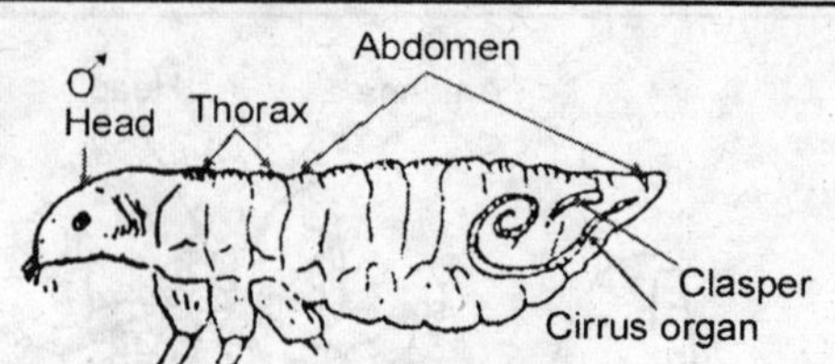

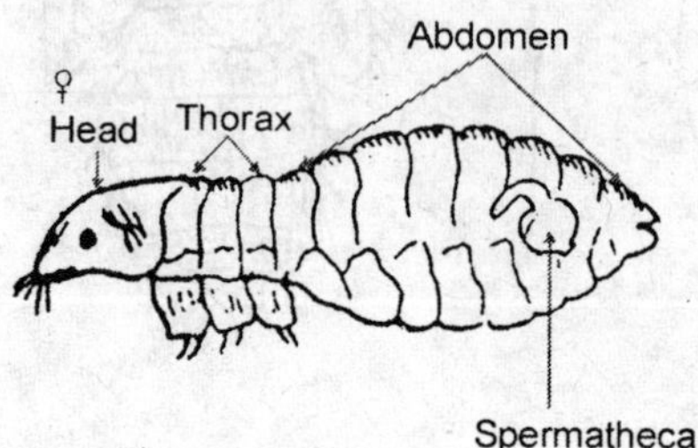

Fig. 5.37: Differentiation of sex in rat flea

Main characteristics of rat flea are presence of soft cushion like structure pygidium and ante-pygidial bristle (Fig. 5.36). Sex is differentiated by the fact that female is bigger and possesses spermatheca which is roughly shaped like letter a (in astia), letter b (in braziliences) and letter c (in cheopis) (Fig. 5.37).

Other types of flea are:

Human Flea – Pulex irritants
Dog Flea – Ctenocephalus canis
Cat Flea – Ctenocephalus felix
Sand Flea – Tunga penetrans

The body is divisible into head, thorax and abdomen. Life cycle passes through egg, larva, pupa and adult. Life cycle takes about 20 days to complete. Life span is about 40 days in tropical area. Infected flea may have blocked or partially blocked ventriculus and they are dangerous in spreading plague bacilli.

Disease Transmitted

- Plague

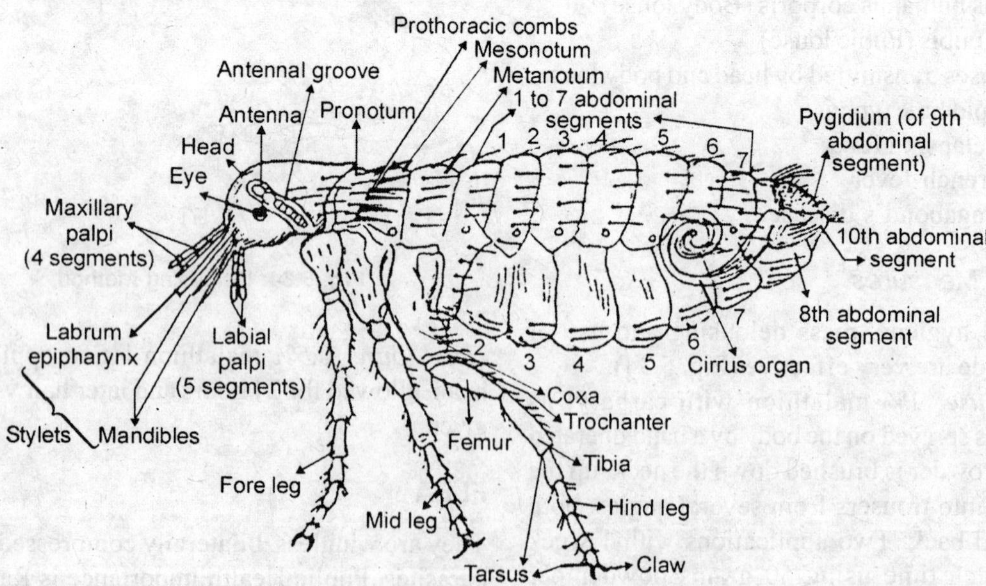

Fig. 5.36: Main character of rat flea xenopsyella

- Endemic typhus.

During entomological survey, following flea indices are used:

1. General flea index (No. of flea per rat).
2. Specific flea index (No. of any one species per rat).
3. Percentage incidence (percentage of each species per rat).
4. Rodent infestation rate:

$$\frac{\text{No. of flea found}}{\text{No. of rats examined}} \times 100$$

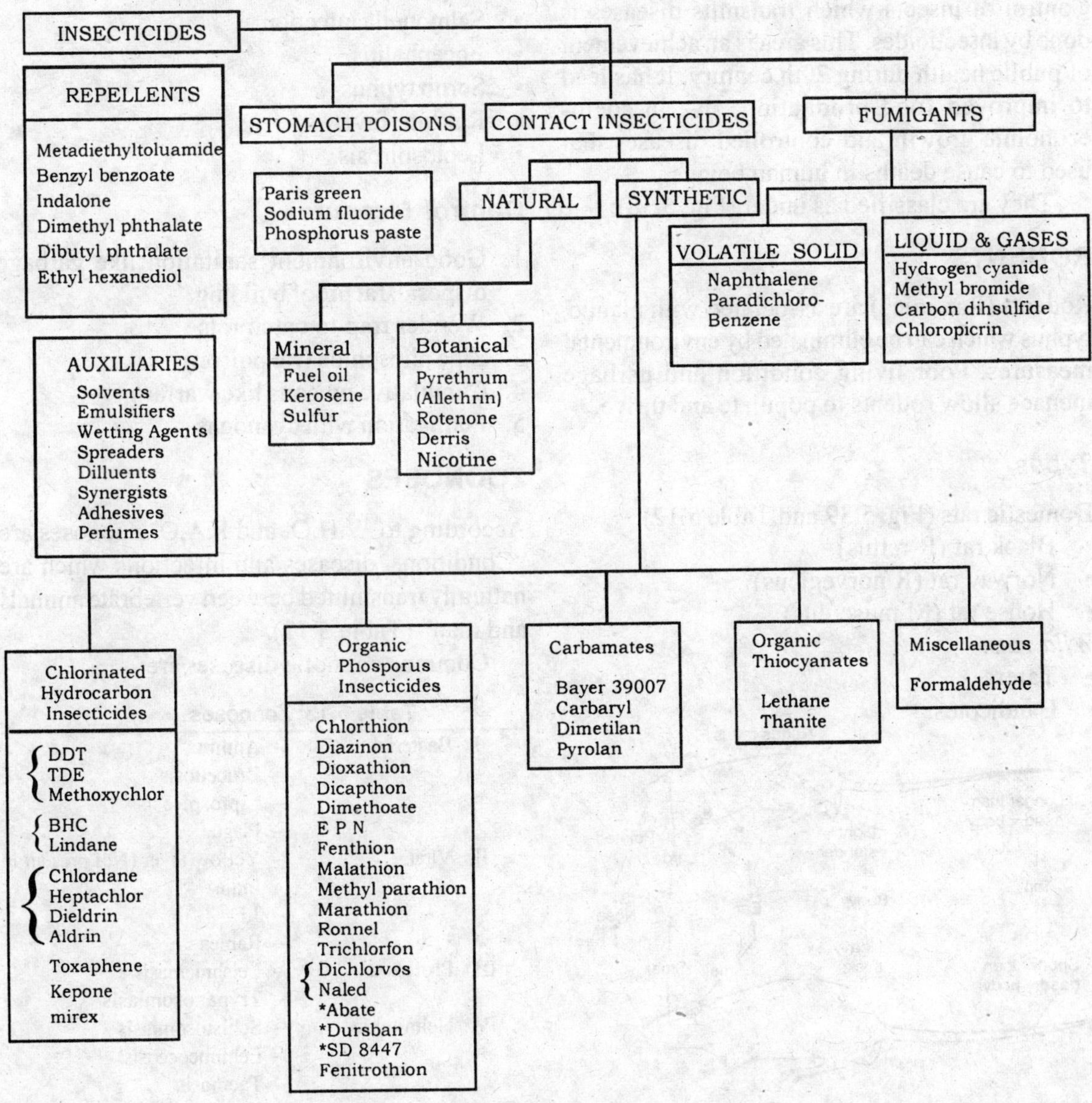

Fig. 5.38: Insecticides

Control Measures

1. Carbaryl or diazinon 2%.
2. Malathion 5%.
3. Rat burrow closure with concrete.
4. Use of repellents (Diethyltoluamide).
5. Rat control measures.

INSECTICIDE

Control of insects which transmits diseases is done by insecticides. This area is an achievement of public health during 20th century. It has lead to improved food production, rise in socio-economic growth and controlled diseases that used to cause deaths in human beings.

They are classified as under (Fig. 5.38):

RODENTS

Rodents (Rat, mice) are associated with plague, typhus which can be eliminated by environmental measures. Poor living condition and garbage menace allow rodents to populate and thrive.

Types

Domestic rats (Fig. 5.39 and Table 5.12):

- Black rat (R rattus)
- Norway rat (R norvegicus)
- House rat (M musculus).

Wild rats:

- Tatera
- Bandicotes.

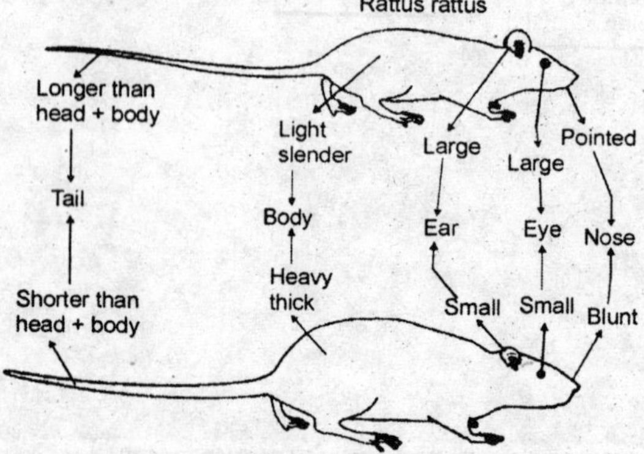

Fig. 5.39 : Black rat and Norvey rat

Table 5.12 : Character differences

R. rattus	*R.norvegieus*
Slender body	Heavy body
Long nose	Blunt nose
Long tail	Short tail
Large eye and ear	Small eye and ear

Disease Transmitted

- Plague
- Salmonella infection
- Encephalitis
- Scrub typhus
- Rat bite fever
- Leptospirosis.

Control Measures

1. Good environment sanitation like garbage disposal, rat proof building.
2. Wonder trap to catch rats
3. Zinc phosphide (rat poison)
4. Cumulative poisons like warfarin
5. Fumigation with cyanogas.

ZOONOSES

According to W.H.O. and F.A.O. Zoonoses are "Conditions, diseases and infections which are naturally transmitted between vertebrate animals and man" (Table 5.13).

Common zoonotic diseases are:

Table 5.13: Zoonoses

I. Bacterial	– Anthrax – Brucellosis – Liptospirosis – Plague
II. Viral	– Yellow fever (Not present in India) – J.E – Rabies
III. Protozoa	– Leishmaniasis – Trypanosomiasis
IV. Helminthic	– Schistosomiasis – Echinococcosis – Taeniasis – Trichinellosis

Components of Control of Zoonoses

i. Diagnosis and treatment in animals
ii. Sanitation of wool, hide, horn and fats
iii. Protection of man from animal bites
iv. International, national and state programme implementations like:

UNEP (United Nations Environmental Programme)
MAB (Man and Biosphere Programme)
EHCP (Environmental Health Criteria Programme).

CHAPTER SIX

Nutrition

IMPORTANCE

The pattern of infection, disability, growth and development depends on nutritional status of an individual. It is also influenced by women's educational status, changes in agricultural practice and provision of hygienic food. Malnutrition in measles, whooping cough and other infections is known to cause serious complications in children. Diet and hygiene determine child's mortality. Knowledge of infection (Germ Theory) helped in understanding the relevance of proper food hygiene. Discovery of vitamins, their benefits to growth and health have reemphasized the importance of diet for the health of an individual. It was for the first time, Head of NIN Hyderabad in 1920; Dr. Mc Carrison found that rat fed by Indian traditional diet showed good growth than rat fed by European diet. This unravelled the knowledge "Protective factor" of vitamins. However early study goes to 1750 when scurvy was treated by lime juice.

Presently nutrition has proved to be associated with socio-economic development of a nation. Infection, immunity, fertility, maternal health, child health and health of sick all depend on nourishment they get. We have nutritional indicators to monitor community nutritional status.

DEFINITION

Nutrition is a science of food and nutrients and their relation to human health.

Nutrient is specific dietary constituent.

Dietetics is the practical application of principles of nutrition.

Diet is the food article in consumable form.

Therapeutic diet is modification of diet for therapeutic purpose.

Food

Foods are grouped under following category for feasible explanation and comparison:

1. Cereals and millets
2. Pulses (legumes)
3. Vegetables
4. Nuts and oil seeds
5. Fruits
6. Animal foods
7. Fats and oils
8. Sugar and jaggery
9. Condiments and spices
10. Miscellaneous foods.

Major Food Sources of Nutrients are tabulated below:

Table 6.1: Source of food for nutrients

Nutrient	*Food*
Energy	Cereals, pulses, roots, tubers, fats, oils, sugar, jaggery
Protein	Milk, egg, fish, meat, liver, pulses, nuts, oilseeds.
Fat	Butter, ghee, vegetable oils, hydrogenated fats, nuts and oilseeds
Carbohydrate	Cereals, pulses, sugar, jaggery, roots, tubers
Fibre	Green leafy vegetables, fruits, unrefined cereals, pulses, legumes

Contd.

Contd.

Calcium	Milk, milk products, ragi, green leafy vegetables.
Iron	Liver, green leafy vegetables, rice flakes, whole-wheat flour, ragi, pulses
Vitamin A	Fish, liver oil, butter, ghee, milk, carrot, Green leafy vegetables, papaya, mango.
B' complex	Milk, egg, liver, home-pound rice, whole wheat, whole gram, pulses, green leafy vegetables, nuts, oil seeds.
Vitamin C	Gooseberry, lime, orange, guava, tomato, lettuce, sprouted gram
Vitamin D	Milk, sunlight

Nutritive Value of Food

Very often we need the availability of proximate principles and available calories in food/food raw materials. They can be tabulated for every 100 grams by their weight as under Table 6.2:

Nutritional Profile of Food

Each food has its own profile. This knowledge is important for formulating diet composition and supplementation.

i. Cereals:

They form bulk of diet. It is deficient in Lysine (Limiting Amino acid). Milling of rice takes off nutritive element. Parboiled rice has good high Vitamin B quantity. Parboiling (Partial cooking in steam) is a method of preserving nutrient. Paddy is soaked in hot water at 70°C for 3 hours; drying and steaming follows; later dried and milled (CFTRI Process). Protein content of wheat is 16%.

ii. Millet:

Smaller grains jowar, bajra, ragi are examples. In jowar limiting amino acids are lysine and threonine. Ragi is rich in calcium.

iii. Pulses:

All pulses have 20% protein except soyabean which has 40%. Germinated pulses have higher content of vitamins. Kesaridhal is associated with Lathyrism.

Table 6.2: Nutritive value of common foods

Food stuff	*Protein*	*Fat*	*Carbohydrate*	*Calories*
Cereal	9.9	2.3	71.0	344
Bread	7.8	0.7	51.9	245
Salt Biscuit	6.6	32.4	54.6	534
Sweet Biscuit	6.4	15.2	71.9	450
Pulses	22.6	2.0	58.4	342
Green Leafy Vegetables	3.8	0.6	6.0	45
Roots, Tubers	1.2	0.2	16.0	70
Other Vegetables	2.2	0.3	6.3	36
Nuts, Oilseed	15.2	46.6	20.4	578
Condiment, spice	9.8	6.6	40.6	261
Fruit	1.1	0.4	7.6	79
Meat	21.0	4.9	0.8	131
Egg	13.3	13.3	0.0	173
Milk	3.6	5.8	4.7	85
Curd	3.1	4.0	3.0	60
Butter	0.0	81.0	0.0	729
Ghee	0.0	100.0	0.0	900
Oil	0.0	100.0	0.0	900
Sugar	0.1	0.0	99.4	398
Honey	0.3	0.0	79.5	319
Jaggery	0.4	0.1	95.0	383
Sago	0.2	0.2	87.1	351

iv. **Vegetables:**
They are grouped under greens, roots, tubers and other vegetables. They yield low calorie, form bulky food; but provide vitamins and minerals.

v. **Nuts, Oilseeds:**
Nuts contribute minerals, essential fatty acids. Acceptable balance food are MPF, Balahar, Malt food.

vi. **Fruits:**
They are protective foods. Since they are eaten raw they provide good amount of vitamins and minerals.

vii. **Animal Food:**
They provide high quality protein. Reference proteins are milk and egg which are nearly perfect food.
   a. **Milk:** Casein is the chief protein. Buffalo milk contains high fat content (8.8%). Skimming removes fat. Toning means 1 part water 1 part natural milk and 1/8 part skim milk powder. Vegetable milk is prepared from groundnut, soyabean etc.
   b. **Egg:** About 60 gram egg has 6G. Protein, 6G. Fat, 30 mg calcium, 1.5 mg iron and provide 70 calories. Boiled eggs are nutritionally superior (Boiling destroys avidin a vitamin preventing factor). Cholesterol content of egg is related to CHD.
   c. **Fish:** It is food of good biological value and a food with balanced amino acids. They are richest source of Vitamin A. Sea fish is rich in iodine.
   d. **Meat:** Flesh of cattle, sheep and goat are commonly used. They give 20% protein. They are source of zinc and vitamin B.

viii. **Fat, Oil:**
They are source of energy and vitamin A, D, coconut and palm contain polysaturated fatty acids. Hydrogenated fat is called vanaspati.

ix. **Sugar, Jaggery:**
They are source of natural sugars.

x. **Condiment, Spice:**
Mustard, ginger, garlic, cardamom, hing, clove, pepper are examples. They stimulate appetite and increase palatability.

xi. **Miscellaneous:**
Coffee, tea, cocoa, aerated waters, alcohol i.e. beverages are examples.

PROXIMATE PRINCIPLES

Protein

They are nitrogenous compounds. They form 20% of body weight in adult. Dietary protein provide essential amino acids viz., leucine, isoleucine, lysine, methionine, phenylalamine, threonine, valine, tryptophan and histidine. They help in new tissue formation. Biologically complete protein is one which contains all essential amino acids.

Functions

- Repair of tissues
- Maintain osmotic pressure
- Antibodies produced.

Sources

Animal source like milk, meat, egg , fish etc. Plant source; pulses, oilseeds.

Evaluation

By NPU (Net protein utilisation).

Requirement

1 G. per kg body weight.

Fat

They are of 3 types; simple, compound and derived. Lauric, palmitic and stearic acid form saturated fatty acids.

Oleic acid, linoleic acid form unsaturated fatty acids; unsaturated fatty acids are found in vegetable oils.

Sources

- Animal source like ghee, butter, cheese, egg etc.
- Vegetable source like (oilseeds) groundnut and coconut etc.

Functions

- Yield calorie
- Support body viscera
- Act as local hormones.

Visible and Invisible Fats

Major intake is from invisible fat and their measurement is difficult.

Hydrogenation

It is a process of converting oil to semisolid form in presence of a catalyst.

Refining

Process of removing rancid material of oil.

Health Effect

- Obesity
- Thick skin, other changes of skin
- Heart disease
- Cancer of some organs.

Requirement

15-20% of total calories (Indian diet provide 30-40 % total calories).

Carbohydrate

- Starch sugar, cellulose are forms of carbohydrate.
- Requirement–60 to 70% of total calories.

Vitamins

They are essential nutrients made up of organic compounds. Their deficiency leads to various disorders.

Water Soluble Vitamins

i. *Thiamine:* It is called vitamin $B_1$and helps in utilisation of carbohydrate.
Source: Cereal, wheat, pulses, nuts, fish.
Loss: By Milling, prevention by parboiling.
Deficiency: Dry beriberi, wet beriberi and infantile beriberi.
R.D.A.: 0.5 mg/1000 calories.

ii. *Riboflavin:* It is vitamin B_2 helps in cellular oxidation.
Source: Milk, egg, liver, green leafy vegetables.
Deficiency: Angular stomatitis, glossitis.
Requirement: 0.6 mg/1000 calories.

iii. *Niacin:* It helps in metabolism of proximate principles.
Source: Liver, meat, fish, groundnut.
Deficiency: Pellagra.
Prevention: By supplementation.
Requirement: 6.6 mg/1000 calories.

iv. *Pyridoxine:* It is called B_6.
Source: Milk, liver, meat, egg yolk, fish, legumes.
Deficiency: Peripheral neuritis.
Requirement: 2 mg per day.

v. *Pantothenic acid:* It helps in adrenal gland function and in synthesis of corticosteroids.
Requirement: 10 mg per day.

vi. *Folic acid:* This helps in synthesis of nucleic acids.
Source: Liver, meat, egg, milk, fruit and leafy vegetables.
Deficiency: Megaloblastic anaemia, glossitis.
Requirement: 100 micrograms per day.

vii. *Vitamin B_{12}:* This helps in synthesis of DNA, along with folic acid.

Source: Liver, meat, egg, milk, cheese.
Deficiency: Megaloblastic anaemia.
Requirement: 1 microgram per day.

viii. *Vitamin C:* It is called ascorbic acid. It is needed for collagen formation.
Source: Fresh fruits and green leafy vegetables.
Deficiency: Scurvy.
Requirement: 40 mg per day.

Fat Soluble Vitamins

i. *Vitamin A:* It is required for vision, for glandular and epithelial tissue functioning, for skeletal growth, as facilitator.
Source: Animal source: Liver, egg, butter, fish, meat.
Plant source: Spinach, amaranth, green leafy vegetables, papaya, mango, pumpkin.
Fortified foods: Vanaspathi, margarine, milk.
Deficiency: Night blindness, Bitot's spots, dryness and eye softening.
Correction: Early deficiency is corrected by 2,00,000 iu of vitamin A orally on 2 successive days.
For community based intervention 2,00,000 iu orally once in 6 months to preschool children.

Criteria for Eye Problem in Community

Eye problem is said to exist if prevalence in population at risk 6 months to 6 years is:

1 %	Night blindness
0.5%	Bitot's spot
0.01%	Corneal xerosis
0.05%	Corneal ulcer
5.0%	Serum retinol level below 10 micrograms per dl.

Requirement: Adult requires 600 mg of retinol.
Hypervitaminosis: It is associated with Vitamin A.

ii. *Vitamin D:* It helps in calcium and phosphorous absorption, stimulates bone formation and permit normal growth of tissues.
Source: Sunlight, liver, egg, butter, fish.
Deficiency: Rickets, osteomalacia.
Requirement: 2.5 micrograms per day.

iii. *Vitamin E:* It is called tocopherol.
Source: Cottonseed, Sunflower seed, egg yolk, butter.
Deficiency: Not specific.

iv. *Vitamin K*: It stimulates the production and release of coagulation factors.
Source: Green leafy vegetables, fruits, milk.
Deficiency: Bleeding tendency.
Requirement: 0.03 mg/kg per day.

Minerals

Minerals are chemical elements that are required for growth, repair and regulation of body functions.

Major Minerals

Calcium: It helps in formation of bones, teeth, helps in muscular contraction, in coagulation of blood.
Source: Milk, milk products, ragi, sitaphal.
Deficiency: Not demonstrated.
Requirement: 500 mg per day.

Other Major Minerals

Phosphorous, sodium, potassium and magnesium.

Trace Elements

They are chemical elements that are required by the body in small quantities.

i. *Iodine:* It is required for the synthesis of thyroid hormones.
Source: Sea foods, cod liver oil, milk, meat and some vegetables. Cabbage, cauliflower interfere with iodine utilisation and hence are called goitrogens.

Deficiency: Hypothyroidism, growth retardation, abortion, stillbirth, cretinism, deaf mutism.

Requirement: 150 microgram per day.

ii. *Iron:* This is present in human body both in circulating form and in storage form.

Functions: Formation of haemoglobin, brain development and function, temperature regulation, muscular activity.

Source: Liver, meat, fish, cereal, green leafy vegetables, legume, nuts, jaggery, dried fruits.

Iron has vital importance during pregnancy, lactation and young children.

Deficiency: Anaemia.

Requirement: 30 mg dietary iron (0.9 mg absorbable form).

iii. *Fluorine:* It is essential for bone and teeth function.

Source: Water , sea foods, tea, cheese.

Deficiency: Dental fluorosis, skeletal fluorosis.

Requirement: 0.5-0.8 mg per litre in drinking water.

iv. *Other trace elements are:* Zinc, copper, cobalt, chromium, selenium and molybdenum.

Calorie

It is the prime requisite of the body for effective growth and development. It is expressed by calories (in terms of kilo calorie). For international comparison calorie is replaced by Joule. For purpose of conversion: 1 calorie (Kcal) = 4184 Joule. The energy available by proximate principle are as under:

Protein	4 calories per gram	(17 Joule)
Fat	9 calories per gram	(37 Joule)
Carbohydrate	4 calories per gram	(17 Joule)

In view of the currently recommended adult body weight, the reference man and reference woman are redefined as under.

REFERENCE MAN

He is between 20-39 years age weight 60 kg, is free from disease and physically fit for active work. On each working day he is employed for 8 hours in occupation that usually involves moderate activity. While not at work he spends 8 hours in bed, 4-6 hours sitting and moving about, and 2 hours walking and in active recreation or household duties.

REFERENCE WOMAN

She is between 20-39 years age healthy, weight 50 kg. She may be engaged for 8 hours in general household work, in light industry or in any other moderately active work. Apart from 8 hours in bed, she spends 4-6 hours sitting or moving around in light activity, and 2 hours walking or active recreation or household chores.

CALORIC REQUIREMENT

For B.M.R.–1 calorie per hour per kg.

For daily activity–additional.

For occupation–additional.

Energy Requirement of Reference Person:

Sex	*Body weight*	*Activity*		
		Sedentary	*Moderate*	*Heavy*
Male	60 kg	2425	2875	3800
Female	50 kg	1875	2225	2925

BALANCED DIET

Balanced diet is an accepted means to safeguard population from nutritional deficiencies. It is defined as a diet containing required proximate principles, calorie, vitamins, minerals and trace elements that can meet the requirement for healthy life. This also allows provision of extra nutrients for given situations like pregnancy, lactation and sickness. In constructing the balanced diet following guidelines are used as base line (adult):

Protein	– 1 G per kg body weight
Fat	– 15-20% of total calories
Carbohydrate	– 50-60% of total calories
Iron	– 28 mg
Retinol	– 600 mg (2400 Iμ)
Thiamine	– 1.2 mg
Riboflavin	– 1.4 mg
Nicotinic acid	– 16 mg
Pyridoxine	– 2.0 mg
Vitamin C	– 40 mg
Folic acid	– 100 micrograms
Vitamin B_{12}	– 1 microgram

Following tables give balanced diet for given specific situations (Tables 6.3 to 6.9):

Adult Man

Table 6.3: Balanced diet for adult man

Items (Grams)	*Sedentary*	*Moderate work*	*Heavy work*
Cereals	460	520	670
Pulses	40	50	60
Leafy vegetables	40	40	40
Other vegetables	60	70	80
Roots and tubers	50	60	80
Milk	150	200	250
Oil and fat	40	45	65
Sugar or jaggery	30	35	55

Adult Woman

Table 6.4: Balanced diet for adult woman

Item (grams)	*Sedentary*	*Moderate work*	*Heavy work*
Cereals	410	440	575
Pulses	40	45	50
Leafy vegetables	100	100	50
Other vegetables	40	40	100
Roots and tubers	50	50	60
Milk	100	150	200
Oil and fat	20	25	40
Sugar or jaggery	20	20	40

Children

Table 6.5: Balanced diet for children

Item (grams)	*1-3 years*	*4-6 years*
Cereals	175	270
Pulses	35	35
Leafy vegetables	40	50
Other vegetables	20	30
Roots and tubers	10	20
Milk	300	250
Oil and fat	15	25
Sugar or jaggery	30	40

Adolescence

Table 6.6: Balanced diet for adolescence

Item (Grams)	*Boys 10-12 years*	*Girls 10-12 years*
Cereals	420	380
Pulses	45	45
Leafy vegetables	50	50
Other vegetables	50	50
Roots and tubers	30	30
Milk	250	250
Oil and fat	40	35
Sugar or jaggery	45	45

ALLOWANCE DURING PREGNANCY

Table 6.7: Additional allowance during pregnancy

Cereals	35 grams	Yield 292 calories
Pulses	15 grams	
Milk	100 grams	
Sugar	10 grams	

Allowance During Lactation

Table 6.8: Additional allowance during lactation

Cereals	60 grams	Yield 521 calories
Pulses	30 grams	
Milk	100 grams	
Fat	10 grams	
Sugar	10 grams	

Balanced diet for elderly people above 65 years.

Table 6.9: Balanced diet for elderly

	Woman > 65 years	Man > 65 years
Cereals	225	350
Pulses	40	50
Vegetables	150	200
Green leafy vegetables	50	50
Roots and tubers	100	100
Fruits	200	200
Milk, milk products	300	300
Sugar	20	20
Fats and oils	20	25

Prudent Diet

This is the diet developed by National Nutrition and Food Policy to achieve highest level of health. It is called prudent diet if following criteria are adopted in a diet:

a. Fat intake below 20-30% of total calories
b. Saturated Fat below 10% of total calories
c. Carbohydrate should contain high fibre
d. Fats, alcohol restricted
e. Salt below 5 grams per day
f. Protein below 15-20% of daily intake
g. Junk foods avoided (Ketchup, cola).

NUTRITION AND HEALTH

There are many health problems which are due to nutritional deficiency, adulteration or harmful excesses. Major concerns are detailed below;

P.E.M.

This is commonly seen during infancy. It affects growth, development and mental outlook of a child. Kwashiorkor and marasmus are two clinical types of P.E.M. Among preschool children, it is 2 percent. Among malnourished, 20% are severely malnourished (Grade III and IV) and remaining are mild and moderate (Grade I and II).

Earlier it was called PCM (Protein Calorie Malnutrition) because of concept of protein gap. Now since energy gap is there, the cause is taken over to food gap in causation of PEM.

Other environment causes are:

- Poor R.C.H.
- Failure of lactation
- No exclusive breastfeeding
- Child rearing practice
- Weaning practice
- Overcrowding in family (Fig. 6.1A and B).

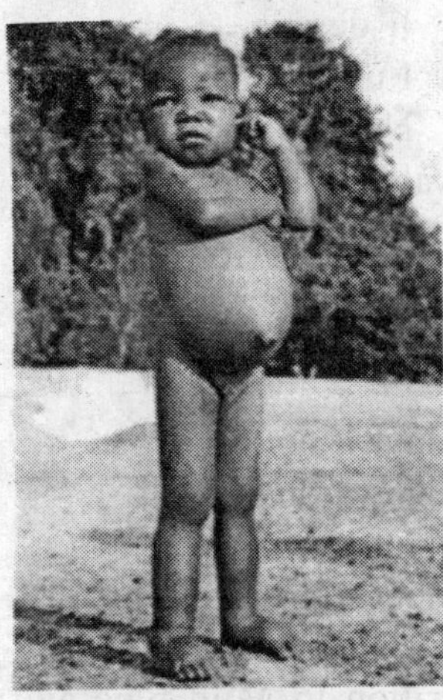

Fig. 6.1A: Kwashiorkor

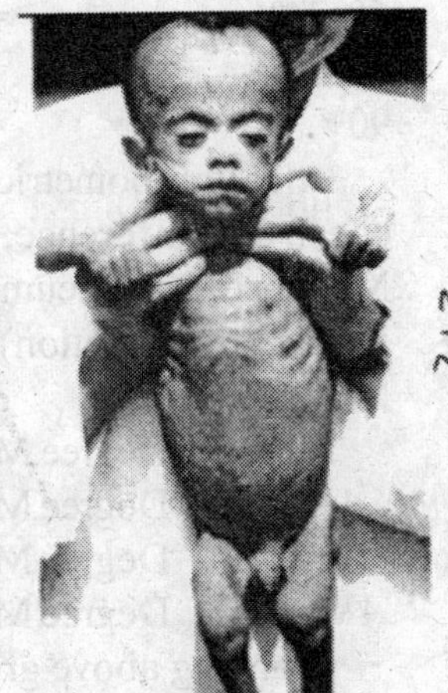

Fig. 6.1B: Marasmus

Difference Between Kwashiorkor and Marasmus (Table 6.10):

Table 6.10: Difference between Kwashiorkor and Marasmus

	Kwashiorkor	*Marasmus*
Muscle Wasting	Not obvious	Obvious
Fat wasting	Not obvious	Obvious
Oedema	Present	Absent
Weight/Height ratio	Low	Very low
Mental change	Irritable	Quiet
Appetite	Poor	Good
Diarrhoea	Present	Present
Skin change	Flaky paint dermatosis	Nil
Hair change	Silky, Pluckable	Nil
Liver change	Enlarged	Nil
Serum albumin	Low	Normal
Plasma amino acid ratio	Raised	Normal

Types of P.E.M.

According to Gomez the degree of P.E.M is classified in terms of weight retardation as under, by a coefficient value:

$$\text{Weight in \%} = \frac{\text{Weight of child}}{\text{Weight of normal for same age}} \times 100$$

Below 60% = III degree
60-74% = II degree
75-89% = I degree
90+ = Normal

All anthropometric values like weight, height, chest circumference, head circumference and Mid upper arm circumference are used to classify P.E.M. (Malnutrition) into following categories.

Normal

I	Degree Malnutrition	
II	Degree Malnutrition	Mild
III	Degree Malnutrition	
IV	Degree Malnutrition	Severe

Planning above grouping is of practical help for supplementary nutrition to Mild type and therapeutic nutrition (Double the dose of supplementary nutrition) to severe degree.

Ecology of Malnutrition (P.E.M.)

According to Jelliffe it is man-made and related to environmental factors which are preventable in nature. They are:

a. *Conditioning influences:* Measles, diarrhoea, helminthic infestation, malaria, tuberculosis.
b. *Cultural influences:* Food habit, religious taboos, food fads, child rearing practices.
c. *Socioeconomic influences:* Poverty, low income, illiteracy, overcrowding.
d. *Food production:* Reduced food production, misdistribution, spoiling due to improper storage.
e. Accessibility of health services.

Role of Protein Assessment in P.E.M.

The quality protein (Reference protein) is a determining force in the causation of PEM. It is the product of digestibility coefficient and biological value divided by 100. It indirectly shows the ratio of Nitrogen retained to nitrogen intake.

If a food has low NPU, the protein requirement is high and accordingly the quantity of food also to be increased.

Prevention of P.E.M.

It needs multidimensional activities which can be tabulated in Table 6.11.

Table 6.11: Prevention of P.E.M.

Primary prevention		*Secondary prevention*	*Tertiary prevention*	
Health promotion	Specific protection	Early diagnosis prompt treatment	Disability limitation	Rehabilitation
MCH nutrition Supplementation Exclusive Breastfeeding	High protein rich diet	Nutrition Surveillance	Hospital Treatment	Nutrition
	Immunisation Rehabilitation	Diagnosis of PEM	Case follow up	
Nutrition Education Family planning	Food Fortification	Supplementary Nutrition Therapeutic Nutrition Deworming		

L.B.W. (Low Birth Weight)

It is defined as birth weight of newborn below 2500 grams, its prevalence is 28-30% in developing countries. Main cause has been growth retardation due to poor socio-economic conditions. In India the national goal to achieve 10% by 2010 is aggregated in the National Health Policy.

According to gestational age LBW can be grouped under 3 categories:

- Preterm (less that 259 days)
- Term (259 to 293 days)
- Postterm (294 days above).

Three main causes that need attention to overcome L.B.W are:

- Malnutrition
- Infection
- Unregulated fertility.

Preventive Measures

- Identification of risk cases and attending to Medical and Nursing care
- Dietary improvement of pregnant women
- Control of maternal infections
- Control of PET, Toxaemia, Diabetes, Hypertension
- Family planning
- Improvement of socioeconomic condition.

Treatment of L.B.W.

Here, there is a great role of nursing care which includes:

- Incubatory care for regulation of temperature, humidity, oxygen supply.
- Nasal feeding since baby cannot suck properly.
- Antibiotic to prevent neonatal infection.

Neonatal Intensive Care Unit (NICU): The role of nursing care is utmost important in a NICU for the prevention of neonatal death by attending to intervention of the following conditions:

- Lung collapse (atelectasis)
- Malformation (Where paediatric surgery are suggested)
- Pulmonary haemorrhage
- Birth trauma leading to brain haemorrhage
- Pneumonia.

Vitamin A Deficiency (Figs 6.2 and 6.3)

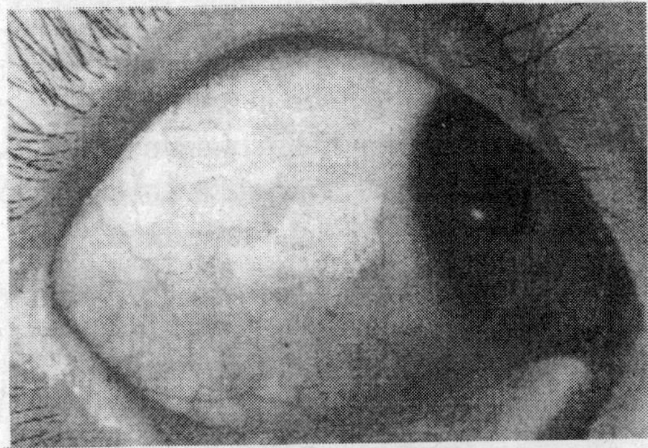

Fig. 6.2: Bitot's spot (foamy)

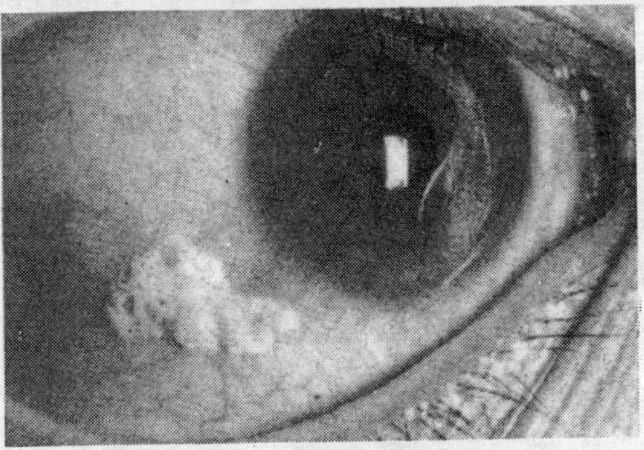

Fig. 6.3: Bitot's spot (cheesy)

Vitamin A deficiency is one of the causes of preventable blindness in India. Young children are susceptible for xerophthalmia. This is associated with faulty feeding practice and ignorance. South India show higher incidence of Vitamin A deficiency than North India.

Prevention and control is done under three strategies (Vitamin A Therapy).

i. *Longterm strategy:* Nutrition education, treatment of infections, immunisation, and periodic massive dose (2 lakh unit) of retinol in oil every 6 months.

ii. *Medium term strategy:* Fortification of foods with vitamin A (Dalda, sugar, tea, margarine, skimmed milk).

iii. *Shortterm strategy:* (Oral dose of retinol palmitate):
To pregnant—2.75 mg per day.
To lactating—11 mg once a week.
Newborn—27.5 mg at birth.
Infants—110 mg once in 6 months.
Young children—55 mg once in 6 months.

Anaemia

Anaemia is a condition in which haemoglobin content of blood is lower than normal as a result of deficiency. Very commonly iron deficiency is the cause of anaemia (Table 6.12).

Table 6.12: Hb% in anaemia diagnosis

W.H.O. criteria for anaemia

Adult male	13 G%
Adult female	12 G%
Pregnancy	11 G%
Children upto 6 years	11 G %
Children above 6 years	12 G %

Cause:

- Inadequate intake.
- Poor bioavailability of dietary iron.
- Loss by haemorrhage.

Effect:

- Maternal mortality
- Foetal mortality
- Abortion
- P.P.H.
- L.B.W.

Prevention of Anaemia

i. In severe anaemia (8 G%) blood transfusion.

ii. In mild and moderate anaemia:
- I.F.A. 100 mg Iron, 0.5 mg Folic acid daily to mothers till Hb% is corrected.
- I.F.A. 100 mg Iron, 0.5 mg Folic acid daily for 3 months to pregnant woman.
- I.F.A. 20 mg Iron, 0.1 mg Folic acid daily to children till Hb% is corrected.

Other measures

- Fortification of salt with iron.

Iodine Deficiency

Iodine deficiency is increasingly becoming public health problem since it is giving wide spectrum of disorders. They can be enumerated as under (Fig. 6.4):

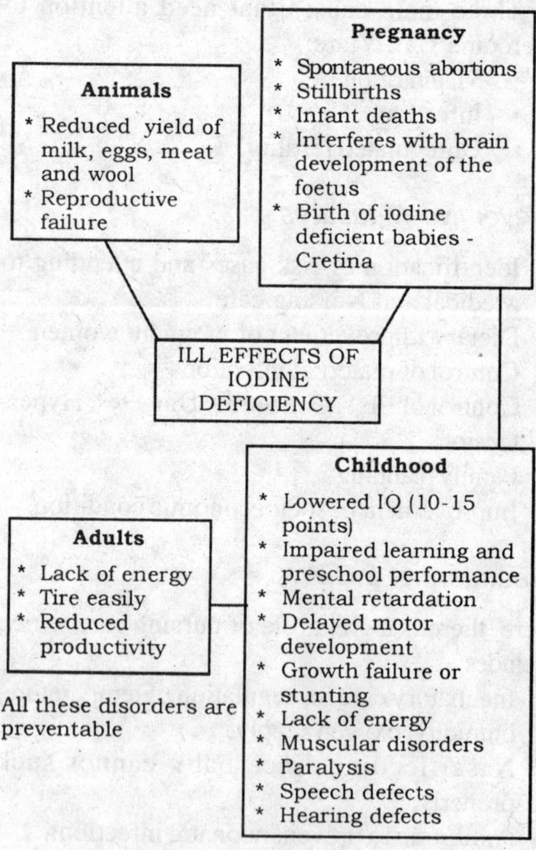

Fig. 6.4: Ill effects of iodine deficiency

Goitre and cretinism are greatly associated with iodine deficiency. "Himalaya goitre belt" is biggest goitre belt in the world.

Epidemiological studies have shown the following observations:

- 140 million people are living in endemic area.
- In endemic belt, goitre is nearly 36% in prevalence.
- In endemic belt, 15% are neonatal hypothyroidism.

Control Programme

- Iodised salt (15 PPM I_2 at consumer level).
- Iodine monitoring and surveillance.
- Manpower engaging in health work is trained on goitre control.
- Health education.

Fluorosis

In India common occurrence of dental fluorosis, skeletal fluorosis and genu valgum indicate the prevalence of fluorosis. This is largely attributed to excessive fluorine content in drinking water. The normal range is 0.5 to 0.8 mg per litre of water.

Dental fluorosis is manifested by white and yellow patches on teeth, corrosion in teeth and mottling of teeth.

Skeletal fluorosis is manifested by fracture and indisposition to move which cripples the individual.

Recent studies have shown that jowar eating area has higher retention of ingested fluoride leading to Genu Valgum.

Control Measures

- Changing the water source.
- Chemical treatment by Nalagonda Technique.

Lathyrism

It is called neurolathyrism, a paralytic disease caused by consuming contaminated non edible pulse "Lathyrus Sativus" (Kesari dhal). It is high in middle part of India when compared to peripheral states of the country. The toxin identified is BOAA (Beta oxalyl amino alanine) which produce neuroparalysis. Clinically it shows following stages:

- Latent stage
- No stick stage
- One stick stage
- Two stick stage
- Crawler stage.

Control Measures

- Banning the crop
- Removal of toxin
  - By steeping method
  - By parboiling
  - Genetic approach
- Health education
- Socio-economic changes.

Cardiovascular Diseases

Nutrition is associated with coronary heart disease. There are supported studies that have shown that elevated blood level of cholesterol and elevated blood level of low density lipoprotein (LDL) result in the development of atherosclerosis.

Dietary changes allowing greater intake of poly unsaturated fatty acids (PUFA) and lesser intake of saturated fat will reduce the risk of heart diseases.

Diabetes

This is one of the common metabolic disorders directly governed by the nutrition and diet component of human beings. Impaired glucose metabolism leads to hyperglycaemia and glycosuria. Non manual occupations, deficiency of zinc, copper, chromium have been added to the evidence of causation of diabetes.

Recently, malnutrition related diabetes is observed. Protein deficiency seems to evolve diabetic state. Excessive consumption of alcohol also increases the risk of diabetes.

Obesity

It is also called hyper alimentation and is known to cause premature death from diabetes, hypertension and coronary heart diseases. Diet containing more calorie lead to post prandial hyperlipidaemia and deposition of triglycerides in adipose tissue resulting in obesity.

Balanced diet, regular exercise, health awareness can control obesity.

Cancer

There are two main observations noted in community survey. One is that dietary intake of fat is associated with cancer of colon, the other is high consumption of fat (per capita consumption of fat) is associated with breast cancer.

Aflatoxin, saccharin and a few food additives and food contaminants are blamed to be carcinogenic.

Since nutrition has shown to influence cancer, great care is to be taken in its primary prevention.

THERAPEUTIC DIET

Hospital Diet

Dietary service in hospitals is as important as therapeutic service. The main objective of the dietary services is to provide better patient-care through properly planned and executed diets.

It is to:

- Serve appetizing and nourishing meal to patients.
- Plan and execute suitable diet which in addition becomes therapeutic.
- Make economical diet.

Following Are Common Hospital Diets

Normal Full Diet (All in Grams except otherwise mentioned):

Item	*Veg*	*Nonveg*
Cereal	350	350
Bread	50	50
Pulses	50	25
Milk/curd	550 ml	300 ml
Greens	300	300
Potato	100	100
Butter	10	10
Oil	20	30
Sugar	50	50
Fruit	150	150
Meat/Fish/Chicken	—	100
Or		
Egg	—	Two
Tea or Coffee	7/15	7/15
Salt	10	10
Condiments	15	15
Yield:		
Calorie	2500	2500
Protein	75	80
Fat	60	70
CHO	420	400

Full Liquid Diet (All Acute Illness)

Item	*Amount (g.)*
Milk	1 litre
Bread	100
Butter	20
Egg	One
Greens (for soup)	150
Potato	100
Sugar	50
Fruit	150
Tea/Coffee	7/15
Salt	10
Provide :	
Calorie	1500
Protein	45
Fat	60
CHO	190

Liquid diet for Fever, Diarrhoea, Post operative, Diabetes, Jejunostomy, Ca-Oesophagus, Anorexia nervosa, Cannot chew, Severe burns, Gastric surgery:

Item	*Quantity (g.)*
Cow's milk	500 m l
Sugar	100
Orange juice	250 ml (six)
Dal for soup/Cereal Kanji	25
Tea/Coffee	7/15
Provide:	
Calorie	1000
Protein	20
Fat	20
CHO	180
Sodium	285 mg

Obesity Diet

Item	*Quantity (g.)*
Skimmed milk	500 ml
Bread	25
Cereal	100
Curds	200
Channa	50
Dhal	25
Greens	500
Oil	10
Tea/Coffee	7/15
Salt	10
Condiment	15
Fruit	2 portions
Provide:	
Calorie	1200
Protein	47 G
Fat	30 G
CHO	183 G

Foods to Avoid

Whole milk, cream , butter, oil, ghee, fried food, honey, sugar, sweets, ovaltine, horlicks, cocoa, cheese, banana, mangoes, grape, jam, arvi, potato, soda, alcohol, dried fruits and nuts.

Foods Allowed Liberally

All vegetables, lime juice, clear soup, pepper water, skimmed milk and all fruits.

Low Cholesterol diet for coronary heart disease, athero-sclerosis, hypercholestemia:

Item	*Quantity (g.)*
Skimmed milk	600 ml
Bread	25
Cereal	100
Curds	300
Channa	50
Dal	25
Veg	400
Fruit	150
Honey	20
Sugar	10
Oil	10
Tea/Coffee	7/15
Provide:	
calories	1200
Protein	54 G
Fat	13 G
CHO	214 G

Peptic Ulcer Diet

Item	*Quantity (g.)*
Milk	1.5 litre
Egg	One
Cream	25
Sugar	50
(1 Egg can replace 100 ml milk)	
Provide:	
Calorie	1375
Protein	54 G
Fat	76 G
CHO	115 G

Bland Diet for Gastric Ulcer, Gastritis, Diarrhoea, Haemorrhoids:

Item	*Quantity (g.)*
Milk	1 litre
Crustless white bread	50
Butter	25
Egg	One
Or ·	
Channa	25
Or Chicken/Fish	100
Rice	150
Dal	25
Cooked veg.	200

Contd.

Contd.

Potato	50
Banana	1
Sugar	50
Tea/Coffee	7/15
Yield:	
Calorie	2075
Protein	58 G
Fat	68 G
CHO	305 G

Guidelines in Diabetic Diet

Free Foods—Leafy veg, tomato, cucumber, radish, lime, clear soup, black coffee/tea, butter milk, sour chutney, pickle, pepper, jeera water, Jamun fruit.

Foods to avoid—Potato, yam, arvi, mango, grape, banana, alcohol, wine.

Foods prohibited—Glucose, sugar, honey, all sweets.

Food Equivalents

50 G rice=any one	Bread	75 G
	Wheat Porridge	50 G
	Dosa	2
	Idli	2
	Potato	150 G
	Biscuit	4
1 portion fruit= 10 Grams CHO = Anyone	100 grams of apple, guava, green, mango, Orange, Musambi, Plum, Papaya, Pear, Peach, Leechies, Pomegranate, 150 grams of grape, yellow melon. 300 grams of Watermelon 50 grams of Banana, Grape, Mango	

Protein free and sodium free diet for hepatic coma, acute anuria:

Sago Kanji

Sago	*50 ml*
a. Water	500 ml
Sugar	50

Contd.

Contd.

b. Lemon	10 ml
c. Orange	200 ml
d. Glucose	100
Water	500 ml
e. Tea/Coffee	7/15

Feeds once in 2 hour provide

Calorie	–	900
Protein	–	2 G.
Fat	–	1 G.
CHO	–	215 G.
Sodium	–	Nil

High Protein Diet for Liver Cirrhosis:

Item	*Quantity (gms)*
Skimmed milk	1 litre
Channa	100
Curds	200
Rice	300
Dal	50
Veg	200
Potato	100
Salt free butter	10
Sugar	100

Provide:

Calorie	–	2500
Protein	–	100 G
Fat	–	40 G
CHO	–	430 G
Sodium	–	730 mg

Gluten Free Diet for Coeliac Disease

Foods allowed : Rice, cornflour, soya products, lean meat, fish, egg, milk, milk product, sugar, honey, all veg, fruit, butter, ghee, oil

Foods prohibited : Wheat products-atta, sooji, maida, biscuit, bread, ragi, oat, rye.

Low Purine Diet for Gout:

Item	*Quantity (g.)*
Milk	200 ml
Bread (white)	50
Butter	10
Channa	50
Curds	200
Rice	150
Oil	10
Greens	300
Fruit	2 portion
Salt	10
Sugar	25
Tea/Coffee	7/15

Yield:		
Calorie	–	1800
Protein	–	40 G
Fat	–	45 G
CHO	–	240 G

Dietary Recommendation in Renal Calculi

If stone is uric acid, urate—Eliminate

Meat, meat product, shellfish, dal, wholegrain cereal, oat meal, dried pea, bean, spinach. (Give alkaline ash and neutral)

If stone is oxalate, eliminate

Green plantain, spinach, arvi (colocasia root), sweet, beet, currants, figs, almond, Cashewnut, grape.

If stone is phosphate—Carbonate

Give acid ash diet.

High ash foods are:

Wholegrain cereal, meat, fish, egg, nut.

High alkaline foods are:

Dal, greens, roots, milk, milk product, fruit, coconut.

Neutral foods are:

Tea, coffee, sugar, butter, oil.

NUTRITIONAL ASSESSMENT

It is a community health device to assess individual and group nutritional status by available field methods. This gives the prevalence and distribution of nutritional problem in a community.

Clinical Examination

It is clinical assessment of nutritional deficiencies. ICMR has formulated a schematic proforma for this type of clinical assessment, which is as under:

CLINICAL

1. General : Normal Built/thin built/sickly
2. Hair : Normal/dull and dry/dry-pigmented/thin and sparse/easily pluckable/flag sign
3. Face : Diffuse depigmentation/naso-labial dyssebacea/moon face
4. Eyes : Conjunctiva—normal/dry on exposure for ½ min/dry and wrinked/bitot's spots/brown pigmentation/angular conjunctivitis/pale conjunctiva
   Cornea—normal /dry/hazy or opaque
5. Lips : Normal/angular stomtitis/cheilosis
6. Tongue : Normal/pale and flabby /red and raw/fissured/geographic
7. Teeth : Mottled enamel/caries/attrition
8. Gums : Normal/bleeding
9. Glands : Thyroid enlargement/Parotid enlargement
10. Skin : Normal/dry and scaly/follicular hyperkeratosis
11. Nails : Koilonychia
12. Oedema : In dependent parts
13. Rachitic changes : Knock-knees or bow legs/epiphyseal enlargement/beading of the ribs /pigeon chest
14. Internal system : Hepatomegaly/psycho-motor change/mental confusion/sensory loss/motor weakness /loss of position sense/loss of vibration sense / loss of ankle and knee jerks/calf tenderness/cardiac enlargement/tachycardia.

ANTHROPOMETRIC:
Weight (kg) : Head circumference (cm):
Height (cm) : Chest circumference (cm):
Mid-upper-arm circumference (cm): Skinfold:

Anthropometry

This is measurement of following on individuals:

- Height
- Weight Adult
- Skin fold
- Head circumference
- Chest circumference Paediatric
- Mid upper arm circumference

Laboratory Assessment

They are:

- Hb % (Anaemia)
- Stool exam (worms)
- Urine exam (diabetes)
- Serum level for metabolites
- (Serum retinol, folate).

Assessment of Functional Indices

- Capillary fragility (Vitamin C)
- Cutaneous hypersensitivity (Zinc)
- Prothrombin Time (Vitamin K)
- Sperm count (Zinc)
- EEG (Nerve function)
- Vaso pressor response (Vitamin C).

Diet Survey

By enquiry and data collection on personal visit, information on food consumption is done in the following ways:

- Weighment of raw food
- Weighment of cooked food
- Oral questionnaire
- Stock inventory.

Minimum of 7 days or 3 days data gives average value for:

i. Per capita consumption of calories
ii. Per capita consumption of nutrient.

Other Methods

They are morbidity data, mortality data and data on ecology and health education services.

NUTRITIONAL SURVEILLANCE

It is defined as keeping a watch over nutrition of a community to take decision on required improvement for better nutrition. It helps in long term planning, management, evaluation and to get over nutrition crisis.

Difference Between Nutritional Surveillance and Growth Monitoring (Table 6.13):

Table 6.13: Difference between surveillance and Monitoring

Nutritional surveillance	*Growth monitoring*
Detect under-nutrition by diagnosis	Preserve normal growth by health education
A sample study	All 0-6 age children
By trained worker	By educating mothers
Precise instrument used	Simple instrument used
Referal to hospital	Referral to P.H.C.

Following indicators are used in nutrition surveillance:

- Birth weight
- Proportion of breast feed
- Proportion of weaned feed
- Height for age
- Weight for age
- Weight for height
- Clinical signs.

The above indicators are used in nutrition surveillance. Each state has a unit to monitor this surveillance called state level National Nutrition Monitoring Bureau.

SOCIAL NUTRITION

Food and nutrition is part of civilization which endorse the security and safety of a society and when it comes to individual it endorses survival.

Social interaction influences under-nutrition, over-nutrition, imbalances and specific nutritional deficiency.

Food habit, custom, belief and tradition make people to develop an attitude which determines the nutritional status of a community. Psychological aspect of love, affection, social prestige is shown through food. Family passion like rice eaters, wheat eaters shapes dietary habits, foods which are avoided, tabulated below, depict food fad which can influence nutritional status.

Table 6.14: Foods avoided under the pretext of hot, cold and other beliefs

Pregnancy	*Lactation*	*Children*	*Elderly*	*Sick*
Papaya	Dhal	Sugar	Rice	Solid food
Carrot	Greens	Banana	Oil	Rice
Leafy vegetables	Rice, fruits	Curds	Spices	
Iron	Banana	Cucumber	Meat	

Cooking practices like direct cooking, boiling, frying, pressure cooking influence the content of nutrient of the diet.

Alcoholism in a society also influences nutrition in a negative way.

FOOD HYGIENE

With the understanding of germ theory, protection of food from contamination by pathogens resulted in an awareness of food hygiene. It is the status of how food in its different placement is maintained. Production, handling, distribution and serving apart from storage decide the quality of food. Bacterial toxin and bacterial contamination hallmark the illness due to food borne diseases.

Food borne disease is an illness either by toxins or pathogens caused by their entry to body through food. This has become a major relevance in the days of mass catering era. They are classified as under:

A. Toxins:

a. Natural toxin: Lathyrism, endemic ascites.
b. Produced toxin: Botulism, staphylocci
c. Chemical toxin: Mercury, lead, DDT.

B. Infections:

a. Bacterial—Typhoid, paratyphoid, botulism, diarrhoea, infantile diarrhoea.
b. Viral—Hepatitis, GE.
c. Parasite—Tapeworm, round worm, amoebiasis, thread worm.

Milk Hygiene

Next to water, milk is a major vehicle of transmission of diseases. Main diseases which are transmitted through milk are:

- Tuberculosis
- Brucellosis
- Anthrax
- Leptospirosis

It is possible to maintain milk hygiene in the prevention of milk borne diseases. They are:

- Measures on positive health of cows and buffalos.
- Dairy sanitation
- Pasteurisation

Methods of Pasteurisation are:

i. HTST method (High temperature and short time method) where milk is rapidly heated to 72°C, held for 15 seconds and rapidly cooled to 4°C.
ii. Holder (Vat) method where milk is kept at 66°C for 30 minutes and then quickly cooled to 5°C.
iii. UHT (Ultra high temperature) method where milk is rapidly heated in 2 stages, first heated to 125°C, cooled rapidly to room temperature followed by heating to 125°C under pressure. In both stage heating is for 10 seconds. Rapid cooling to room temperature and bottling is followed.

To test the effect of pasteurisation Methylene Blue reduction test is done; when methylene blue is added to 10 ml milk and kept at 37^0C and observed for disappearance of blue colour. Quick disappearance is an index of poor pasteurisation.

Meat Hygiene

Animal food which is also an important part of diet can cause disease like tape worm infestation (Beef tapeworm, pork tapeworm), bacterial infection (anthrax, actinomycosis, tuberculosis) and food poisoning.

Procedures that are followed in meat hygiene are:

- Veterinary examination of animals brought to slaughter house.
- Slaughter house sanitation.

Fish Hygiene

Traditionally stiffness, bright red gills and clear permanent eyes are known to exhibit good eatable fish.

After death of fishes, autolysis by bacteria causes concern and should be taken care of in avoiding hepatitis, and fish tape worm infestation. Of late tinned fish are being adjudged best if they posses following criteria:

- No rusting
- No leakage
- No evidence of tampering
- No bloom out phenomenon at opening.

Egg Hygiene

Eggs are sterile inside and are bound to get contaminated by soil, faecal matter in the environment. Bacteria including typhoid organism can penetrate a cracked shell which can cause food poisoning.

Inspection and good preservation technique help in overcoming disease by poor egg hygiene.

Fruits and Vegetables

Sanitation of fruit and vegetables is a challenge to modern society.

Disposal of garbage is public health problem in market place, particularly so in corporation areas, since garbage is a source of transmission of amoebiasis and worm infestation. Since fruits and vegetables are eaten raw, it poses problem with poor food sanitation.

For an effective hygiene of fruits and vegetables, actions on following are relevant:

- Proper sanitation in handling of fresh fruits and vegetables.
- Washing fresh fruits/vegetables especially leafy vegetables with potassium permanganate solution.
- Proper disposal of garbage.
- Proper storage methods of perishables.

FOOD TOXINS

Food toxins are common causes of food poisoning. Epidemics of gastroenteritis are traced, most often, to food toxins. Common toxins are described below:

Epidemic Dropsy

Outbreaks of epidemic dropsy with the manifestation of non-inflammatory bilateral swelling of legs, diarrhoea, cardiac failure and death, and even glaucoma used to occur and the cause was discovered in 1926 when it was attributed to contamination of mustard oil with argemone oil. In 1941 "Sanguinarine" the toxin was identified for causing dropsy. Contamination was by ignorance (accidental) and also for commerce (deliberate).

Toxin prevention is possible by avoiding seed contamination and enforcement of PFA Act.

Aflatoxin

It is fungal toxin by *Aspergillus flavus* which infest foodgrains particularly ground nut. Many deaths have occurred because of liver failure. Among children, the clinical condition is described under "Indian childhood cirrhosis".

Prevention of toxin is possible by health education for not consuming the contaminated foodgrain. One has to ensure proper storage after drying. If moisture content is maintained below 10 percent, toxin formation is prevented totally.

Ergot

Ergot is a field fungus known as *Claviceps fusiformis*, which grows as black mass. Consumption of ergot causes ergotism.

Nausea, vomiting, giddiness, drowsiness, cramps of limbs, gangrene of limbs are usual manifestation of ergotism.

Control is possible by health education and removal of infested grains by hand-picking. Infested grains can be removed by floating in 20% salt water.

Neurolathyrism

Contamination of edible dal with non-edible harmful dal viz. Kesaridal (Lathyrus sativus) which produce a neuro-toxin BOAA (Beta oxalyl Amino Alanine). Neuroparalysis starts with difficult gait to crawling. The clinical stages are described according to ambulatory condition of the patient.

- Latent stage
- No stick stage
- One stick stage
- Two stick stage
- Crawler stage.

Prevention is possible by banning the crop, parboiling, health education and genetic approach.

Endemic Ascites

Millet (Panicum miliare = Gondhli) is contaminated with crotalaria seeds (Jhunjhunia) which contain hepatotoxin called pyrrolizidine alkaloid. Ascites and jaundice are common clinical manifestations.

Prevention is by health education and deweeding crotalaria plants.

Fusarium Toxin

Sorghum and rice gets infested with fusarium fungi. G.I. manifestations are common. Control of grain contamination and disallowing the use of contaminated grains prevent toxic effect.

FOOD ADDITIVES

Many chemicals used as additives to increase shelf life of food, improve taste, to change the texture, to give a colour, are called food additives. All junk foods like (Biscuit, cake, confectionery, jam, jelly, coke, ketchup) contain food additives. Food additives are not nutritious, and are added intentionally.

Indiscriminate use of additive pose health problems. Contaminants incidental through packing, insecticides and environmental conditions also pose a threat to public health.

Permitted Food Additives are:

- Colouring agents (Saffron, turmeric).
- Flavouring agents (Vanilla).
- Sweetening agent (Saccharine).
- Preservative agent (Sorbic acid, acetic acid).

These additives are controlled by G.O.I. through:

- F.P.O. (Fruit Products Order).
- P.F.A. Act (Prevention of Food Adulterations Act).
- B.I.S. (Bureau of Indian Standards).

FOOD FORTIFICATION

Reinforcement of nutrients with additional supplies to prevent deficiency is called *food fortification*.

This is mainly to improve the quality of diet of a community.

Examples:

- Fluoridation of water
- Iodization of salt
- Vitamin A and D to vanaspathi
- Vitamin A and D to milk

- Salt with iodine and iron.

Food fortification is a long term nutritional measure in the control of nutritional health problem.

FOOD ENRICHMENT

This process is the restoration of nutrient value of a food to its normal level. It is not a feasible process that can be adopted for a community nutrition programme. Mainly because of its temporary addition which can wean off again, enrichment is possible at the distribution level.

Example of vegetable oil when looses its vitamin content, enrichment with vitamin A and D is done at the source of distribution.

FOOD ADULTERATION

Food adulteration causes concern because it allows the food to lose its quality and at the same time, it may be injurious to health.

Common types of adulteration are noted in the following Table 6.15:

Table 6.15: Common food adulterants

Asfoetida (Hing)	–	*Resin, gum, grit*
Butter	–	Starch, animal fat
Black pepper	–	Papaya seed
Cereals	–	Soapstone bits
Chilli powder	–	Brick powder
Coffee powder	–	Chicory, Tamarind husk
Dal	–	Kesaridal
Dhania powder	–	Cow dung powder
Ghee	–	Vanaspati
Haldi	–	Lead chromate powder
Icecream	–	Starch, cellulose
Milk	–	Water, starch
Mustard seed	–	Argemone seed

Common Food Standards

i. The Agmark standard (By Directorate of Marketing and Inspection).
ii. ISI Mark (By Bureau of Indian Standards).
iii. PFA Standards (By Central Committee for Food Standards).
iv. Codex Alimentarius (By Commission from FAO/WHO).

P.F.A. Act 1954:

To ensure pure food and to avoid deceptive trade practices; Prevention of Food Adulteration Act was enacted in 1954. Recently in 1986 it was amended for the third time giving it a more coverage. Food adultration is punishable by life imprisonment and or fine. Food laboratories help in final decision in this regard.

NATIONAL NUTRITIONAL PROGRAMMES

In the early part of post independence due to high prevalence of malnutrition, Government of India launched several nutritional programmes. Early emphasis has been on increased food production and supplementary feeding to the vulnerable groups. The aim of all nutrition programmes is to provide additional nutrients to target groups to fill the gap between intake and requirement.

These can be described under following heads:

For Overall Nutritional Status

-A.N.P.

Applied Nutrition Programme was introduced in 1960 to make people conscious of their nutritional needs and to increase production of foods for required consumption. Evaluation showed no desired awareness could be generated in the public. The community kitchen and school garden could not function properly. The programme lacked effective supervision and has become defunct.

S.N.P.

Major beneficiaries of special nutrition programme which was started in 1970 were preschool children, pregnant women and lactating mothers. This provided supplementary nutrition, supply of vitamin A solution and IFA tablets. The aim was for:

- 300 calories and 12 grams protein for a child.
- 600 calories and 20 grams protein for women and is for 300 days a year.

Because of lack of infrastructure it is not efficiently functioning.

Balwadi Nutrition Programme

This was started in 1970 for 3-6 aged children in rural areas, under social welfare department. This provided pre-primary education along with providing 300 calories and 10 grams protein per day.

Mid Day Meal Programme

Mid Day Meal Programme (Centre)

It was launched in 1961 throughout the country, to improve children school attendance. The meal as a supplement supplying 1/3 of total calorie and half of protein need with local preparation and as low cost meal is an added attraction to school children. A model meal is to contain the following:

Cereal/millet	–	75 grams
Pulses	–	30 grams
Oil	–	8 grams
Leafy vegetable	–	30 grams
Non leafy vegetable	–	30 grams

Now mid day meal programme is a part of Minimum Needs Programme.

Mid Day Meal Programme (States)

Few states have taken up their own state level budgetary schemes to provide mid day school meal. Major examples are, Chief Minister's Noon Meal Programme" in Tamil Nadu, Chief Minister's mid day school meal "Akshara Dasoha" in Karnataka.

Specific Disease Prevention Programmes

Vitamin A Prophylaxis Programme

This was started in 1970, by administering massive single dose of all preparation of Vitamin A (2 Lakhs IU) orally to all preschool children every 6 months through health workers.

Prophylaxis Against Nutritional Anaemia

It was started under the name National Nutritional Anaemia Prophylaxis Programme (NNAPP) with an objective of assessment, treatment, prophylaxis and monitoring anaemia among mothers. Distribution of IFA Tablets to Mothers and Children (1-12 years) was taken up through RCH centres, PHC's and ICDS Anganwadies.

Control of Iodine Deficiency Disorders

Started in 1962, widened to national network, mounted in 1986 to replace plain edible salt by iodised salt in a phased manner. This is helping a lot in bringing down Iodine Deficiency Disorders. The programme is called NIDDCP (National Iodine Deficiency Disorders Control Programme).

Other Indirect Programmes

ICDS

Integrated Child Development Service programme started in 1975 to help ICDS beneficiaries namely 0-6 age children, pregnant, lactating and women of reproductive age group. Supplementary nutrition and therapeutic nutrition are being carried out at Anganwadi level which is evaluated by growth monitoring.

IPP

India population project is an indirect nutritional programme through Family Welfare Schemes in selected places.

CHAPTER SEVEN

Maternal and Child Health (Reproductive Child Health) Including School Health and Geriatric

INTRODUCTION

Pregnant women, lactating mothers and children below 14 years have been the vulnerable group in a community. Their health indicates and determines the community health.

Total women population of India as per 2001 census is 495, 738 and 169 which constitute 48.27 % of the total population.

Among this 15-45-year age group women constitute 22% of total population.

45 to 49-year age group women constitute 1.67 % of total population.

Thus total of women15-49-age group form 23.67 % of total population.

Children below 14 years form 42% of the total population.

Definition

Under RCH programme, Govt. of India, Ministry of Health and Family Welfare has defined the term as under:

"People have the ability to reproduce and regulate fertility. Women are able to go through pregnancy, child birth safely; the outcome of pregnancies is successful in terms of maternal and infant survival and well-being. And couples are able to have sexual relations free from fear of pregnancy and of contracting disease."

Concept of RCH

It is an integrated approach of service which provides health services to young women and young children through family welfare programmes like UIP, ORT, CSSM, ARI control, emergency and essential obstetric care, MTP services, RTI and STD control, essential newborn care and vitamin A prophylaxis.

RCH Package

As mentioned under concept of RCH, the components under RCH are depicted as below (Fig. 7.1):

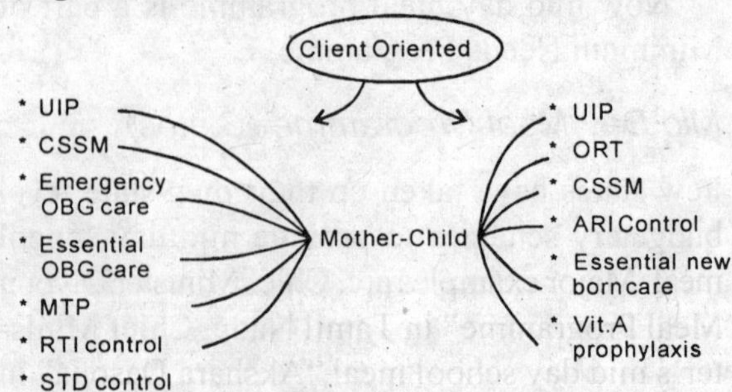

Fig. 7.1: R.C.H. package

C.S.S.M.

Child survival and safe motherhood programme (CSSM) initiated in 1992 which later got integrated to RCH in 1997 has major public health interventions like essential obstetric care, 24 hours delivery services at PHC, emergency obstetric care, MTP, prevention of RTI and STD and survey of districts. Following services are specified in RCH programme:

- Registration of all pregnancies, at the early period.
- Providing minimum 3 ANC check ups.
- 100% coverage of TT to pregnant women.
- Nutrition education and advice.
- Detection of risk pregnancies
- Immediate and prompt referral of risk cases.
- Training of all indigenous dais.
- Safe delivery by trained Dai, MPW in the community.
- Advice on birth spacing.
- Provision of institutional deliveries.

Delivery Service at PHC

To promote and provide institutional deliveries, 24 hours delivery facility at PHC and provision for additional honorarium to attending staff are provided at primary health centre.

MTP (Medical Termination of Pregnancy)

On indication like unintended and unwanted pregnancies, when women select MTP, it is allowed and conducted at PHC on fixed dates. Manpower training and provision of MTP equipment are attended under the scheme. This is mainly to reduce morbidity and mortality due to unsafe abortions.

Control of RTI/STI

With the collaboration of NACO (National AIDS Control Organisation) which provides assistance to set up clinics, a link with HIV/AIDS control is an ongoing programme. Training of manpower, supply of drug kit is attended under the scheme. This scheme provides provision of contract technician (two) to each district.

U.I.P.

This was earlier a part of CSSM and is now under RCH. Since 1997, provides immunisation against 6 preventable diseases. Supply of DPT, DT, OPV, measles, BCG and cold chain establishment and additional items supporting UIP.

Drug and Equipment Kits

Drug kit and equipment kit to sub centre, PHC under RCH activities are given in Chapter 4.

ORT

Under the RCH programme ORS packets are supplied to the states. Along with drug kit, 300 packets per year, in 2 lots are supplied by the Central Government. Rational use of drug, nutritional care and ORT are motivated to reduce child mortality.

A.R.I. Control

Acute Respiratory Infections are to be prevented to prevent deaths due to pneumonia. Training health workers for recognition and management is undertaken. Through drug kit cotrimoxazole is supplied under the scheme.

Vitamin A Prophylaxis

Below 3 years of age all children are provided with 5 doses of Vitamin A as follows:

9 months	–	I dose 1 lakh units
18 months	–	II dose 2 lakh units
24 months	–	III dose 2 lakh units
30 months	–	IV dose 2 lakh units
36 months	–	V dose 2 lakh units

Emergency Obstetric Care

Many deliveries are home deliveries and if they are associated with complications, maternal morbidity and mortality rate will go up. Thousands of referral units are identified under RCH programme. They are strengthened with emergency obstetric kit, equipment kit and skilled health professional. Involvement of NGO for decentralising activities is another novel idea under RCH scheme.

Essential Obstetric Care

This refers to basic maternity service to all pregnant women in the country. This ensures the following:

- Registration of pregnancy at 16 weeks or as early as possible
- 3 ANC check ups by (ANM) MPW
- Safe delivery (Home or Health Centre)
- 3 PNC check ups.

This component is greatly intended at home visiting and hence a specific criteria of domiciliary care.

Essential Newborn Care

This component reduces the perinatal and neonatal mortality in the community. Services extended under following areas:

- Resuscitation of newborn with birth asphyxia
- Prevention of hypothermia
- Prevention of infection
- Exclusive breastfeeding
- Referral of sick newborn
- Care of LBW babies.

RCH KEY INDICATORS

a. Currently married women
- Percent married females to total females in the age

10-14 years –	4.5 %
15-19 years –	35.3 %
20-24 years –	81.8 %
15-44 years –	79.5 %

b. Mean age at marriage–17.7 years
c. No. of children per married women aged 45-49 years
   - Ever born – 4.3
   - Surviving – 3.7
d. Currently married women with any ANC - 67.2 %. (Any one or two of ANC check up, TT, IFA)
e. Currently married women with full ANC – 14.8 % (all had 3 ANC check up + TT + 100 IFA tablets)
f. Institutional delivery—35.0 %
g. Safe delivery (by trained)—41.9 %
h. Women with pregnancy complications—34.8% (Swelling hand, feet visual disturbance bleeding convulsions weak or no foetal movement abnormal presentation).
i. Delivery complications—36.4 % (Premature births obstructed labour prolonged labour)
j. Post delivery complications—42.0% (High Fever Lower abdominal pain Foul smelling Vaginal discharge Excessive bleeding Dizziness Severe Headache
k. Currently married women 15-44 age with symptoms of RTI/STD—28.8%
l. Currently married women 15-44 age who are aware of AIDS—41.1%
m. Males aged 20-54 years with symptoms of RTI/STD—12.7%
n. Males aged 20-54 years who are aware of AIDS—57.4%.

MATERNITY CYCLE

Study of maternity cycle is important in understanding physiological basis of pregnancy, delivery and lactation. These periods influence the health of mother and child. Any pathology leads to maternal and infant morbidity and mortality.

RCH PROBLEMS (MCH PROBLEMS)

Malnutrition

Pregnant woman, lactating mothers and children are affected by malnutrition in developing countries. They cause LBW, Anaemia, Toxaemia, PPH. Intrauterine period influence foetal growth and weaning period influence childhood malnutrition. Direct interventions like supplementation, indirect interventions like environmental sanitation prove effective anchor in the prevention of malnutrition.

Infection

Foetal growth retardation, puerperal sepsis, LBW are due to maternal infections. Women infected with toxoplasmosis and cytomegalovirus are increasing. On the other hand, diarrhoea, ARI, skin infections of infants are seen to a great extent. Malaria and tuberculosis are serious infection of childhood. Programmes under RCH are aimed at the prevention of these infections.

Uncontrolled Reproduction

Repeated child births have seen their association with anaemia, abortion, LBW and APH. There is need for small family norm to safeguard mother and child health. High birth rate is associated with high IMR and under five death rates (Table 7.1) as per observations by UNICEF and UNDP:

Table 7.1: BR, IMR, UFMR in developed and developing countries

	Developed Countries	*Developing Countries*
Birth rate/1000 population	14	25
IMR/1000 LB	7	69
Under five MR/1000 LB	8	96

INDICATORS OF RCH CARE (INDICATORS OF MCH CARE)

M.M.R. (Maternal Mortality Rate)

Pregnancy related death is sometimes used to denote the death of woman while pregnant or within 42 days of termination of pregnancy irrespective of cause of death.

WHO has defined MMR as "the death of woman while pregnant or within 42 days of termination of pregnancy irrespective of duration and site of pregnancy from any cause related to or aggravated by the pregnancy or its management but not from accidental or incidental causes."

$$\text{M.M.R.} = \frac{\text{Female death due to complications of pregnancy, child birth or within 42 days of delivery from puerperal causes in an area during a year}}{\text{Total live births in that area for a year}} \times 1000$$

It is 3.9/1000 live births in India.

Infection and bleeding are common causes of maternal mortality. While hepatitis, heart disorders and endocrine causes are more in developed countries, in developing countries the causes are mostly infection, anaemia, jaundice and malaria.

Other influencing causes of maternal mortality have been:

- Women's age
- Birth interval
- Parity
- Socio-economic status
- Cultural practices
- Nutritional status
- Environmental sanitation.

Causes of MMR in India Are

Obstetric cause :	Haemorrhage, infection, unsafe abortion
Non-obstetric :	Anaemia, renal disease, hepatic cause diseases
Social causes :	Age at childbirth, parity, malnutrition, poor transport, social custom.

Prevention of Maternal Mortality

Tackling obstetric, non-obstetric and social causes reduces the M.M.R.

R.C.H. programme detailed earlier with its components like early registration, anaemia correction, essential obstetric care, emergency obstetric care and preventing complications have an impact on M.M.R.

Foetal Deaths

This is a crude indicator of RCH. No reliable informations are available and if available they are usually after 28 weeks of gestation. Hence foetal deaths are redefined under still births.

Still Birth Rate

It is death of foetus weighing 1000 grams or more occurring during one year in every 1000 total births.

$$\text{Still Birth Rate} = \frac{\text{Foetal deaths weighing above 1000 grams at birth}}{\text{Total LB + Still births weighing above 1000 grams at birth}} \times 1000$$

Present estimate of still birth rate in India is 8, urban areas showing around 5.

Perinatal Mortality Rate

This includes still births and early neonatal deaths.

$$\text{Perinatal mortality rate} = \frac{\text{Late foetal and early neonatal deaths weighing above 1000 grams at birth}}{\text{Total LB above 1000 grams at birth}} \times 1000$$

Perinatal mortality rate is a significant yardstick of measuring obstetric and paediatric care in the country. National goal to achieve 35 is postponed to beyond 2000.

Table 7.2: Perinatal mortality rates

Japan	5/1000
U.S.A.	10/1000
Thailand	20/1000
India	40/1000

Following risk groups are identified in influencing high perinatal mortality. They are:

- Elderly mothers
- Young mothers
- Parity 5 and above
- Heavy smoking
- Severe anaemia
- Multiple pregnancies.

Causes of perinatal mortality can be grouped under 3 categories:

1. *Antenatal causes:* Maternal diseases, pelvic diseases, birth defects of reproductive organs, Rh incompatibility, Toxaemia of pregnancy, APH.
2. *Intranatal causes:* Birth injury, Asphyxia, obstetric complications.
3. *Postnatal causes:* Premature baby, respiratory distress syndrome, congenital anomalies.

Preventive Steps

Tackling above 3 causes at appropriate time and existing RCH programme include catering TT, IFA, essential obstetric care, emergency obstetric care, safe delivery practice, essential newborn care.

Neonatal Mortality Rate

Deaths of newborn occurring from birth till 28 days after birth are called neonatal mortality. It is calculated by:

Neonatal Mortality Rate:

$$= \frac{\text{No. of deaths of newborn before 28 days after birth in a year}}{\text{Total LB in that year}} \times 1000$$

Neonatal mortality reflects endogenous factors like LBW, birth injury, etc., which affect newborn. It is directly related to gestational age and birth weight. In India 60% of infant deaths are occurring before 28 days after birth of newborn babies. It is approximately estimated at present as 49 per 1000 live births.

Post Neonatal Mortality Rate

It is the ratio of post neonatal deaths in a given year to the total number of live births in the same year. It is calculated by:

$$\text{Post neonatal mortality rate} = \frac{\text{No. of deaths of children between 28 days to 1 year in a year}}{\text{Total LB in that year}} \times 1000$$

This mortality is influenced by exogenous factors like diarrhoea, ARI, malnutrition. Large family and high birth order are found significantly related to this mortality. It is estimated to be, at present, 25 per 1000 live birth.(26 Rural; 16 Urban)

Infant Mortality Rate (IMR)

It is the ratio of infant deaths registered in a given year to the total number of live births of the same year. It is calculated by :

$$\text{I.M.R.} = \frac{\text{No. of deaths of children below 1 year of age in a year}}{\text{Total LB in that year}} \times 1000$$

It is one of the most important and sensitive indicator of RCH. It is a unique rate because it covers a large 1 year age population, when they suffer from disease or condition which is specific to that age and intervention brings out *remarkable decline of IMR.*

Table 7.3: IMR in developed and developing countries

Developed countries		*Developing countries (per 1000 live births)*	
Japan	3	Bangladesh	51
USA	7	India	67

I.M.R. of India is estimated, at present, at 67 per 1000 live births. Most of urban studies have shown a declined rate of IMR when compared to rural areas.

I.M.R. is greatly related and influenced by female literacy rate and birth rate.

Causes of I.M.R.

i. Neonatal causes:
- L.B.W.
- Birth injury
- Birth defect
- Rh incompatibility
- Diarrhoea
- A.R.I.
- N.N.T.

ii. Post neonatal causes:
- Diarrhoea
- A.R.I.
- Malnutrition
- Birth defect
- Other infections.

I.M.R. is influenced by following factors:

Table 7.4: Factors influencing I.M.R.

Biological	*Economical*	*Socio-cultural*
Birth weight	Income of family	Early marriage
Mother's age	Standard of living	Sex of child
Birth order	Purchasing power of family	Breastfeeding
Multiple pregnancy	Affordability	Planned motherhood
Family size	Possessions	Mother's education
High fertility		Broken family
		Unwed mother
		Overcrowding

Prevention of I.M.R.

i. Good antenatal care
ii. U.I.P.
iii. Exclusive breastfeeding
iv. Growth monitoring

v. Small family norm
vi. Good sanitation
vii. Essential obstetric care
viii. Essential paediatric care
ix. Female literacy
x. Socio-economic development.

Child Death Rate

It is calculated by $= \frac{\text{No. of deaths of children 1-4 age in a year}}{\text{Total No. of children 1-4 age (MYP)}} \times 1000$

Child death rate reflects environmental conditions and socio-cultural conditions of the family. A child has high risk of dying at 2nd year of life.

It is estimated, at present, at 10 percent of total deaths.

Common Causes of Child Death Rate in India Are

- Diarrhoea
- A.R.I.
- Malnutrition
- Other infectious diseases
- Accidents.

Prevention of 1-4 years mortality lies on the specific control measures against causes mentioned above.

Child Mortality Rate (Under 5 Mortality)

It is the annual number of deaths of children under 5 years expressed as a rate per 1000 live births.

$$\text{C.M.R.} = \frac{\text{No. of deaths of children below 5 years in a year}}{\text{No. of LB in that year}} \times 1000$$

Table 7.5: CMR of selected countries (per 1000 LB)

Japan	–	4
U.S.A.	–	6
Sri Lanka	–	19
Thailand	–	29
India	–	95
Pakistan	–	110

Causes of Child Mortality Rate

- A.R.I.
- Neonatal infections
- Diarrhoea
- Measles, malaria
- Malnutrition
- Accidents.

Note

C.M.R. estimate, at present, is at
95/1000 live births
OR
23.7/1000 under five-year population.

Prevention is action on noted causes and control of influencing factors.

Child Survival Index

It is calculated by:

$$\text{C.S.I.} \frac{(1000)\text{–Child mortality rate}}{10} = \frac{(1000)–95}{10}$$

$$= 90.5$$

Note the calculation: 95-Child mortality rate That means 95 children die out of 1000 children. Remaining who are alive are (1000-95) = 905 children.

For 1000 children..........905 children survive.
For 100 children........90.5 children survive (rounded off to 91.0).

SOCIAL WELFARE PROGRAMMES FOR RCH

They are grouped under 3 heads:

1. Programmes for women
2. Programmes for children
3. Combined programmes.

I.C.D.S. (Integrated Child Development Services)

In pursuance of the national policy for children, I.C.D.S. scheme was initiated in 1975. It is an integrated package of:

a. Supplementary nutrition
b. Immunisation
c. Health check up
d. Medical referral service
e. Nutrition education
f. Health education and
g. Non-informal education of 0-6 children.

Administration of I.C.D.S.

Under Ministry of Social and Women Welfare, Integrated Child Development Service is being undertaken through state directorate. There are urban, rural and tribal blocks which are administered by CDPO; under CDPO 4 Mukhya Sevikas each controlling 20–25 anganwadies acts as mentor to AWWs. Each anganwadi has an AWW who is a community woman who helps in AW functionaries. 1978 and 1982 surveys gave good results which allowed great expansions. At present there are 4368 ICDS projects operating. Of late adolescent girl scheme was sanctioned to 507 blocks as a special intervention to 11–18 years age girls. Some blocks were sponsored by NGOs and few others were sponsored by World Bank.

Recently we have proposal for:

a. Universalisation of I.C.D.S. scheme.
b. Setting up of community nutrition centres, and
c. Sanction of Indira Mahila Yojana are under consideration.

I.C.D.S. coverage is considered good based on the fact that:

a. There is reduction in severe malnutrition among children.
b. Birth weight is gained among beneficiaries.
c. Good immunisation coverage.
d. Reduced I.M.R. and
e. Reduced child mortality rate in the area under ICDS coverage.

Objectives of I.C.D.S.

a. To improve the nutritional and health status of children in the age group 0–6 years.
b. To lay the foundations for psychological, physical and social development of the child.
c. To reduce mortality and morbidity, malnutrition and school dropout.
d. To achieve an effective coordination of policy and implementation among the various departments working for the promotion of child development; and
e. To enhance the capability of the mother and nutritional needs of the child through proper nutrition and health education.

Package of services in I.C.D.S.

Pregnant women	Health check up TT Supplementary nutrition Nutrition Education Health Education
Lactating mothers	Health check up Supplementary nutrition Nutrition Education Health Education
Women 15–45 age	Nutrition Education Health Education
0–3 children	Supplementary nutrition Immunisation Health check up Referral
3–6 children	Supplementary nutrition Immunisation Health check up Referral Non formal education

Supplementary Nutrition

This programme is mainly targeted towards pregnant, lactating and 0-6 children group. It provides 200 calories and 10 gm protein for infants; 300 calories and 15 gm protein for 1-6 children; 500 calories 25 gm protein to pregnant and lactating women. It is given for 300 days a year. For severe malnutrition therapeutic nutrition (double quantity) is given.

Nutrition and Health Education

Topics are given and workers are trained for this aspect.

Immunisation

Children and mothers are covered for U.I.P.

Health Check-up

This programme covers pregnant ANC, lactating PNC, IFA to lactating along with supplementary nutrition. Minimum 3 check-ups are done. Children will have (a) Weight record (b) Milestone observation (c) Immunisation (d) Every 3-6 months check-up (e) Treatment for Diarrhoea, ARI (f) Deworming (g) Vit A prophylaxis and (h) Referral service.

Non Formal Education

This is for 3-6 age children to reduce dropouts from schooling.

SCHOOL HEALTH

IMPORTANCE

For raising health status of a nation, school age group children are to be given special care. Being future generation, school children form an economic group of the country.

HISTORICAL DEVELOPMENT

1909	First school medical examination at Baroda city
1946	Bhore Committee recommend its importance.
1953	Secondary education committee emphasises need of examination and school feeding.
1960	G.O.I. Constituted a school health committee which suggested means of improving school health.
1997-2002	9th five-year plans envisaged the progress of school health care.
2003-2007	Formal documents have been prepared and are waiting for clearance which include widened version of school health care.

HEALTH PROBLEMS IN SCHOOL CHILDREN

Main problems noticed are malnutrition and infectious diseases. Emphasis is laid on following illnesses among school children.

- Skin infection including scabies and louse infestation
- Dental caries
- Measles, mumps and chickenpox
- Round worm and Hook worm infestations
- Vision alteration
- Hearing impairment
- A.R.I.
- Diarrhoea.

Role of nursing profession is in provision of comprehensive nursing care as educator, counsellor, organizer and co-ordinator. They include:

i. Health appraisal—General examination and risk child identification.
ii. Treatment and follow-up.
iii. Advice on healthful school environment:
    - Good floor space of more than 10 sq ft per school child and not more than 40 students in a class.
    - Proper sitting desk arrangement.
      Door and window should be 25% of floor space.
    - Good lighting.
    - Good protected water supply.
    - Urinals and latrine at 1 per 60 and 1 per 100 respectively.

iv. Preventive immunisation like child T.T. as per schedule, cholera, typhoid at requirement.

v. *Nutrition:*

- Arrangement of mid day meal programme providing 250 days of feeding with supplementary food which should provide.

75G	Cereals and millet
30G	Pulses
8G	Oil
30G	Leafy vegetables
30G	Non-leafy vegetables.

- Broad principle of mid day meal is to supply 1/3 daily calorie and half of daily protein. They are prepared as home foods. It is advisable to adopt low cost meal. Range of calorie and protein can be adjusted to 350-570 calories and 13-32 grams protein per day.
- It can be alternated with snack called "Meal Snack" days.

vi. *First Aid:*
Teacher training for first aid is a requisite.

vii. *Mental Health:*
To maintain positive mental health and to overcome behavioural deviation.

viii. *Dental Health:*
To control dental disease and defects.

ix. *Eye Health:*
For correction of refractive error, squint treatment, trachoma treatment and Vitamin A administration.

x. *Health Education:*
On personal hygiene, health awareness, first aid.

xi. *Health Appraisal*:
Teacher to be educated to note and to take action on:
Skin rash
Respiratory symptoms
Neck rigidity
Eye redness

Menu for North Indian School Children

Menu	*Programme*	*Calorie*	*Protein*	*Cost (Rs.)*
1. Maize roti+ rape leaves + buttermilk	3 days	380	16	1.25
2. Bajra cooked + curry	a	430	15	1.60
3. Tandoori roti+ aalu chole	week	420	16	1.80
4. Missi roti+ curd		560	17	1.50
1. Aalu chole+ bread	2 days	370	14	1.80
2. Marunda+Khaman Dhokla	a week	560	27	2.40

Menu for South Indian School Children

Menu	*Programme*	*Calorie*	*Protein*	*Cost (Rs.)*
1. Rice + Sambar + Buttermilk	3 days	550	15	1.80
2. Pongal + Curry + Buttermilk	a	500	15	1.75
3. Veg Chapaties	week	500	21	1.60
4. Wheat Pulse Porridge + Buttermilk		450	14	2.00
1. Sundal+ Buttermilk	2 days	36	13	1.75
2. Laddu+Buttermilk	a week	500	19	2.00

Diarrhoea
Fever and chills
Headache
Vision defect
Hearing defect
Behaving rudely
Flushed face
Swollen face.

INITIATION OF SCHOOL HEALTH BY NURSE

- Know the setup of school (Administration)
- Establish rapport with teachers
- Make periodic visits to school
- Check physical facilities at school
- Arrange parent teacher counselling
- Arrange meetings for school improvement
- Arrange and help physical check-up of children
- Take care to observe chronic defects among school children
- Help in their treatment and referral.

COMPONENTS OF SCHOOL HEALTH SERVICES

- Medical examination
- Follow-up
- Disease prevention
- First aid and emergency
- Health counselling
- Records
- Psychological services
- Cooperation from parents.

SCHOOL HEALTH RECORDS

Along with cumulative card, health card should also be maintained for each student. That should contain the following:

- Identification data.
- Past health history
- Family history of any illness
- Findings of medical check-up
- Information on care given.

NURSING ROLE IN HANDICAP CHILDREN

Special attention is required for a school child which is handicapped because education of handicapped child is not an easy task. It requires special nursing care and a good interaction with parents and school management.

GERIATRICS

IMPORTANCE

Now that expectation of life is increased, geriatric age group is widening and we have nearing 3.8% of the population being above 65 years age. This comes to nearly 39 million people above the age of 65 years as per 2001 census.

HEALTH STATUS

Various studies have shown that illness among old age is multifactorial and multiorgan. Main illnesses seen are loss of vision (cataract), non ambulatory (arthritis), bronchitis, vitamin deficiencies, Ear infections, diabetes, hypertension and accidents. ICMR study has shown that reported sicknesses are as under by proportion (pooled observations):

- Gradual loss of vision 88
- Muscle joint disorders 40
- Neurological 18.69
- Cardiovascular 17.44
- Respiratory 16.13
- Skin infections 13.35
- G.I. tract 9.10
- Mental ill health 8.5
- Loss of hearing 8.2
- Genitourinary disorder 3.5

COMMON HEALTH PROBLEMS

Old Age Problems

The change in old age is called senescence which is a natural process. Common effects of old age are:

- Senile cataract
- Nerve deafness
- Osteoporotic changes
- Bronchitis with emphysema
- Changes in mental outlook, and
- Many more old age changes.

Chronic Illness

Old people are prone to a few known chronic diseases. Of particular importance are:

- Atherosclerosis
- Heart attacks
- Hypertension
- Stroke
- Cancer
- Diabetes
- Accident and fractures
- Gout
- Rheumatoid arthritis
- Fibrocystic
- Neuritis
- Chronic bronchitis
- Asthma
- Prostate enlargement
- Fibroid of uterus.

Psychological Disturbances

Dependency, retired life and loneliness aggravate mental changes; cessation of reproductive activity lead to jealousy; social maladjustment leads to emotional disorders.

PUBLIC HEALTH ASPECT OF OLD AGE

1. **Primary Level:**
   Good health habits like
   - Good sleep
   - Good and required nutrition
   - Curtailing smoking, alcohol and fatty foods
   - Avoidance of overeating (Obesity control).

   Avoiding risk factors like:
   - Care at routine to avoid accident, fracture.
   - Diet restrictions.
   - Periodic health checksup.
2. **Secondary Level:**
   - Screening for hypertension
   - Early diagnosis and prompt treatment for infections.
3. **Tertiary Level:**
   - Rehabilitation for physical defects
   - Rehabilitation for cognitive defects
   - Rehabilitation for functional defects
   - Use of caretaker for support.

NURSING RESPONSIBILITIES OF OLD AGE CARE

- Advice, counselling, help for safe housing, good diet and happy surroundings.
- Help old person to overcome infection, mental strain and frustration.
- In case of bed-ridden, there is a need for frequent visit for careful attention. She helps in bed sore prevention.
- Demonstrate feeding, bath and back care to the family in case of chronic patients (e.g. Stroke)
- Help in development of favourable attitude towards elderly by youngsters.

NUTRITION OF ELDERLY

During ageing process, certain inevitable degenerative changes occur that will result in functional decline. They are usually influenced by nutrition followed by genetics, psychosocial and economic conditions. Hence proper nutrition and health care are necessary for elders to lead a normal life.

Balance Diet for Geriatric Age

Foodstuff	*Requirement (Grams)*	
	Male	*Female*
Cereals	350	225
Pulses	50	40
Vegetables	200	150
Leafy vegetables	50	50
Roots, tubers	100	100
Fruits	200	200
Milk and milk products	300	300
Sugar	20	20
Fats and Oils	25	25

Nutrient Required for the Old Age

Foodstuff	*Requirement (Grams)*	
	Male	*Female*
Calorie	2200	1700
Protein	65 G	50 G
Fat	50 G	40 G
Calcium	1 G	0.9 G
Iron	38 mg	30 mg
Vitamin A(retinol)	1030 µg	930 µg
Thiamine	1.96 mg	1.45 mg
Riboflavin	1.78 mg	1.51 mg

Some Dietary Tips for the Elderly

The diet of the elders may be modified according to physical activity of the individual and general health condition. The following tips are suggested for dietary management of the elders. They are:

1. Take simple but nutritious diet.
2. Improve the quality of diet by adding liberal quantity of green leafy vegetables, fruits and whole cereals.
3. Take frequent but small meals.
4. Take plenty of fluids and semisolids.
5. Avoid dry foods.
6. Reduce total fat.
7. Reduce refined carbohydrate.
8. Reduce salt intake.
9. Avoid fasting.

SOCIAL WELFARE FOR ELDERLY

There are many social welfare schemes that are helpful to the positive health of elders. They are:

- Old age homes when no dependents are there for security, food and shelter.
- Social assistance like pension, old age pension etc.
- Home services for attending to all physical requirements.
- Home care services for attending to all biological requirements.
- Meals on wheels services to supply fresh, hot food to home supply at appropriate time and at required frequent timings.
- Health checkup camps for elders for screening their health.
- Socio-economic benefits to elders like concession in rail, bus, and other benefits to senior citizens.

CHAPTER EIGHT

Human Sexuality

IMPORTANCE

Sex, a wide term, which do not mean aptly, play a dominant role in human life. It is an accepted creative and pleasurable force shaping human behaviour. It is not just equal to reproduction, but more than a bio-psychosocial function.

It has positive aspects like:

- Pair bonding
- Fostering intimacy
- Providing pleasure
- Bolstering self-esteem
- Reduction in tension etc.

It has negative aspects like:

- Asserting masculinity
- Asserting femininity
- Exploitation of sex
- Expression of hostility
- Psychological turmoil
- Emotional turmoil etc.

DEFINITION

According to W.H.O. it is defined as "the whole range of behaviour associated with psychobiological phenomenon of sex."

It is dealt under family health where disciplines like psychology, gynaecology, urology, nursing, sociology interact in its problem management.

COMPONENTS

Biological

It is a biological component dealing right from birth till death through infancy, childhood, adolescence, adulthood and old age. It deals with sexual desire, male and female sex differences, sexual response, sexual behaviour and sexual functioning.

Psychological

Development of gender, sex identity, emotions, thoughts, feelings and personality traits are covered under psychological component.

Socio-Cultural

It covers regulation of sex socialisation, regulation of sexual behaviour, sex role play, family practices and social pressures in sex life.

Understanding of human sexuality requires the study of these factors and their interaction and inter-relationships.

Socio-cultural component of human sexuality:

They influence sexual development through social learning. Subsequently it gives rise to sexual behaviour of an individual in a society. Culture approves certain norms of sexual behaviour to assure peace, to stabilise domestic relations and to facilitate procreation. Historical, ethical, economic and educational subcultures are packed up constraints in human sexuality. Culture moulds the expression of sexual drive. Some major factors influencing human sexuality are:

- Marriage and family
- Religion
- Social class
- Media and advertisement
- Contraception and abortion services
- Technological development
- Educational status
- Revolutions.

SEX EDUCATION

As a component of population education it was introduced in India through National Family Welfare Planning Programme during 1960. It includes mostly education on reproduction; however, it should also impart positive attitude to sex behaviour. Sex education can motivate people to change or to modify the existing negative attitude and misbehaviours.

Main goal of sex education is to develop an ability to merge biological impulses with socially acceptable norms of sex behaviour conducive to a satisfying family life as adult men and women.

It is going on as a learning process without our knowledge both in informal form (Home, peer group) and formal form (School, University). Feeling of love and affection that has to be from parents in role modelling and also by siblings is not a true sex in human sexuality. It is the learning of sex attitude, sex emotion which is responsible for family relation and family responsibility that needed to be imparted in sex education.

Parents need to attempt to satisfy the natural and anxious curiosities of their child from where sex education starts. During adolescence, physiology of body, sexually transmitted diseases are to be made understandable. Sex education and counselling for adult men and women is managed by family physicians.

Content of sex education in nursing care are:

i. Anatomy and physiology of reproduction.
ii. Physical and emotional changes during puberty.
iii. Behaviour towards opposite sex.
iv. Moral codes and cultural standards.
v. Responsibility of marriage and family.
vi. Planned parenthood.
vii. Small family norms.

Common health problems associated with human sexuality are:

i. Masturbation
ii. Emotional inadequacy
iii. Unwanted pregnancy
iv. S.T.D.
v. HIV/AIDS
vi. Infertility, sterility
vii. Divorce.

SEX THERAPY

The care of sex problems which needs treatment is multidimensional. They are:

a. *Somatic therapy:* Drug, hormone or surgical treatment for certain conditions (e.g., genital tract infection, impotency).
b. *Behavioural therapy:* Required for changing attitude of patient.
c. *Psychoanalysis*: For cases of imagination and fantasies.
d. *Hypnosis:* It is to induce relaxation.
e. *Psychotherapy:* Emotional treatment.

COUNSELLING

Nursing profession has been giving guidance and advice on all matters of health problems associated with human sexuality. In family planning, sterilisations, abortions, S.T.D. it is part of general health service. Educational and counselling techniques are to be learnt to impart the art of communication and good listening. From this we can remove erroneous beliefs and taboos to promote positive attitude in human sexuality.

CHAPTER NINE

Personal Hygiene

IMPORTANCE

The word hygiene has come from Hygiea (The Goddess of Health) who was the daughter of a leader of Greek Medicine Aesculapius. "Personal hygiene" is appropriately called as "personal health" mainly because it is not just cleanliness of body. It has other factors equally important to maintain the health of the individual. Positive health is something more than cleanliness and absence of disease. It is a positive state of well being of whole body which will enable the body to grow and develop normally to its full capacity and have the ability to enjoy all the opportunities that life may present.

DEFINITION

It deals with practices of an individual which help in maintaining and promoting his health physically, mentally, socially and spiritually.

Benefits of Personal Hygiene

- Helps in maintaining good clean physique
- Helps in muscular and bony strength
- Helps in keeping health of oral cavity, tongue, teeth
- Helps in maintaining skin integrity
- Helps in the control of:
  - Genitourinary infections
  - Skin infections
  - Gastrointestinal disorders
  - Musculoskeletal disorders.
- Helps in building up resistance.

COMPONENTS

Skin

It is a delicate organ. Apart from protection and insulation it helps in the process of excretion. Perspiration contains thrown out waste products which is evident after an act of heavy exercise. The sebaceous gland secretion acts as a natural coat to the skin. In high temperate climate and tropical countries where perspiration is high, skin cleaning becomes a paramount importance.

Skin needs regular bathing and appropriate clothing. If sebaceous glands are blocked with dirt, it leads to many complications like sebaceous cyst, impetigo, scabies, prickly heat and ringworm infection.

Bath with hard soaps is routine in human habits. Bathing cleans, increases circulation, give muscle tone, improve appetite, make free from infection and gives a sense of freshness and well-being. If water temperature is between 35°C and 36°C it is warm bath, between 33°C and 35°C cold bath and 36°C to 43°C hot bath. Oil bath is common in traditional families which gives coolness and softness to the skin. Turmeric and sandal application has germicidal action.

Ritual bath like after menstruation, after childbirth, after hair cut, after a visit to graveyard are quite interesting to note and to be understood by the nursing community. Bathing in well, swimming pools are attached with exercises.

Sunbath is appropriated to allow sunlight (UV and cosmic rays) in early morning or late evening which is found to increase blood circulation. Care must be taken to avoid sunburn. Before and after seawater bath, sun bath is advocated which has a utility in personal health.

Clothing

It has many fold uses like protection from extreme climate, protection from insect bite; maintain body heat and personal value of decoration. Dress code from health point of view may not be suitable for civilisation point of view.

Material used in clothing has impact on skin. Cotton cloth is a good conductor of heat, absorbs moisture, easily washable and suitable for tropics. Khadi hand-woven is economical and durable cotton. Wool is best for winter, it being bad conductor of heat. Silk is bad conductor of heat. Rayon and other synthetics are slightly warmer but are found to produce skin allergy.

Care of the Hand

Care of the hand is of paramount importance because it is an agent to contaminate food. Washing hands before eating is the first lesson of personal hygiene to avoid food borne infections. After visiting toilet and latrine, hands must be washed with soap and water.

In nursing care, washing hands is a must before any procedure. Nursing hand wash is to be followed as under:

"Wet the hands from elbow towards finger tips, soap well, wash the tips of fingers and thumbs turned in, then wash between fingers and arms with rotary motion. Then rinse from elbow downwards. This helps to remove dirt. It is repeated in case adherent dirt is there."

Care of the Hair

Hair is an outgrowth of epidermis. It grows from hair follicle which will be situated in dermis. The composition of hair is dead thorny cell. The colour of the hair is due to pigment between the cells during its growth. Softness of hair is due to sebaceous gland secretions. The hair is reflection of personal health, which is seen as streaked yellowish brown among malnourished individuals.

Each person should have his/her own comb and brush for a better personal hygiene.

Care is needed at hair-cut, for; it may cause injury, infection or infestation.

In case of head louse infestation, application of 5% benzyl benzoate overnight, head bath and proper grooming is advocated *(also refer page 80 and page 85 for B.B. emulsion application).*

Body Sweating

Sweating affects the adolescent, who is inclined to be nervous, especially girls who get excited. It is not only embarrassing but also ruins clothes. Cheap and unreliable deodorants cause skin problem. A good anti-perspirant when used though takes off perspiration; it causes irritation in the skin (if not used properly). Sweat allowed to decompose in woollen material is offensive. Repeated bath and hygienic practice are the only answer for bad excessive sweating.

Blackheads and Acne

This is common among adolescents. It particularly affects those with a greasy type of skin. The pores from sebaceous glands become blocked with sebum and a hard head forms on the top (Comedo). At the top infection may occur. Regular wash with soap, careful rinsing and drying, exposure to fresh air and sunlight, and evacuation of blocked pore by gentle pressure or by comedo remover will help to some extent in controlling acne and black heads. They may have to limit sweet and starchy foods since there is significant association of acne and diet.

Hygiene of Toilet

The kidneys excrete about 4 pints of water per day which helps in the excretion of urea, uric acid, creatinine and inorganic salts from the body. One to 1½ litre of water consumed per day help in good elimination process. Bladder control as an outcome of civilised life and social inhibitions should be avoided. It should be treated as a physiological function of the body (excretion).

Bowel Habit

Regular bowel habit avoids constipation. Too much or too little rigid regulations are harmful and emotionally put an individual in a dangerous position. Diet with high fibre help to overcome constipation. Since constipation is known to cause headache, tension, abdominal discomfort, gastro intestinal infections, it is advisable to develop a good and routine bowel habit.

Care must be taken at advice for flexible attitude in case where a person is on liquid diet, on fasting etc. Where passing stool once in 3-4 days may be normal (for the given individual). In females, since there are chances to infect urethra or vaginal area from the bowel, it is advisable to educate them to clean from the vagina to rectum.

Menstrual Hygiene

This aspect is surrounded by taboos and superstitions. It should be looked as a physiological process in all female human beings. A young girl usually gets instructions from her mother. Recently, mass media is playing a very important role in educating the girls about menstrual hygiene. Traditionally, taking bath is considered as not advisable during menses. Actually washing and cleaning of groin and vulva is mandatory. Woman hygiene kit (natural or sanitary pad) should be changed regularly and should be disposed off hygienically. There is no need to feel unwell while girls are menstruating. Intravaginal tampons can be used if found comfortable. Vaginal douching is not necessary at the end of cycle. Nature takes care to see by itself by clearing all menstrual debris. It is the habit of cleanliness that accounts most in menstrual hygiene. For healthy couple (regarding intercourse) there is no sound medical reason for advising against intercourse during menstruation.

Care of Special Sensory Organ

Eyes

Eyes reflect health and is found dull when ill or fatigued. Eyes need correction and use of glass when there is impairment of vision. Care is needed at beautification of eyelash, eyelid and eyebrow. The colour, the chemical, the lotion, the substance used must be harmless. It is advisable to avoid common stick to apply kajal since eye infection can spread very easily.

Light from above and left is advocated for reading and not to strain eyes. Whenever a touch or cleaning of eye is needed, hands and fingers must be washed thoroughly with a detergent soap. Washed hand and finger should not be dried *with dirty* cloth.

Any headache, watering of eyes, fatigue on reading, eyes must be got tested.

Protective goggle at work and while riding a two wheeler avoids accidental injury to the eye by foreign body or avoids pterygium which is an exposure effect.

Ears

There are no specific criteria that wax should be removed as a ritual. Since it is a normal secretion process and a protective phenomenon wax formation in the ear do not call for attention. In case of excess secretion it may need to be attended with wax solvent and ear syringing by a trained person. No external material including dirty finger be put inside ear lest it may cause otitis media. Cleaning the outer ear during bath is found sufficient. No hard substance is put to ear lest it may cause rupture of tympanum. In case of entry of an insect like ant, use of oil is preferred to make it flow and remove.

Care of the Nose

Breathing, air entry, dust entry and pathogen by air cause health hazards. Enlarged adenoids can lead to mouth breathing, which is found associated with frequent cold and frequent sore throat. Taking off the hair from nostril is not advisable because hair is necessary as a natural filtering agent.

While sneezing one should use handkerchief to avoid discharge at air which can cause air pollution.

At swimming blowing the nose gently is advocated.

Oral Hygiene

It implies good teeth, good gum and good healthy buccal cavity. Mastication produces and promotes saliva and gastric secretion which help in digestion. Emotional satisfaction of eating is associated with good oral hygiene.

Mouth

Mouth cleansing or rinsing is a good habit after each act of food consumption. Very hot, very spicy and extraneous substances like tobacco leaves irritates and produce ulcer and even malignancy. Poor oral hygiene can lead to periodontal diseases (Pyorrhoea) and loss of tooth. Halitosis (bad breath) is an indication of oral cavity fermented smell which can be totally avoided by good oral hygiene.

Mouth rinsing with drinking water is more than sufficient in 99 percent cases. In 1% of cases sodium bicarbonate gargling, desensitising oral rinse with either potassium nitrate or sodium fluoride, may be needed.

A very inexpensive dentifrice can be made by warm water with a pinch of salt (hypo saline) as a wash to mouth and gullet. Mouth can be a seat of many organisms. If care is not taken for oral hygiene septic tonsils, infected sinus can produce widespread mouth sickness and are preventable.

Teeth

Dental caries is common and worldwide problem. This can lead to cavity formation and tooth decay. Decay is by acids of mouth bacteria acting upon food particles in the mouth. Sweets, chocolates, biscuits are seen associated with occurrence of dental caries. Sweet as sticky substance and increased sugar consumption enhances dental caries. Soft proteinous materials accumulating around neck of teeth constitute dental plaques which are to be removed by daily habit of tooth brushing. It is seen that caries is dependent on fluoride content of water. Optimal level of fluoride in drinking water (0.5-0.8 mg per litre) prevents dental caries. Fluoride containing dentifrices can reduce dental caries by 20%.

Limiting refined carbohydrates, avoiding frequent chewing of snacks in between meal, disallowing smoking, alcohol and tobacco leaves bring about an improved dental hygiene in the coming days.

Patient's denture also need wash under running water, placed in a tooth mug of cold water and returned to the patient. In addition to regular cleaning, the patient should be given antiseptic mouthwash last thing at night and a bowl of antiseptic for dentures if they are not worn at night.

Nutrition

Knowledge of balanced diet, to suit the body needs in anabolism and catabolism is judged best under personal health. Roughage consisting of high fibre diet can reduce many gastrointestinal problems like constipation, mucous diarrhoea, intussusceptions and intestinal polyposis. Junk foods are *better avoided* and a traditional food can help to increase a man's life expectancy.

Exercise

Depending on one's age regular exercise is a must for a good personal health. At home active engagement in household duties, social useful productive work and ritual inevitable exercises do as much good as an exercise by a sportsman or gymnast. It is a tool to restore strength, correct deformity and to reduce body weight.

In hospital practice post-operative exercises, postnatal exercises and physiotherapeutic exercises are well-known in keeping the body and mind fit for a positive personal hygiene.

Posture

Good posture in standing, walking, sitting and recumbent has an active role for positive health. Round shouldered position, dropped chest, protruding abdomen, are indication of ill health or deformity. Poor nutrition, chronic infection, bone defect, emotional maladjustment can cause poor as well as bad exposure. Personal hygiene in posture is meant to well adjusted emotional life and free from physical defects.

Sleeping Habit

The amount of sleep needed varies with age, occupation and habit. Physiologically 8 hours of sleep (1/3 of active life) is found sufficient for regaining bodily and mental fatigue. "Early to bed and early to rise" is a dictum found useful for an active life. There is no use in sleeping for 12-16 hours which are full of dreams and is superficial. Deep sleep of 4 hours without bodily strain by dreams is found healthy for active life.

Sleep is a natural process to overcome fatigue and to recuperate the energy, strength and vigour spent during day's work. Developing good sleeping habit can reduce tiredness, body ache, headache, nausea and discomfort, provided it is undisturbed deep sleep for a limited time.

Other Aspects

Other aspects of personal hygiene for a better personal health:

- Wearing footwear while walking in an open field where open field defecation prevails can prevent hookworm infection.
- Observing *purdha*, avoiding even sunrays prone to cause certain respiratory infections like tuberculosis.
- Alcoholism, smoking and gambling do not allow cultivating good health habit in an individual. He also lacks in personal hygiene.
- Awareness at traditional barbering, tattooing and circumcision can allow personal hygiene which can reduce the incidence of skin infection, AIDS, tetanus and scabies.
- Personal hygiene in the form of no spitting, no urination etc. in swimming pool can bring down certain infections. This needs an idea of swimming pool sanitation.
- Ritual purifications if not harmful, have an equal effect on a good personal hygiene.
- Poor personal hygiene can cause (auto grade) thread worm infection which is overcome by cleanliness after defecation and drug treatment.
- Care and observation of meat to be eaten can prevent tape worm infection, is a part of personal hygiene.
- Louse infestation and scabies are known fundamentals to personal hygiene.
- Worm infestations are avoidable if raw fruits and vegetables are washed and used at eating.

CONCLUSION

Personal hygiene, personal habits and personal health are interwoven in such a way that they are not separable from one another. Good habits and personal hygiene for health are known since age old days. But health by habits and health by hygiene needs culture imbibed motto in an individual for a positive health.

CHAPTER TEN

Preventive Obstetrics and Preventive Paediatrics

REVIEW OF REPRODUCTIVE SYSTEM

Pelvis harbour female organ of generation. It is designed for its work of child-bearing. For anatomical purpose it is upper part a shallow cavity formed by the iliac fossae which is called *false pelvis* and bony basin lower portion containing organs of generation called *true pelvis.*

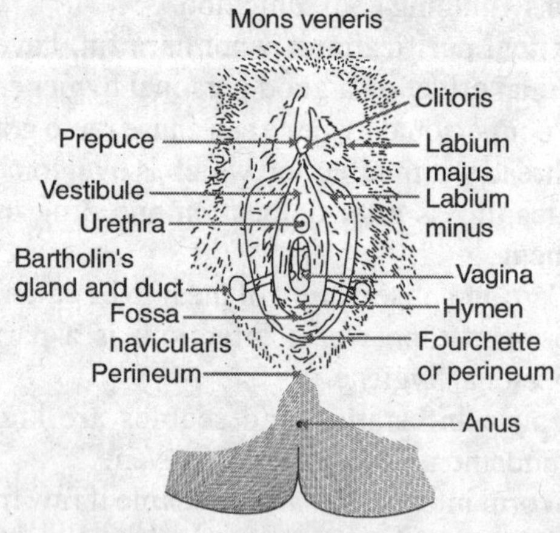

Fig. 10.1: External organs of generation

External organs of generation are mons pubis and vulva. Mons pubis is pad fat covering pubic bone and is covered with pubic hair. Vulva consists of labia majora, labia minora. Clitoris is situated at meeting point of labia minora. Urinary meatus is in the centre of a triangular surface 'vestibule'. Below this is the orifice entrance to vagina.

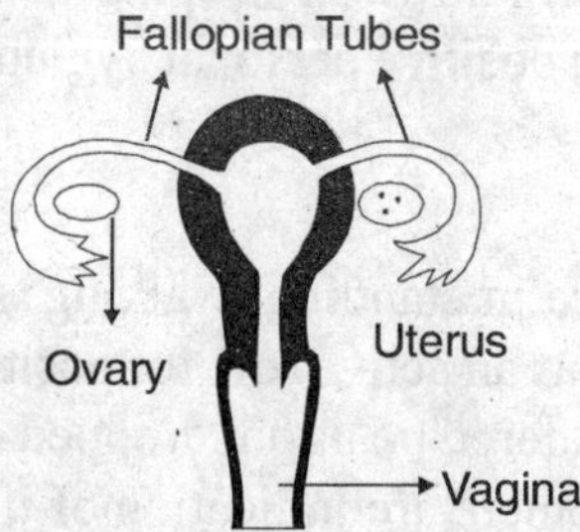

Fig. 10.2: Internal organs of generation

Internal organs of generation consist of vagina, uterus, fallopian tube and ovaries (Fig. 10.2).

Vagina is a passage about 4" long sloping upwards and backwards from vulva to the cervix uteri. Its wall allows great expansion during labour. Uterus is pear shaped 3" × 2" × 1" with notable parts; body and cervix. It is tilted forward on the vagina and hence is antevertion in normal occurrence. Inner layer is endometrium, invests the fallopian tube and ovaries in the form of broad ligament. The fallopian tubes leave the fundus of the uterus by tiny opening at either side. The cilia in the lining help the passage of ova along. Two ovaries on either side about the size and shape of almonds have 2 functions:

1. Produces internal secretions
2. Produces ova.

Female Pelvis

The pelvic bone is made of 2 innominate bones, a sacrum and a coccyx (Fig. 10.3).

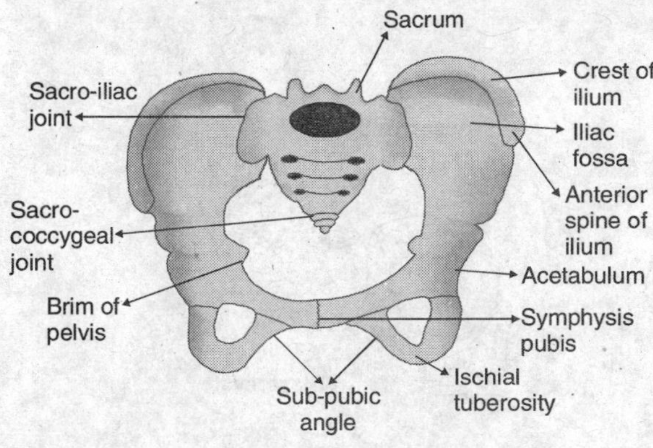

Fig. 10.3 : Pelvic bone

Innominate bone is large, strong, irregular bone which has parts (a) Ilium (b) Ischium and (c) Pubis. Upper expanded part of ilium is hip bone which presents a bony crest, iliac fossa, anterior prominence and posterior prominence. Ischium has large tuberosity which carry total load of body at rest. United front portion by a pad of cartilage form symphysis pubis. The sacrum which forms posterior wall of pelvis is a wedge shaped bone with five fused vertebrae. Extreme end of vertebral column is coccyx.

The relations of pelvic organs of reproduction enlarge as pregnancy advances and passes out to abdomen where they lie in relation to other abdominal organs.

Nursing care invites the following attention:

- Thorough clean of area before examination to avoid infection from rectum and bladder.
- Care in external/local infection to protect the spread of infection to peritoneal cavity through fallopian tube.
- Tear of vagina and cervix during labour can create fistulae.
- For correct, easy and painless introduction of vaginal speculum, upward and backward slope of vagina should be remembered.
- Illegal abortion instruments in rural area can pierce posterior fornix of vagina to cause peritonitis.

Menstrual Cycle

After attaining menarche, ovarian follicle ripen and secrete oestrogen which causes endometrial changes during menstrual cycle along with secondary sex characteristics like development of breast, widening of hips, the rounded curves, growth of axillary and pubic hairs (Fig. 10.4).

Anterior lobe of pituitary gland stimulates ovary by FSH to ripen and to produce oestrogen which cause endometrium to grow and thicken. Fully ripe follicle bursts on 14th day of menses. At that time, LH of anterior lobe of pituitary gland stimulates (along with oestrogen) the development of blood vessels and glands in endometrium. This is called premenstrual period which is ready to take up fertilised egg, if available. If there is no fertilisation, endometrium breaks down again causing menstrual flow which contains mucus and shreds of endometrium and unfertilised ovum.

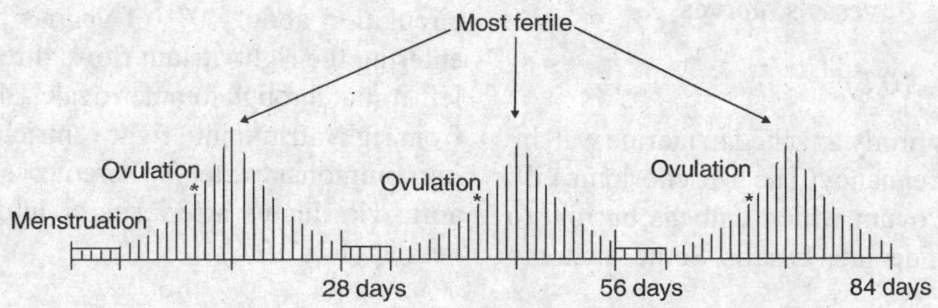

Fig. 10.4: Menstrual cycle

Average blood loss will be 100 to 300 ml lasting for 3-5 days.

Fertilisation

By sexual intercourse, semen is deposited in vagina, sperm enters uterus through fallopian tube and fertilisation (union of ovum and sperm) occur in fallopian tube. When fertilisation takes place, sperm penetrates ovum usually in fallopian tube. Each of these cells contains 24 chromosomes. The result of union is the formation of a single cell containing 48 chromosomes (24 from sperm 24 from ovum). The fertilised cell enters uterus and gets implanted there; cell's differentiating stages like morula, tryphoblast and eventually embryo develops.

Foetal Development

Fertilised cell undergoes cell division. At this stage it appears like mulberry and is called a morula. Further cell differentiation leads to outer layer tryphoblast concerning with absorbing nutrition and inner cells eventually become the embryo. Tryphoblast grows to primitive chorionic villi. Its surface is called syncitium. Two small vesicles appear, one with clear fluid (amniotic sac) and the other with opaque material (yolk sac). Between them the embryonic disc gets located with 3 distinguished layers:

1. Ectoderm • to form skin and appendages.
2. Entoderm • to alimentary tract.
3. Mesoderm • to connective tissue, muscle, vessels, nerves.

Placenta (Fig. 10.5)

The placenta is firmly attached to uterine wall by 12th week of pregnancy. The true chorionic villi on the part of ovum which embeds burrow to spongy layer of decidua basalis. Some anchor to placental tissue and other dip to maternal blood spaces where blood is free. All nutrient and oxygen required by foetus is passed by osmosis. The placenta will be as large as a dinner plate, one inch thick and is extended with umbilical cord to foetus. There are chances of extra small placenta and hence after III stage of labour careful examination is needed to ensure all placental tissue has come away. Functions of placenta are:

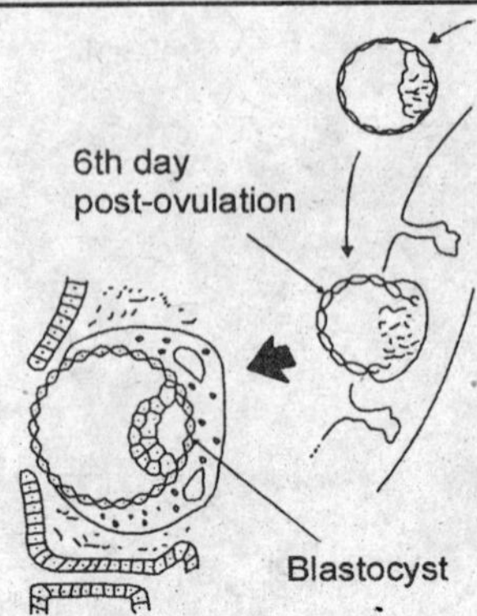

Fig.10.5: Placenta

- Supply nutrient
- Carry waste material
- Supply oxygen and remove CO_2
- Acts as a barrier to infection
- Acts as endocrine to secrete hormone.

Foetal Circulation

Heart as a single tube initially develops by 5th week and produce heart beat of 65/minute. By 11weeks definite circulation with heart beat of 140/min is established. In the mature foetal circulation about 40% of venous blood return entering the right atrium flows directly into the left atrium through foramen ovale. Blood pumped from right atrium into right ventricle is expelled into pulmonary artery where it passes either to aorta via ductus arteriosus or into pulmonary vessels (Fig. 10.6).

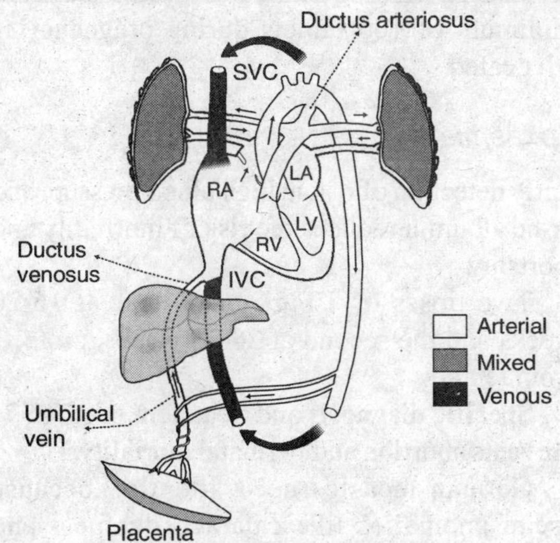

Fig. 10.6: Foetal circulation

NORMAL PREGNANCY AND MANAGEMENT

Pregnancy Changes

Pregnancy is a normal physiological condition and **should never be referred as patient.** With our earlier knowledge of anatomy and physiology of human reproductive system, let us study the intricate changes on a woman who is pregnant. Pregnancy changes are referable to signs and symptoms of pregnancy.

Amenorrhoea: This is a common sign of pregnancy. But for nursing care it is a relative sign because menstruation may still continue with pregnancy and amenorrhoea may be due to some gynaecological conditions. In nursing management threatened abortion should be remembered.

Breast changes: By 6th week of pregnancy breasts are seen to be enlarging and the woman is conscious of sensation of fullness. Area around nipple becomes pigmented. By 20th week, secondary areola occurs by whitish spots. It is a reliable sign in primigravida. But in nursing care pseudocyesis (false pregnancy) is to be noted.

Genitalia: Cervix becomes more secretary, vagina and vulva become purple. It is due to extra venous blood in 2nd month onwards.

Morning sickness: Nausea and vomiting from 4th week which may be due to changing metabolism and extra cellular activity.

Frequency of micturition: This is due to pressure on urinary bladder from 3rd month onwards. This also continues in late pregnancy when bladder is displaced upwards.

Abdomen: Per abdominal examination for the height of uterus which usually correspond to the period of amenorrhoea. It is obvious from 18th week onwards. About 12.5 kg will be the contribution to weight gain in pregnancy.

Foetal movement: After 18 weeks the foetal movement "quickening" is felt. From 6th month foetal heart sound is heard. The uterine "soufflé" a soft swishing sound as the blood enters the uterine arteries can be heard just above the pubes to the left of the midline.

Pregnancy test: Urine examination for pregnancy test will be positive, usually on or after 40 days of conception.

Antenatal Care (ANC)

ANC is for achieving normal delivery with a healthy baby. This helps in high risk identification to foresee complications, remove anxiety of mother, teach element of mother care and personal hygiene. Minimum of 3 antenatal visits, 1 at 20 weeks, second at 32 weeks and third at 36 weeks are required. In first visit history taking, physical examination, examination of urine, blood and stool, blood grouping and Rh typing are done. On subsequent visits physical examination and laboratory test are done. The visits are used for IFA advice, TT immunisation and nutrition advice. Following conditions are considered high risk:

- Elderly primi
- Short stature primi

- Malpresentation
- APH
- Threatened abortion
- PET and toxaemia
- Anaemia
- Twins and hydromnios
- Previous bad obstetrical history
- Pregnancy with systemic disorders.

Above normal or away from normal findings are notable and have to be put in ANC record along with identification data.

Home visiting will win women's confidence which also help to observe social and environmental conditions.

Prenatal Advice

Nutrition: Average weight increase during pregnancy is around 12 kg. Her diet needs extra calorie and extra protein which is highlighted in nutrition chapter.

Food for pregnant women		*(Additional Calories)*
Cereal	35 g	118
Pulses	15 g	52
Sugar	10 g	10
Milk	100 g	83
	Total	293 calories

Personal Hygiene

It includes cleanliness, good bowel habit and regular household work.

Drugs should be used only when essentially required but under doctor's supervision.

Pregnant woman should not be exposed to unnecessary x-ray.

Any warning sign like swelling feet, fits, headache, blurring vision, bleeding per vagina are to be reported for emergency obstetric care.

Specific Health Protection

Anaemia

I.F.A. containing 60 mg elemental iron and 500 microgram folic acid should be advised and minimum of 100 tablets during pregnancy is advocated.

Toxaemia

Early detection of risk in high blood pressure and urine albumin reduces the risk of morbidity and mortality.

Two doses of TT given, 1 dose at 16-20 weeks and the second at 20-24 weeks, protects from tetanus.

Specific diagnosis and treatment of RTI/STI prevents abortion and perinatal mortality.

German measles need attention because foetal anomalies like cataract, deafness and congenital heart disease are associated with rubella in early pregnancy.

If the mother is Rh –ve and the child is +ve, it provokes an immune response in her so that she forms antibodies to Rh which can cross placenta and produce foetal haemolysis. Routine test and timely intervention prevents this Rh iso-immune response.

HIV +ve mother can transmit disease to growing foetus. Precaution to check mother to child transmission is possible by specific protective measure.

Mental Preparation

Time and opportunity are given to mother for acceptance and cooperation for fruitful outcome of pregnancy.

Family Planning

In indicated cases small family norm through post partum centre is undertaken.

Child Component

In ANC check up presence of paediatrician help in paying attention to accompanied children, which boosts the morale of the RCH activities.

Intra Natal Care (INC)

Effective intra-natal care is required to overcome complications of labour. Prevention of maternal and neonatal sepsis is overcome by:

a. *Five clean practice:*
   - Clean surface for delivery
   - Clean hands for cutting cord
   - New blade for cutting cord
   - Clean tie for cord
   - No application on cord stump.

b. Issue of disposable delivery kit (DDK) which contain:
   - A piece of soap
   - A new razor blade
   - Two pieces of thread
   - Two cotton swabs.

Domiciliary Care

Confinement at home by trained traditional birth attendant or health worker female M.P.W. (Female) in majority of cases where normal obstetric history exist, is ideal. Out reach domiciliary care is an extension of good intra-natal care to the community. There is a need of referral in cases of :

- High temperature during labour
- Heavy bleeding and collapse
- Placenta not separated within 30 minutes after delivery
- Cord prolapse
- Prolonged labour.

LABOUR

It is a series of increasingly strong and painful rhythmical contraction of the uterine cavity, assisted in the later stages by the abdominal muscles, which expel the foetus. Uterine contraction in labour is painful and not painful in pregnancy (before labour).

Nursing care need the understanding of terms used for an act in an emergency. Foetus lies in uterus in an attitude of universal flexion with the head at the lower pole and the back lying against the anterior abdominal wall. Head presentation is normal and all other presentations like occiput, face, brow, breech, cord are abnormal presentations.

LOA (left occipito-anterior) where vertex presentation is the most common and the one is described in normal labour.

Stages of Labour

First Stage: It is from the onset of labour to full dilatation of cervix. Per vaginal examination is done to ascertain if the cervix has begun to dilate. There is little bleeding from torn capillaries, in the beginning then with mucus "The show" starts with fore water in front of head (liquor omni). When tension rises, membrane ruptures, fluid escapes by which time foetal head starts getting brunt of the pressure. This may produce "Caput succedaneum" which, however is soon reabsorbed. The interval between the pains gives the mother rest and allows free flow of blood, through the uterine muscle to the placental site. The stage is 24 hours in primi and lesser (6-12 hours) in multi.

Second Stage: It is from full dilatation of cervix to the birth of baby. This takes 2 hours in primi and lesser in multi. Retraction of uterine muscle presses down from above and advances with each pain. Head descends through vagina, perineum is stretched, head passes through vulva and is delivered between contractions. The shoulders rotate and are born with the next contraction and rest of the body is delivered at the same time.

Third stage: It is from the birth to the delivery of placenta. The baby breathes and often cries lustily immediately after it is born and the cord may be cut as soon as convenient. There is no need to wait until it has ceased to pulsate (Table 10.1).

Table 10.1: Apgar scoring system

Sign	Score 0	1	2
Heart rate	Absent	<100/min	>100/min
Respiration rate	Absent	Weak cry	Strong cry
Muscle tone	Limp	Some flexion	Good flexion
Reflex irritability	No response	Some motion	Cry
Colour	White	Blue periphery	Pink all over

Interpretation of Apgar Score:
A normal score at 1 min is 7-10.

Score of 4-6 at 1 min = moderately depressed baby.

Score of 0-3 at 1 min = severe depression.

Hypothermia Prevention

Neonatal death can occur by hypothermia which is due to fall in body temperature since ambient temperature to which they are born is always by several degrees cooler than temperature in the womb. Newborn body temperature is 99.5° F and hypothermia occurs if room temperature is below 97.5°F.

Measures suggested are:

1. After birth, baby is quickly dried with clean cloth and wrapped with cotton clothing (Turkey towel) (Two-towel method).
2. Skin to skin contact with mother at breast feeding is allowed.
3. Avoid bath to newborn for one week.

Strong contraction which causes expulsion of foetus also results in separation of central area of placenta. The centre is bunched up and behind it is a pool of blood from maternal sinuses forming haematoma. Abdominal palpation revealing soft uterus concludes that contraction is over.

Nursing care should be vigilant on the following complications of labour:

- C.P.D. (Cephalo Pelvic Disproportion)
- Foetal abnormalities like breech, hydrocephalus
- Uterine inertia
- P.P.H. (Postpartum haemorrhage)
- Retained placenta.

Rooming In

For mental stability, self confidence and for early breast feeding baby is kept by the side of mother's bed. This is called "Rooming-in".

Post Natal Care

Care of the mother and the newborn is attended as Post Natal Care services. This is combined area of perinatology which involves both obstetrical care and paediatrician care.

The puerperium is the time, approximately 42 days during which time the genital organs are returning to normal in their size and position after pregnancy and labour. This is called involution. The nursing responsibility includes:

- Checking healing of placental site.
- Checking involution of uterus.
- Establishment of lactation
- Care of the newborn.
- Teaching the mother, mother craft.

Routine observations are made and recorded daily at nursing duty. They include:

- Temperature, pulse, respiration
- Lochia
- Involution of uterus
- Excretions.

Establishment of Lactation (Exclusive Breastfeeding)

The advantage of breastfeeding to mother and newborn are emphasised to mother and at her earliest, she should start breastfeeding. No other feed is allowed and there is no restriction to collostrum. Only breast feeding till 4 months and no other feed at that time constitute "Exclusive Breastfeeding".

Nursing profession play a key role in ensuring 100 percent exclusive breast feeding and make their institution a "Centre of Excellence".

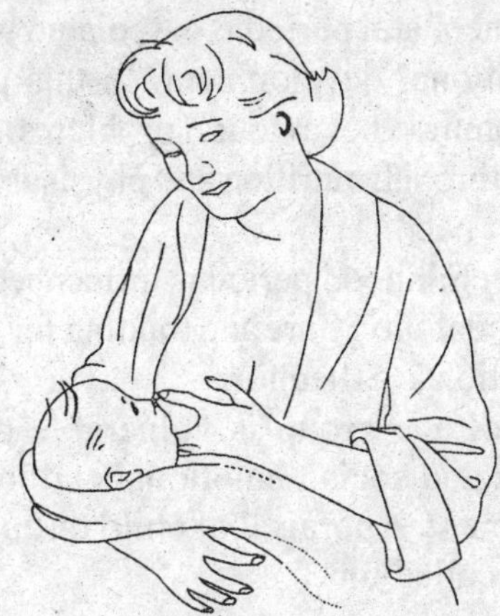

Fig. 10.7: Position at breastfeeding

Advice on postnatal exercise will build up muscular strength and early recovery from brunt of pregnancy and labour.

Nursing care include a vigilance on common puerperal complications. They are:

- Traumatic-perineal tears and fistulae.
- Puerperal sepsis.
- Breast complications.

Good postnatal care takes care of the following:

- Prevention of complication of postnatal period.
- Care for recovering mother.
- Check exclusive breastfeeding.
- Provide PPC service.
- Give health education.
- To control puerperal sepsis, thrombo-plebitis and secondary haemorrhages.

Postnatal Care Measure

PNC Examination

Postnatal care involves examination twice a day during first 3 days, later once a day till cord drops off. Each examination should cover pulse, respiration, temperature recording, breast examination, uterus involution, examination of lochia, excretion position. At the end of 6 weeks, follow up for involution of uterus is done. Later monthly post-natal examination for first 6 months, thereafter once in 3 months till 1 year, is done. In rural area, effort must be made to have minimum 3 post natal visits.

Anaemia is kept in mind and if found, correction with supplementation is advocated. Nutrition is looked after with additional allowance of calorie and protein (Table 10.2):

Table 10.2 : Additional calorie to lactating mother

	Additional	*Allowance (Calories)*
Cereals	60 G	203
Pulses	30 G	105
Milk	100 G	83
Fat	10 G	90
Sugar	10 G	40
Total Calories		521

Postnatal exercises are necessary to bring muscles back to normal as early as possible. Many known exercises are displayed in postnatal wards, which need to be appreciated by nursing students during ward work.

Psychological assurance to allay fear and insecurity help the mother to come to normal, which otherwise would have precipitated by pregnancy and labour.

Social assurance by good family atmosphere is another requisite for women to have smooth and eventful post delivery period.

Basic education on health is given to mother for personal hygiene, environmental hygiene, infant feeding, pregnancy spacing, health check-ups and birth registration.

PREVENTIVE PAEDIATRICS

IMPORTANCE

This area takes care of children from conception to adolescence by averting diseases and disabilities among children. Prevention of disease and promotion of physical, mental and social well-being of children are key success in preventive paediatrics. A strategy of primary health care to paediatric age group through Growth monitoring, ORS, nutritional surveillance, promotion of exclusive breastfeeding, UIP and regular health check is aimed at.

Child Rights

During 1974 Government of India adopted a National Policy for children which declare:

"It shall be the policy of the state to provide adequate service to children, both before and after birth and through the period of growth, to ensure their full physical, mental and social development. The state shall progressively increase the scope of such services so that, within a reasonable time, all children in the country enjoy optimum conditions for their balanced growth."

Following this, many programmes like ICDS, supplementary feeding. Nutrition education, national children award, welfare of the handicapped, CSSM, RCH etc., were introduced.

HUMAN CYCLE

Fertilised egg (Embryo) 14-63 days
Foetus 9th week to birth

	Early neonate birth to 7 days	
Infant	Late neonate 7 days to 28 days	
Neonate		
	Post neonate 28 days to 1 year	
	Preschool age 1 year to 5 years	
	School age 5 to 14 years	
	Adolescent	14 – 18 years
	Adult	18 – 45 years
	Middle age	45 – 64 years
	Old age	65 – 100 years

Biological Principles

During 1 month of neonatal period natural adjustment to biological growth is seen. Nutritional needs in terms of breastfeeding and human activity for neonatal problems are attended.

Late neonatal period is associated with social and emotional development. In this period we notice common behavioural problems. Appraisal of infant through nutrition and physical protection is the felt need.

Early childhood period is influenced by nutritional availability. Care and training for the proper socialisation is called for.

School age group is vulnerable period for infection and social, emotional and intellectual development. Appraisal of child through school health is called for.

Adolescent and adult period is filled with social, emotional and intellectual development. Puberty changes allow changes in behaviour. Guidance during puberty and sex education has been found useful in human society. Recreation and vocational interest are added burden during this period. Special problems for the adolescent in society, if not tackled, leads to delinquent changes.

Adult life is period of getting acquaintance of maturity from all angles. There is little maladjustment which has medical answers. Preparation for marriage and planned parenthood for the job of good family pattern calls for attention.

Middle age and old age have their own events which are tackled in human geriatrics (Chapter 7).

Development of Personality

Hereditary plays a part in personality development. Environment plays a greater role in this aspect. It is difficult to get an ideal situation for all. Consequently we develop personality, strong in some aspect and weak in others. If it is socially acceptable it is judged as normal.

According to Erick Erickson, human development takes place in 8 stages. Through these stages physical, mental, social and spiritual developments go together. Certain situations illustrate how human development is intricate with social interaction.

- A girl overprotected, not given a choice to face difficulties, all wants are attended, no chance given to learn the art of housekeeping and house management; she breaks down with "marriage".
- Basic need of a family like food, cloth, shelter, love affection is zero; then children become deviants.
- A boy who lost his father, brought up by overanxious mother reacts like hostile dissatisfied.

Nursing role in human development has an obligation to work for the overall development of man.

Infancy

They are completely dependent for feeding, elimination, cleanliness, warmth and protection. Love and protection are needed for proper development.

Food satisfaction is fused with infection and malnutrition which severely affect mental growth and development.

Preschool (Toddler)

Rapid physical growth, muscular coordination and control over physical functions are seen. Family pattern and social regulation have an impact on their health. Foundation of future life, the basic blocks for a future personality are laid at this stage. Socialisation and spiritual health implicit good development.

School Age (5-14 years)

Rapid physical and mental growth is seen; proper nutrition protection from infection and injury are made available. Encouragement and help are need for emotional development. Life long attitudes and habits are formed at this stage. They are prone to fantasies; strong attachment is seen with same age groups irrespective of sex. Teachers also help in secondary socialisation. At this stage they are sexually latent.

Adolescent (15-18 years)

This is a crucial stage of development. There's transition from childhood to adulthood. Secondary sexual characteristics develop. Emotionally they are very sensitive to criticism and correction. At the same time they are insecure and unsure of themselves. To overcome inferiority they put up a show in dress, speech. Sexual feelings cause fantasies and attention seeking.

Early Adulthood (18-25 years)

They are at the zenith of strength and energy. Socially they are ready to assume competent role in life. Physical health and mental health make them to assure their role play in life.

Adulthood (25-45 years)

This is the height of productive life and achievements. Emotionally and spiritually they will be stable.

Late Adulthood (45-64 years)

Physical strength and attractiveness gets reduced. They are prone to sickness and infirmities if move for health is not obviated. Depressive episodes are common in this phase of human cycle.

Old Age (65 +)

Failing physical strength and sickness produce emotional insecurity. Geriatric problems make them upset at every stage and even they are worried about death.

An insight into the above eight stages of human development will help to get an insight to the nursing profession for an effective nursing care in day-to-day practice.

PREVENTIVE PAEDIATRICS

Certain specific biological and psychological needs must be met to ensure the survival and healthy development of a child. It needs recognition, diagnosis and timely management of health problems and rests on paediatric care and Nursing Paediatrics. Childhood period is a vital period for socialisation which transmits attitude, custom and behaviour. Children are susceptible to disease, disability and death.

Perinatology

This calls for professional care to the foetus at risk. Inborn errors of metabolism and birth defects are diagnosed through USG, amniocentesis, chorionic biopsy and foetoscopy. The knowledge gained by perinatology is useful to prevent LBW, birth defects and birth asphyxia. Nursing care allows genetic counselling and planned Parenthood in perinatology. Recent nursing care allows providing care for:

- Limitation of families
- Spacing of births
- Delaying women's first pregnancy
- Ensuring maternal nutrition
- Look to intrauterine infections control.

Overall modern nursing care directs its effort in maternal nutrition, family planning and counselling of young couple.

Neonatology

Neonatal nursing care concentrates on optimum newborn care through priority based scientific approach. Early neonatal period is crucial and hence great care is to be exercised for the prevention of preventable neonatal health problems.

The neonatal care includes cardiopulmonary resuscitation, prevention of hypothermia, chemoprophylaxis and early detection of defects and disorders. Neonatology takes care of TORCHES in daily hospital procedures (Toxoplasmosis, rubella, herpes infection and syphilis).

Immediate natal care includes the following:

Airway

Immediate attention to cardio-pulmonary function is given. Mucus and other secretions are cleared. Positioning of newborn with head low to drain secretions is tried. Intensive measures like suction, oxygen mask, intubations or assisted respiration should be ready.

Labour ward equipments for above items are attended by nursing staff.

Apgar Score

This is a monitor done at 1 minute and 5 minutes after birth. A score of 7-10 normal, 4-7 mild depression and 0-3 severe depression allows for prompt action.

Care of the Cord

As soon as pulsation is stopped the cord is cut by sterilised instrument; there is no necessity to apply any antiseptic over the stump. It shrivels up and separates by necrosis in one week.

Care of the Eyes

Eyes are cleaned. One drop of 1% freshly prepared silver nitrate solution prevents gonococcal conjunctivitis. Any discharge need to be attended by ophthalmologist. Because of immediate and good eye care opthalmia neonatorum is greatly prevented.

Skin Care

To prevent hypothermia, skin bath is avoided till one week. Neonate bath by nurse need special skill and is considered to be a professional gift.

Protection of Body Temperature

Two-towel method and rooming in provide effective maintenance of newborn body temperature. Thermal control may be needed in severe hypothermia.

Breastfeeding

Breast feeding is initiated at the earliest. In case of a caesarean there may be little delay till mother regains consciousness from anaesthetic effect and still then it must be as soon the mother regains her consciousness since, colostrums is most suitable to the neonate.

Special Nursing Care of the Newborn

a. First examination is done by nurse who conducts delivery, for:
   - Any birth injury
   - Any defect
   - State of maturity
   - Any cyanosis of lip, skin
   - Dyspnoea
   - Imperforated anus
   - Persistent vomiting
   - Twitching, neck rigidity, concussion
   - Body temperature variation.

   Any deviation is to be brought to the notice of duty paediatrician for immediate attention.
b. Second examination is done within 24 hours of birth which should follow regular nursing protocol as under:
   - Body length (Crown-head-thoracic)
   - Body weight
   - Body temperature
   - Skin for cyanosis, pallor, jaundice, erythema, bullous lesions.
   - Thoracic cage retraction
   - Respiratory rate over 60 per minute
   - Absence of femoral pulse.
   - Central cyanosis
   - Posture and muscle tone
   - Signs of hydrocephalus
   - Any signs of cataract, coloboma, conjunctivitis
   - Any dysmorphism, accessory auricle, preauricular pits, hare lip, cleft palate.
   - Abdominal mass, distension, imperforate anus.
   - Joints, bones for deformity, dislocation.
   - Hypospadias, undescended testis, hydrocele in male child.
   - Fused labia, enlarged clitoris in female child.
c. Early detection of transplacental infections like:
   - Congenital syphilis
   - Jaundice in childbirth of HBV positive mother
   - Newborn of HIV positive mother
   - N.N.T.

Neonatal Nursing Procedures

Birth Weight Recording

Naked baby on a clean towel on the scale pan is taken. In case of home visiting sling bag using a salter weighing scale is used. The measurement is done to nearest 100 grams.

Height Recording

By infantometer with a fixed head piece on which the newborn is laid supine with legs fully extended, feet flexed at right angles to lower limbs. The measurements are done to nearest to 0.1 cm. At home visiting, one family member can help the nurse and a metallic tape is an appropriate technology.

Head Circumference Recording

With the help of a measuring tape, measure is taken at the maximum circumference of the head in the occipito frontal diameter.

Parameters to be obtained by an attending nurse are:

Weight	– Birth weight
Height	– Total, sitting, knee length
Perimeters	– Head circumference
	Chest circumference
	Abdominal circumference
	Arm circumference
	Calf circumference
Diameter	– BiAcromial
	BiCristal

	BiEpicondylar
	BiStyloid
	BiCondylar
Skinfold Thickness –	Subscapular
	Biceps
	Triceps
	Supra iliac

Neonatal Screening Procedures

- Apgar scoring
- Blood phenylalanine for PKU
- T_4 or TSH assay for hypothyroidism
- Coombs Test for incompatibility
- Agar gel electrophoresis for G_6PD and thalassaemia
- Snap test for congenital dislocation of hip.

Identification of at Risk Infant

- Birth weight below 2.5 kg
- Twins
- Birth order of 5 and 5 +
- Artificial feeding
- Severe malnutrition (Grade III, IV)
- Failure to gain weight
- P.E.M.
- Diarrhoea
- Working mother.

LOW BIRTH WEIGHT

Any infant with a birth weight of less than 2.5 kg regardless of gestational age is called L.B.W. (Table 10.3)

Table 10.3: Difference between preterm baby and small for date baby

	Preterm	*Small for Date*
Birth	Before 27 week of gestation	Preterm or full term
I.U. growth	Normal	Retarded
Prognosis	Easily brought back to normal	Difficult to bring back to normal
Weight	More than 10th percentile for gestational age	Less than 10th percentile for gestational age
Palmar and Plantar crease	Developed	Not developed
Areola of nipple	Developed	Not developed

LBW is calculated by:

$$\frac{\text{LB with} < 2.5 \text{ kg}}{\text{Total LB}} \times 100$$

While it is 4 to 8% in developed countries, in a developing country like India it is 26%. I.C.M.R. quotes that maturity, respiratory distress and feeding problem makes 2.5 kg non-acceptable as LBW among Indian children. But criteria is coming in the way that when applied the percentage comes down to nearing zero. For examples when 2.5 kg is criteria and prevalence is 26% the prevalence comes down to 5.5% with 2.0 kg criteria.

Causes: Malnutrition
Infection
Uncontrolled fertility 2.5 kg

Association: Mental retardation
I.M.R.
Morbidity

Strong Association: Maternal nutrition
Length of pregnancy

Prevention

- Dietary improvement of pregnant women.
- Control of maternal infections, diseases.
- Incubatory care to LBW.
- Proper feeding of LBW.
- Infection control of LBW.

Nursing observation and reporting of the following are called for, since they are leading causes of deaths among LBW babies.

a. Atelectasis
b. Malformation

c. Pulmonary haemorrhage
d. Birth trauma giving rise to intracranial bleeding and anoxia
e. Pneumonia.

INFANT FEEDING

The present paediatric concept is for exclusive breastfeeding of infants. Breast milk is ideal and no other feed is required for the child. On an average Indian mother secrete 600 ml of milk, which yield 6.6 gram of protein which is more than sufficient for the baby. Chances of survival, reduction of infection are known with exclusive breastfeeding (Table 10.4).

Table 10.4: Advantages of breastfeeding

Advantage	*Disadvantage*
Safe	NIL
Clean	
Hygienic	Except among
Cheap	Inverted nipple
Available at body temperature	Crack, fissure
Meets nutritional requirement	
Contain antimicrobial factors	
Easily digestible	
Promotes bonding	
No obesity	
No hypocalcemia	
No hypomagnesaemia	
Natural spacing possible	

Artificial Milk

It is indicated in mother's death, failure to breast feed due to defects of breast. It is done by dried whole milk powder and fresh milk from cow. For planning artificial feeding following principles are kept in mind:

- Calorie required is 100 per kg body weight
- Protein required 2 G. per kg body weight
- Carbohydrate required 10 gram per kg body weight
- After 4 months undiluted boiled cooled milk should be given
- On an average child needs 6-8 feeding per day
- During illness, calorie should be increased (Tables 10.5 and 10.6).

Table 10.5: Notable points in artificial feed

Dried milk powder	*Cow's milk*
Safe	Natural source
Free from bacteria	Need humanization of milk upto 2 months
Fortified	
But expensive	

Table 10.6: Difference between breast milk and cow's milk

	Breast milk	*Cow's milk*
Protein	11 G/L	33 G/L
Non-protein	0.32 G/L	0.32/L
Linoleic acid	3.5 G/L	1.0 G/L
Lactose	62 G/L	50 G/L
Calcium	0.3 G/L	1 G/L
Phosphorus	0.1 G/L	1 G/L
Iron	1.5 mg/L	0.5 mg/L
Vitamin C	60 mg/L	20 mg/L
Vitamin D	50 I U	25 I U
Calorie	640 calories	650 calories

WEANING

It is a gradual process of withdrawal of breast milk and substitution of weaning food. It is advocated after 4 months. They are cow's milk, fruit juice, soft cooked rice, dal soup, vegetable soup. Weaning period is crucial and observation is advisable to prevent malnutrition and infection. At the age of one year supplementation with cereals, pulses, vegetables and fruits is necessary. It is always advisable to have home made weaning foods.

Care of the Preschool Child

By virtue of their number, they need and are entitled to a large share of health service. Malnutrition is common and care for its detection through under five care is accorded. Common morbid conditions are anaemia, Xerophthalmia, diarrhoea, whooping cough, Measles, eruptive fevers, skin infections, eye infections, intestinal parasitism.

Malnutrition and infection influence growth and development at this stage. Toddlers are not easily accessible and hence special inputs like day care centres, play centre, Child Park are needed.

HEALTH PROBLEMS IN CHILDHOOD PERIOD

1. Low birth weight (LBW)
2. P.E.M.
3. Micronutrient malnutrition
   - Vitamin A
   - Iodine
   - Iron
   - Calcium
   - Zinc
4. Nutritional Anaemia
5. Nutritional Blindness
6. I.D.D.
7. Infections
8. Accidents
9. Poisoning
10. Behavioural problems.

CONGENITAL MALFORMATIONS

Congenital malformations are subsequently determined before and during birth and commonly recognisable in early life. It refers to anatomical defects in childhood. In case of biochemical and functional disorders are seen, they are grouped under congenital anomaly.

Incidence of congenital malformations has been estimated to be 30 per 1000 live births, which causes 18% of I.M.R. in the world. As per WHO estimates global incidence of some selected malformations are as under (Table 10.7):

Table 10.7: Global incidence of congenital malformations

Heart defect	6 per 1000 live births
Cleft lip	0.9 per 1000 live births
Cleft palate	0.5 per 1000 live births
Spina bifida	1.0 per 1000 live births
Other defects	17.0 per 1000 live births

Incidence of congenital malformation in India is estimated to be 20-28 per 1000 live births. It is the third leading cause of perinatal mortality in India.

Cause of Congenital Malformations

- Down's syndrome
- Klinefelter's syndrome
- Turner's syndrome
- Phenylketonuria
- Tay Sachs disease
- Galactosemia
- Huntington's chorea
- Thalassaemia
- Sickle cell disease
- Haemophilia
- Rubella
- Cytomegalovirus infection
- Toxoplasmosis
- Drugs induced (Thalidomide).

Possible risk factors are:

- Late marriage of woman
- Consanguineous marriage.

Diagnosis of Congenital Malformations

During Prenatal period following laboratory tests are diagnostic of congenital malformations:

i. Maternal blood sample or amniotic fluid sample for specific protein called α protein detection.
ii. U.S.G. (Ultra Sonography) helps to visualise malformations.
iii. Taping amniotic fluid during second trimester can help diagnosis of Down's syndrome and neural tube defect.
iv. Chorionic villi sampling after 9 to 10 weeks of pregnancy help in determination of chromosomal aberration.

Prevention

a. Prevention of consanguineous marriage
b. Prenatal diagnosis for chromosomal aberration in advanced maternal age

c. Control in the use of teratogenic drugs
d. Attention to environmental improvement than touching heredity for a successful normal reproduction.

Handicapped Children

According to Last it is "the reduction in a person's capacity to fulfil a social role as a consequence of an impairment, inadequate training for the role, or other circumstances. Applied to children, the term usually refers to the presence of impairment or other circumstances that are likely to interfere with normal growth and development or with the capacity to learn" (Table 10.8).

Table 10.8: Handicap differentiated from impairment and disability

Handicapped	*Impaired*	*Disabled*
Cannot perform a social role	Abnormal structure and function	Unable to perform an activity

Current Problem (World)

Mental retardation – 100 million (Estimate)
Hearing loss – 48 million (Estimate)
Polio lameness – 13 million (Estimate)

Current Problem (India)

It is estimated that 2.3 percent of the population (2001 population = 1,027,015247) viz., 23.6 million (23,621,350) are physically handicapped. Among 0-6 age population (2001 census = 157,863,145) developmental delay is estimated to be 1.1% viz., 1.7 lakhs (1,736,494).

Types

Physically Handicapped

Blind, deaf, mute, hair lip, cleft palate, talipes, lame, cardiac defect, Accidents, burns and other injuries.

Mentally Handicapped

Moron, imbecile, mentally retarded.

Socially Handicapped

Orphan child, destitute, delinquent.

Prevention

- Genetic counselling.
- Identification and advice of at risk group in a population.
- I.P.P.I.
- Rubella vaccination.
- Proper nutrition of expectant mother.
- Banning teratogenic drugs.
- Avoiding unnecessary X-ray at early pregnancy.

Control

- Detection and proper management of handicap in the community.
- Training and education of handicapped.

Institutions working for handicaps

1. Occupational Therapy College, New Delhi.
2. Occupational Therapy School, Nagpur.
3. Occupational Therapy School, Mumbai.
4. Physical Therapy School, Mumbai.
5. All India Institute of Physical Medicine and Rehabilitation, Mumbai.
6. Institute of Physical Medicine and Rehabilitation, Vellore.
7. N.I.M.H. (National Institute for Mentally Handicapped), Secunderabad.
8. N.I.O.H. (National Institute for the Orthopaedically Handicapped), Kolkata.
9. Ali Yavar Jung National Institute for the Hearing Handicapped, Mumbai.
10. National Institute for the visually Handicapped, Dehradun.
11. All India Institute of Speech and Hearing, Mysore.
12. Many other Non Government voluntary organisations.

Behavioural Problems in Children

There are many types of behavioural problems in children. They are grouped as under:

Educational

Slow learner, School phobia, Repeat failure.

Habit

Bed wetting, Nail biting, Thumb sucking, Masturbation.

Personality

Jealous, Tantrum, shy, Hysteric.

Psychosomatic

Depression, Delusion, Hallucinations.

Antisocial

Stealing, Cruelty, Sexual offence, destructiveness.

One of the major behaviour problems in India is Juvenile Delinquency. It is described below:

Juvenile Delinquency

It is an offence committed by a boy below 16 years or by a girl below 18 years. It is high among boys between 15-16 years in India.

Causes

- Chromosomal anomalies
- Broken Homes
- Urbanised life with poverty.

Prevention

It is possible to prevent juvenile delinquency through:

a. Proper Schooling to provide education
b. Social welfare activities to facilitate deviation in behaviour and
c. Family life improvement

Others

Some of the concepts in child health are:

i. **Child abuse:**
Physical violence on child, sexual abuse, mental and emotional maltreatment, neglect, Deprivation, Lack of opportunity are included under child abuse. Physical battering has lead to death, blindness and mental retardation.

ii. **Street children:**
Children without family are living and working on the street, are at risk for malnutrition, tuberculosis, drug abuse and criminal exploitation.

iii. **Battered baby syndrome:**
Children below 3 years received inexcusable violence resulting in mental and neurological complications.

iv. **Child labour:**
Children below 15 years are obligated to work and earn.

GROWTH AND DEVELOPMENT

Child grows and develops which include physical growth and intellectual-emotional-social development. With optimal nutrition, optimum growth and development is possible.

Thus growth is defined as increase in physical size of body and development is defined as increase in skills and functions.

Reference Value

For studies and comparison we use standard values as under:

1. Harvard standard
2. WHO standard
3. I.C.M.R. standards.

Measurement of Growth

Weight recording: Beam type weighing scale is used in clinics and hospitals. In the Field (Home visiting) a salter spring machine is used.

Height recording: Upto 2 years infantometer is used. Older children can stand and height is measured by the rod attached to the lever type machine or by anthropometer. In home visiting measuring height against a wall is found quite satisfactory.

Mid upper arm circumference: This measurement is done with a tape while the arm is relaxed at the side of the body.

Head and chest circumference: They are measured with the help of a tape.

Indian Standards

Table 10.9: Mean weight and height of Indian children

	Mean weight (Kg)		*Mean height* (Cms)	
	Boys	*Girls*	*Boys*	*Girls*
Birth	3.1	3.0	49.2	48.8
6 months	7.5	8.9	88.3	84.5
1 years	9.5	8.7	73.4	72.1
2 year	11.7	10.6	84.5	82.1
3 years	13.6	12.6	92.7	90.0
4 years	14.9	14.3	98.1	98.0
5 years	17.0	16.0	106.7	104.4
6 years	19.5	17.2	114.6	109.4

Table 10.10: M.U.A.C. in Indian children

	Mean M.U.A.C. (Cms)	
	Male	*Female*
1 year	14.9	14.4
2 years	15.1	14.5
3 years	15.3	14.8
4 years	15.5	15.0
5 years	15.7	15.4
6 years	16.2	15.7

Table 10.11: Weight increment in infants

Age	*Weight increment per week*
0–3 months	200 G
4–6 months	150 G
7–9 months	100 G
9–12 months	50-75 G

Table 10.12: Weight and height increments from 1 to 5 years

Weight increments per year	
1 – 2 years	2.5 kg
3 – 5 years	2.0 kg
Height increments per year	
1st year	25 cm
2nd year	12 cm
3rd year	9 cm
5th year	6 cm

Growth Pattern

Rapid growth occurs in infancy. All babies loose weight during first 4 days after birth. The same is regained in 8 days. It doubles in 5 months, trebles at 1 year.

Length of baby increases 1½ times by 1 year. Weight, height and M.U.A.C. are given in Table nos. 10.9 and 10.12.

Growth is a natural process and it is a sign of well nourishment. If there is loss of appetite, listlessness, decreased activity and peevishness it is reflection of illness and ill nourishment. Since weight is made up of height and fatness which is recorded in weight, *the weight* is the best indicator for the growth of a child. Each child varies in its weight according to local influencing factors. Hence a range is considered for fixing normal or abnormal. Following is the reference standard by N.C.H.S., USA (National Centre of Health Statistics). They are Harvard values considered as standard by W.H.O.

Age (years)	*Boys*		*Girls*	
	Median	*± 2 SD*	*Median*	*± 2 SD*
Birth	3.3	2.4 – 4.3	3.2	2.2 – 4.0
6 months	7.8	5.9 – 9.8	7.2	5.5 – 9.0
1 year	10.2	8.1 – 12.4	9.5	7.4 – 11.6
2 years	12.69	9.9 – 15.2	11.9	9.4 – 14.5
3 years	14.6	11.4 – 18.3	14.1	11.2 – 18.0
4 years	16.7	12.9 – 20.8	16.0	12.6 – 20.7
5 years	18.7	14.4 – 23.5	17.7	13.8 – 23.2
6 years	20.7	16.0 – 26.6	19.5	15.0 – 26.2

This uses concept of centile. Lower the percentile more the growth retardation and vice versa.

Growth Charts

We have growth charts for recording weight corresponding to a given age. Since less than 6 years are considered for growth monitoring R.C.H., in I.C.D.S. services, weight recording is done for 0-6 age children in the I.C.D.S. (Govt. of India) chart. The I.A.P. has recommended the following classification for child nutrition.

Normal: Upto 80% of median (reference curve).

I Degree: Malnutrition–Between 80-71% of median (reference curve).

II Degree: Malnutrition–Between 70-61% of median (reference curve).

III Degree: Malnutrition–Below 60% of median (reference curve).

When plotted, it is the direction of growth curve that is important and not actual weight. As long as it is upwards it is satisfactory. When remains straight or point downwards it indicates retardation and cause must be asserted at the earliest. Infection, diarrhoea, measles are common reasons for no weight gain or pointing downwards. Regular weight recording (as highlighted under R.C.H chapter) is called *(Growth monitoring)*. Since we monitor, find out cause of growth faltering, discuss with mother for supplementation, it is better to use the word *Growth Monitoring and Promotion.*

Nursing care should make sure of the following in growth monitoring and promotion.

i. Good reliable weighing scale
ii. Growth chart
iii. Knowledge on recording and interpretation of growth on the growth chart
iv. Two way discussion with mother of the child for action.

Growth charts are useful in diagnosis, education, take measure, evaluation, teaching and growth monitoring and promotion.

Commonly used I.C.D.S. Growth Chart used by Anganwadi worker in Anganwadi is given below (Tables 10.13 to 10.18):

I.C.M.R. Standards

Table 10.13: I.C.M.R. Standard for weight (Boys and Girls)

Age (years)	*Male Child Mean Weight Kg*	*Female Child Mean Weight Kg*
1	8.4	7.8
2	10.1	9.6
3	11.8	11.2
4	13.5	12.0
5	14.8	14.5
6	16.3	16.0

Table 10.14: I.C.M.R. standard for height (Boys and Girls)

Age (years)	*Male Mean height (cm)*	*Female Mean Height (cm)*
1	73.9	72.5
2	81.6	80.1
3	88.8	87.2
4	96.0	94.5
5	102.1	101.4
6	108.5	107.4

Table 10.15: I.C.M.R. Standard for head circumference (Boys and Girls)

Age (years)	*Male Mean Head Circumference (cm)*	*Female Mean Head Circumference (cm)*
1	44.4	43.6
2	45.9	45.2
3	47.3	46.2
4	48.0	47.1
5	48.5	47.8
6	49.0	48.3

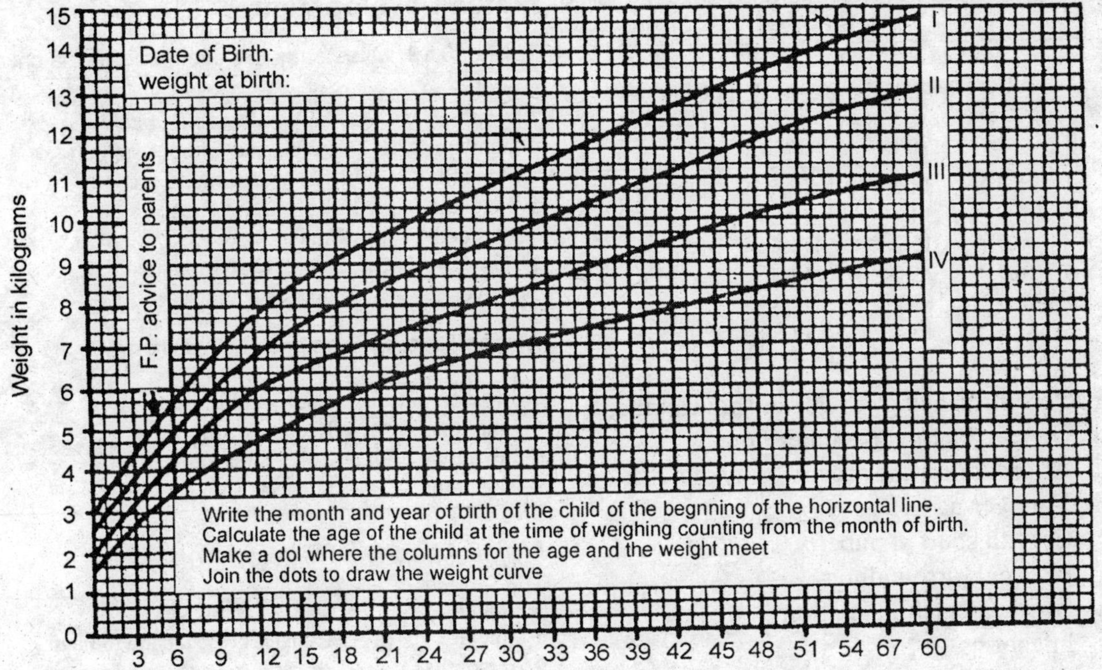

Weights of average of well-fed healthy children should be above the uppermost line I.
Children whose weight falls between lines I and III are under-nourished and require supplementary feeding at home.
Children whose weight falls below line III are severely malnourished. Consult the doctor and follow his advice.
Children whose weight falls below line IV will have to be hospitalized for treatment

Growth chart in use in India, showing use of several reference curves to indicate the nutritional status of the child

Fig. 10.8: I.C.D.S. growth chart used for growth monitoring

Table 10.16: I.C.M.R. Standard for chest circumference (Boys and Girls)

Age (years)	*Male Chest Circumference (cm)*	*Female Chest Circumference (cm)*
1	43.3	42.3
2	45.8	45.1
3	48.0	47.2
4	49.4	48.7
5	50.8	50.1
6	52.5	51.3

Table 10.17: M.U.A.C. circumference standard for boys

Age (years)	*M.U.A.C. WHO Standard (Male)*			*Indian (Shanti Ghosh) (Male)*
	100%	*90%*	*80%*	
1	16.3	14.4	12.8	14.9
2	16.8	14.7	13.0	15.1
3	17.0	15.3	13.6	15.3
4	17.0	15.3	13.6	15.5
5	17.0	15.3	13.6	15.7
6	17.3	15.6	13.8	16.2

Table 10.18: M.U.A.C. circumference standard for girls

Age (years)	*M.U.A.C. WHO Standard (Female)* 100%	90%	80%	*Indian (Shanti Ghosh) (Female)*
1	15.6	14.0	12.5	14.4
2	15.9	14.4	12.8	14.5
3	16.9	15.2	13.5	14.8
4	16.9	15.2	13.5	15.0
5	16.9	15.2	13.5	15.4
6	17.3	15.5	13.8	15.7

Factors influencing growth and development:

i. Genetic factors like inheritance
ii. Affordability and acceptability of nutrition
iii. Younger age
iv. Growth spurt at puberty
v. Physical surroundings
vi. Good parentchild relation
vii. Infections
viii. Parasitism
ix. Standard of living
x. Birth spacing.

Relation of Head and Chest Circumference in Preventive Paediatrics

At birth head circumference is larger than chest circumference. Cross over of these take place around 24th month among Indian children when compared to American children.

Milestones

Behavioural development in terms of (a) Motor (b) Personal (c) Adoptive and (d) Language developments are having specific landmarks of development in human life cycles. These are averages and hence are not absolute. Relative approach of fixing milestones for development is ideal, after studying individual cases, for fixing either normalcy or abnormalcy (Table 10.19 and Fig. 10.9).

Motor Development

Table 10.19: Milestones in development of a child

6 weeks	– Smiles, recognises
3 months	– Holds object deliberately
4 months	– Holds head without support
5-6 months	– Lifts head turns to see
6-8 months	– Sits without support
9-10 months	– Crawls
1 year	– Stands with support
1-1½ years	– Stands without support

Major Sociopersonal Developments

6-8 weeks	– Looks and smiles
4-5 months	– Recognises mother
6-8 months	– Enjoy hide and seek
9-10 months	– Suspects stranger

Major Adoptive Developments

4-5 months	– Reaches for object
6-8 months	– Transfer objects hand to hand
9-10 months	– Releases objects
12-14 months	– Builds the shape

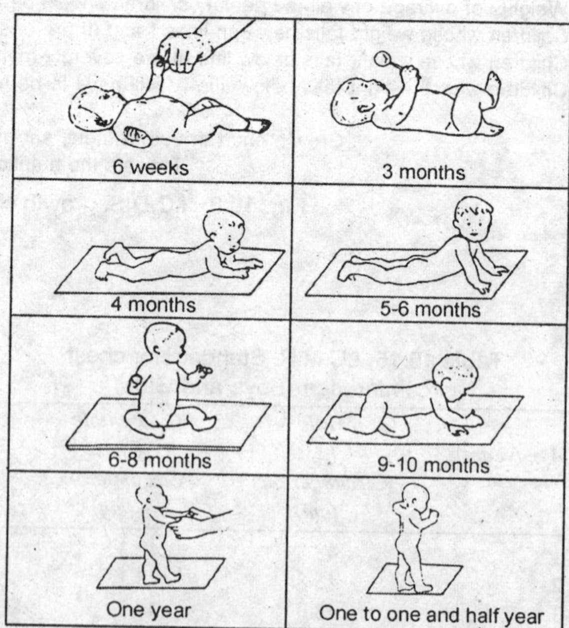

Fig. 10.9: Milestones

Major Language Developments

6-8 months	– Experiments with noise
9-10 months	– High sounding noise
10-11 months	– First word " Ma, ma"
18-21 months	– Joins words

Child Guidance Clinic

It was started in 1909 with an intention to deal juvenile delinquent child. Now other forms of child maladjustments are tackled through child guidance clinic.

Child guidance clinics are run in team spirit by child psychologists, psychiatrists, psychosocial workers, paediatrics speech therapists, neurologists and occupational therapists. Common methods employed in child guidance clinics are :

- Child counselling
- Play therapy
- Parental counselling.

Under Five Clinics

Earlier years well baby clinics were running which took preventive care services. Now, of late, Under Five Clinics have taken up the task of integrating treatment, prevention and surveillance activity in the community (Fig. 10.10).

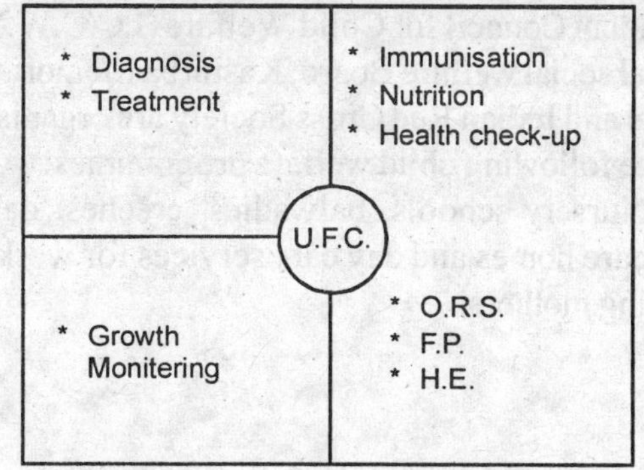

Fig. 10.10: Functions of under five clinics

Child Placement Activities

Problem children and deviants are tackled through child placement procedures. Mainly they are as under:

i. *Adoption:* Childless couple can legally adopt which give a permanent placement for orphans.
ii. *Faster homes:* Social work minded organisations run faster homes which are nearer to a family to provide love and affection.
iii. *Orphanage:* It is an Institution where large number of broken home children, street children, begging children are placed.
iv. *Remand home:* A child is kept under a trained person, psychiatrist and doctor to improve mental and physical well-being of a child. It also has elementary schooling.
v. *Borstal:* Deviant child, misbehaved in a certified school, usually above 16 years of age are sent to borstal for training and reformation.

Legislation for Child Health

1. The Child Labour (Prohibition and Regulation) Act, 1986 to protect the child from child labour.
2. The Child Marriage Restraint Act, 1978, to raise legal age of marriage to 18 years for girls and 21 years for boys.
3. The Children Act, 1960, to provide comprehensive scheme of care, protection and rehabilitation to delinquent child.
4. The Juvenile Justice Act, 1986, to provide comprehensive scheme of care, protection and rehabilitation to delinquent child.

Child Welfare Programmes

This is mainly to cover a wide spectrum of needs of children who are socially, economically, physically or mentally handicapped. These children will be usually under any one of the following categories:

a. Children of working mothers
b. Destitute children
c. Handicapped children.

Indian Council for Child Welfare (I.C.C.W.), central social welfare Board, Kasturba Memorial Trusts and Indian Red Cross Society are organising the following child welfare programmes:

i. Nursery schools, balwadies, crèches, day care homes and day care services for working mothers.
ii. Holiday homes for 12 to 16 age group children for spending holidays for deviated healthy activities.
iii. Recreation facilities like park, children library, balbhavan, children film, children museum, hobby classes etc.

CHAPTER ELEVEN

General and Specific Epidemiology

GENERAL EPIDEMIOLOGY

IMPORTANCE

Epidemiology has its involvement in disease occurrence, causation, transmission and health-related event. Improved knowledge of Epidemiology has brought into focus the risk factors. Separate departments exist in.

Nursing profession at its nursing care process uses the knowledge of disease transmission, disinfection and causation, for efficient nursing. It is inter-connected with the triad of Nurse-Ward-Patient in case of hospitals and Nurse-Health Centre–Community in case of Public Health Nursing activities.

DEFINITION

According to Mac Mohan it is defined as "the study of the distribution and determinants of disease frequency in man."

Twenty-eight years later John M. Last has given new definition to the word epidemiology as "the study of the distribution and determinants of health related states or events in specified populations and the application of this study to the control of health problems."

MAIN AIMS OF EPIDEMIOLOGY

International Epidemiological Association and Indian Epidemiological Association have endorsed 3 aims of Epidemiology as under:

i. To describe the distribution and magnitude of health and disease problems in human populations.
ii. To identify aetiological factors (risk factors) in the pathogenesis of disease.
iii. To provide the data essential to the planning, implementation and evaluation of services for the prevention, control and treatment of disease and to the setting up of priorities among these services.

APPROACHES TO EPIDEMIOLOGY

One approach is to ask questions like What? Where? When? Who? and Why?

Second approach is to make comparison and judge which is better?

Disease Transmission

Dynamics of disease transmission is represented in the Figure 11.1.

Disease transmission depends on source of infection, mode of transmission and susceptibility of man who gets the disease.

Some of the terms that are to be known by their meanings are:

Reservoir: "Any person, animal, arthropod, plant, soil or substance in which disease agent live and multiply."

Case: "A person in the population or study group identified as having a particular disease, condition or disorder which is under investigation."

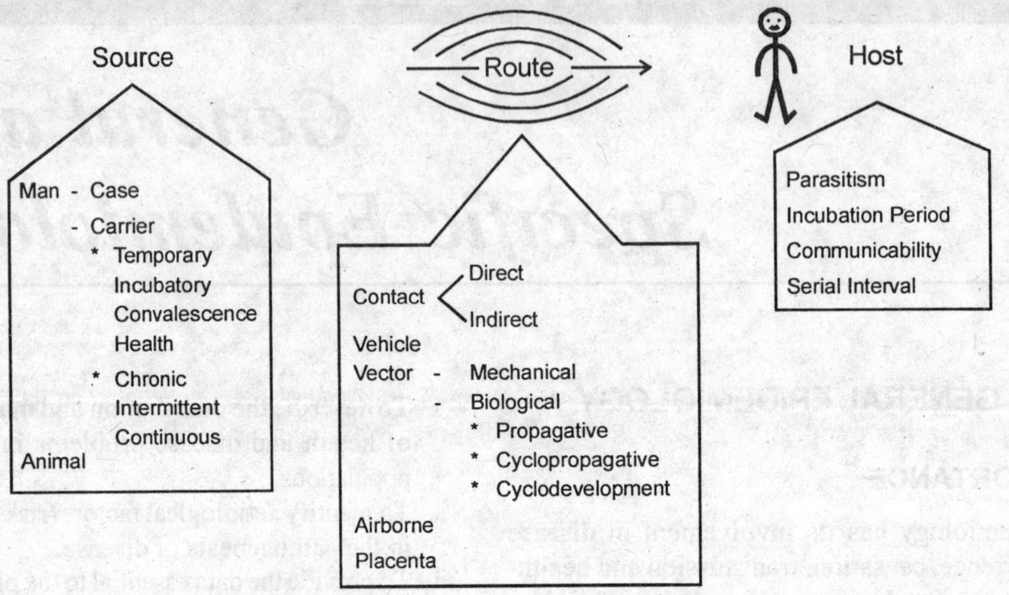

Fig. 11.1: Dynamics of disease transmission

Carrier: "An infected person or animal that harbours a specific infectious agent in the absence of clinical manifestation and which serve as a potential source of infection to others.

Chronic carrier: "Person who excretes disease agent for indefinite period". Chronic carrier state is known with typhoid, malaria, gonorrhoea and hepatitis.

Droplet infection: When droplets of saliva and nasopharyngeal secretions are sprayed to the air, (it is forceful in cough, sneeze) droplet infection occurs. Respiratory infection and tuberculosis are typical droplet infections. If droplet is tiny 1-10 microns it is called droplet nuclei.

Incubation period: "Time interval between invasion by disease agent to disease manifestation by signs symptoms" in non-communicable disease it is called Latent period. If development occurs outside man (e.g., Malaria parasite in mosquito) it is called extrinsic incubation period.

Secondary Attack Rate (SAR): "The number of exposed persons developing the disease within the range of the incubation period following exposure to the primary case."

Immunity

By virtue of infection or immunisation, man develops specific protective antibodies, is called immunity. This can be:

i. Active by humoral or cellular.
ii. Passive by giving immunoglobulin.

Herd Immunity

It means the immunity developed and demonstrated in a group of people against a disease. So herd structure can give protection to an individual in that group by virtue of being a member of that group.

Immunisation

It is one of the most effective Public Health Interventions to reduce childhood mortality and morbidity due to vaccine preventable disease

(VPD). It is very much cost effective. Nursing care lies in effective implementation and supervision of activities of the programme. Knowledge and skills in line with recent advances is required to strengthen nursing care in the field.

In 1992, UIP became part of CSSM (Child Survival and Safe Motherhood programme). In 1997 it becomes component of RCH (Reproductive and Child Health programme).

National Immunisation Schedule

Pregnant		
	Early pregnancy	TT-1 or Booster
	4 week later	TT-2[Y]
Infants		
	At birth[@]	BCG+OPV "O" dose
	6 weeks	[l]BCG[@], DPT 1 , OPV 1
	10 weeks	DPT – 2, OPV 2
	14 weeks	DPT – 3, OPV 3
	9 months	Measles
Children		
	16-24 months	DPT OPV (Booster)
	5-6 years	DT [m]
	10 years	TT [m]
	16 years	TT [m]

Y Last dose of TT should be given at least 1 month prior to expected date of delivery

@ In case of individual delivery/if not given at birth

m 2 doses DT given at interval of 1 month

1 If there is no past history of immunisation

Table 11.1: Syringe and needle specifications

Vaccine	*Syringe*	*Needle*
B.C.G.	1 ml syringe (BCG syringe)	26 gauge
Other vaccine	2 ml syringe	23 gauge
For reconstitution	5 ml syringe	20 gauge

Table 11.1 and Fig.11.2 give an idea of specifications and injection safety management. Fig.11.3 gives idea of injection site and angle of needle.

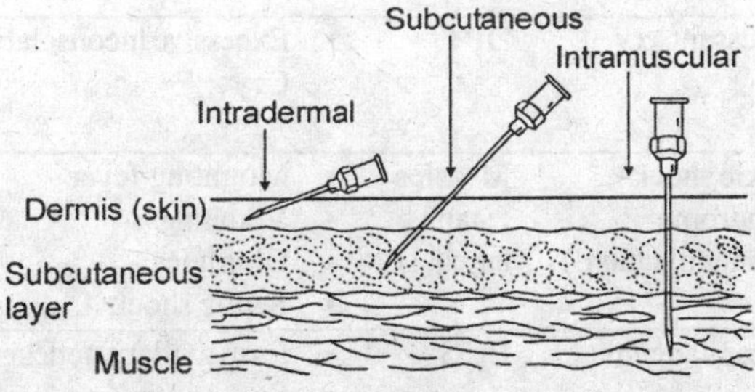

Note: The approximate angle of the needle to the injection site is:
Intra-dermal injection : 15° (BCG)
Sub-cutaneous : 45° (Measles)
Intra-muscular: 90° (DPT, DT,TT, Hepatitis B)

Fig. 11.3: Injection site and angle

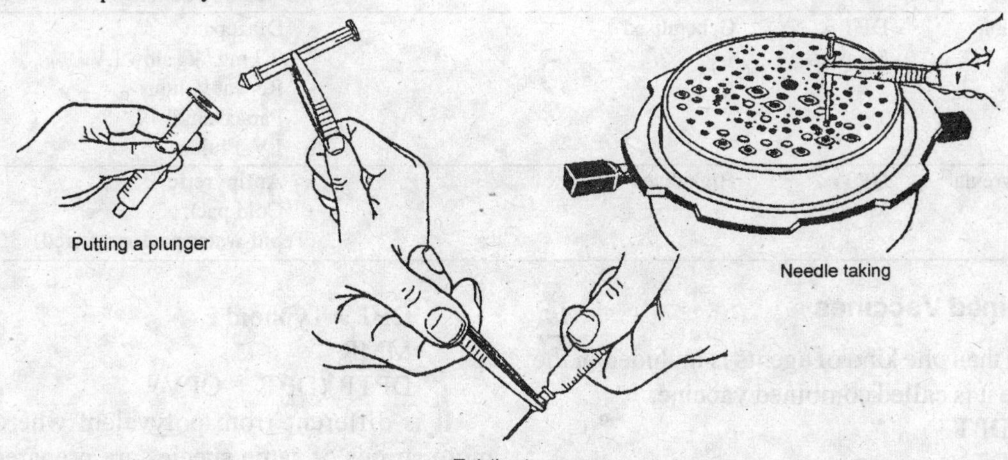

Fig. 11.2: Managing injection safety

Nursing care and nursing management of reactions due to immunisation are tabulated as under:

Event	*Vaccine*	*Symptom*	*Nursing care and nursing management*
Anaphylaxis	Any	• Acute decompensation of CVS • Hypovolemic shock • Altered sensorial • Larynx spasm/Oedema • Acute respiratory distress	• 1:10,000 adrenaline 0.01 ml per kg.(I.M.) • C.P.R. • I.V. volume expanders • Oxygen • I.V. hydrocortisone
Hypotension	DPT	• Acute paleness • Loss of consciousness	• I.V. Fluid • Dexamethasone • Oxygen
Incessant cry	DPT	• Excessive inconsolable Cry	• Oral paracetamol • Advice feeding • Avoid DPT and give DT
Toxic shock Syndrome (Contamination!)	Measles (Staph aureus!)	• Mounting fever • Vomiting • Diarrhoea • Septic shock	• I.V. Fluid • Steroid, Antibiotic • Paracetamol Oral • Supportive Therapy
Lymphadenitis	BCG	• Firm axillary nodes • Soft nodes • Sinus, ulcer	• No treatment • Aspiration • INH 5mg / kg once a day For 3 months
Abscess any Nerve injury	Any	• Abscess • Fever	• Antibiotic • Antipyretic • Drainage
Local reaction	Any	• Swelling • Redness	• Paracetamol < 3 months 1/8 tablets < 3 years ¼ tablet < 5 years ½ tablet
Convulsion	DPT Measles	Generalised	• Diazepam 0.3 mg / kg slow I.V. • Repeat ½ hour • Paracetamol • I.V. Fluids
Hyperpyrexia	DPT Measles	High fever	• Antipyretic • Cold pack (Tepid water pack preferred)

Combined Vaccines

If more than one kind of agents is included in the vaccine it is called combined vaccine.

Eg. DPT
DT
DP
DPT + Typhoid
MMR
DPTP (DPT + OPV)

It is different from polyvalent where 2 or more strains of same species are prepared.

Common immunoglobulins used are:

Rabies (RIG) (Rabies Immunoglobulin)	20 I u/kg body weight	for prevention
Tetanus (TIG)	4000-6000 units for therapy	250 units for prophylaxis
Rh isoimmunisation (RhIG) (Rhesus factor immunoglobulin)	1 vila of 15 ml = 300 μg	for prophylaxis
Severe measles (IG) (Human Immunoglobulin)	0.25 mg per kg body weight	for prevention
Hepatitis B (HBIG) (Hepa B Immunoglobulin)	0.05 ml/kg body weight	for prevention
For newborn-HBIG	0.05 ml at birth, at 3rd month and at 6th month for prevention	

Hazards due to immunisation are:

1. Local reaction–Pain, Swelling, Redness, Tenderness, Nodule, Abscess.
2. General reaction—Fever, Headache, Malaise.
3. Faulty technique to cause infection.
4. Neuritic manifestations.
5. Some latent infection becomes dominant
6. Foetal damage in some cases.

THE COLD CHAIN

It is a system of storage and transport of vaccines at low temperature from the site of manufacture to the site of vaccination. Polio and measles are stored in freezer. Others (DPT, DT, BCG, Diluents) are stored in cold part of fridge. Ice line refrigerator (ILR) and deep freezers (DF) are used at higher level for long duration storage. Vaccine carriers and day carriers are used to carry small dose for short length of time.

Control and Prevention of Disease (Fig. 11.4)

EMPORIATRICS

This is described as a science of health of travellers. They are exposed to malaria, giardiasis, dengue, influenza, SARS, STD, HIV/AIDS, amoebiasis, typhoid, hepatitis. Diagnosis and

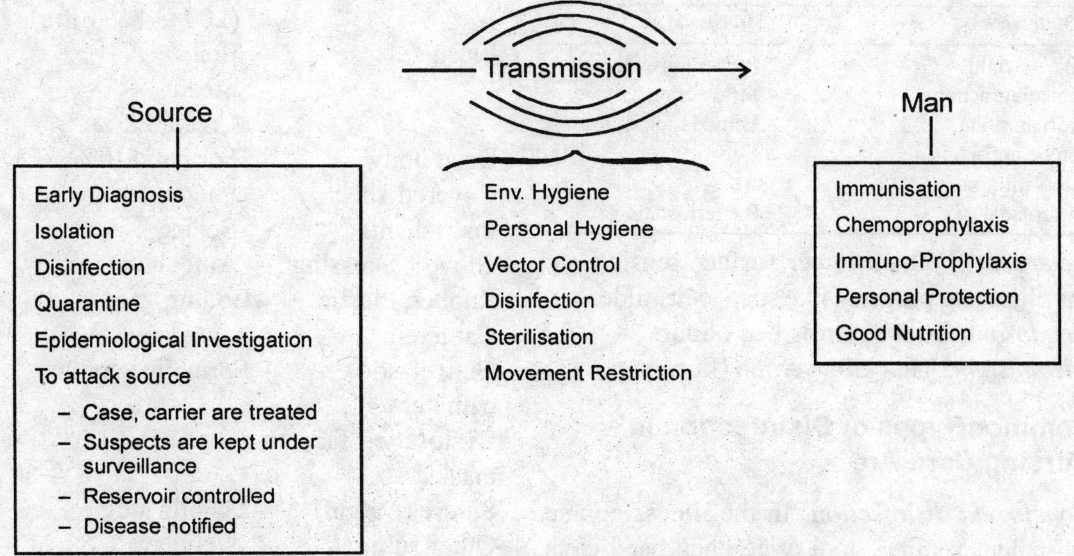

Fig. 11.4: Measures to be taken in the control and prevention of disease

detecting the source help in interventions. Personal protection, health awareness, required immunisation help in preventing diseases of travellers.

EPIDEMIC INVESTIGATION

When an epidemic occurs, which is beyond our imagination, procedure followed to examine, observe and analyse the disease occurrence is called "epidemic investigation". Following actions are taken in public health activities:

- Diagnosis is confirmed
- Innumerable cases occurring are confirmed.
- Geographic area is mapped
- Contact search of cases done.
- Data is analysed for time, place and people involved.
- A cause is suspected (Hypothesis)
- It is tested.
- After report preparation, measures to check spread is continued.

DISINFECTION

A method of killing pathogens is called disinfection (Table 11.2):

Table 11.2: Difference between disinfection and antiseptic

Disinfection	*Antiseptic*
Kills outright	Prevent growth
Immediate action	Mild action
Short duration	Long duration
Can be antiseptic in low dilution	
Bactericidal	Bacteriostatic

Detergents: Which lower surface tension and has cleansing property like soap, cetrimide.
Deodorant: That controls bad odours.
Disinfestant: That kills vermin (lice, bugs).

Common Types of Disinfection in Nursing Care Are

Concurrent disinfection: In the illness course; for sputum, vomitus, stool, urine, linen, hand, cloth, apron and gown.

Terminal disinfection: At discharge or at death.

Prophylactic disinfection: Instruments at hospital, O.T. material, hand scrubbing, etc.

They are classified as under:

I. 1. Physical
 2. Chemical
 3. Natural.

II. 1. Solid
 2. Liquid
 3. Gas.

Hospital disinfection procedure:

Faeces, Urine	– 2-hour contact Phenol 10% Formalin 10% Bleaching powder 8% Cresol 5%
Sputum	– Burning Autoclave (20 min 20 Lb) Cresol 5%
Room	– Soap water wash Cresol 2.5% Phenol 5.0% Formalin 10% Formalin + KMno4 in water (200 G. / ½ Litre)
Linen	– Boil Steam Cresol 2.5%
Dead body	– Formalin 10%
Covered sheet	Phenol 5%
Instruments	– Boiling
Glove + Dressing	– Autoclave
Rubber, Plastic Catheter	–Boiling
Gum elastic catheter	– Formalin vapour
Cystoscope face mask	– Pasteurisation
Suture (Catgut)	– Lygol's iodine
Other suture	– Autoclave
Polythene tubing	– Gamma radiation

Urinals – Hypochlorite solution
Bedpan – Lysol
Blanket – Hot formalin vapour

Operation Theatre Disinfection

i. Soap-water clean, aeration, sunlight
ii. Wash with chlorinated lime (25 PPM)
iii. Wash with 1% Formaldehyde solution
iv. Wash with 2.5% cresol
v. 500 ml formalin in 1 litre per 30 cub.mtr. as fumigation
vi. 200G. KMO_4 in 500 ml formalin in 1 litre water for 30 cub. mtr.

Epidemiology–Measurement

Common measurement like:

i. *Rate:* Birth rate, IMR etc.
ii. *Ratio:* Sex ratio, nurse population ration etc.
iii. *Proportion:* 22% scabies, 6% tuberculosis etc., are used in epidemiological measurements.
iv. *Mortality:* To form a uniform basis, international death certificate is proposed. Its usual format is as follows:

Mortality measurements are:

- Crude death rate
- Specific death rate (to sex, age, disease)
- C.F.R.
- Proportion mortality rate
- Survival rate
- Standardised death rates.

Morbidity measurements are:

- Incidence (New cases in defined population in a given time)
- Prevalence (All current cases (Old + New).

Epidemiology—Uses

There are wide varieties of uses which are applied in day-to-day patient care and public health activities. They are enumerated as under:

- Establish cause of health and disease.
- Help in community diagnosis.
- Gives clinical picture of disease.
- Provides the list of determinants and distribution of disease.
- Help general practice.
- Help in the investigation of an epidemic.
- It is a tool for mass survey.
- It establishes need and methods of control and prevention of disease.
- Chances of risk are measured.
- Syndromes are described by the knowledge of epidemiology.
- Temporal variation (Seasonal) of a disease is established for health care management.
- Helps in establishment of a model of nursing care for any given disease.
- It gives an idea for promoting, protecting and rehabilitating for a given condition/disease/syndrome.

HOSPITAL ACQUIRED INFECTIONS (NOSOCOMIAL INFECTION) (HOSPITAL CROSS INFECTION)

Overcrowding, unhygienic methods and resistant strains of organisms are common causes of Hospital Acquired Infections.

Source

- Patients in hospitals e.g., urinary tract infections, skin infections, viral infections, respiratory infections.
- Hospital staff like doctors, nurses, ward boys who can harbour pathogens in their noses, skin surfaces and mobiles.
- Hospital environment e.g., dust, furniture, any facilities.

  Various types of infections are:
  - Viral infections
  - Skin infections
  - Respiratory infections
  - Urinary tract infections.

  Routes of the infections are:
  - Droplet
  - Direct, and
  - Hospital procedure.

Prevention

The major preventive measures are:

- Isolation of cases
- Judicious use of antibiotics
- Hospital disinfection procedures including CSSD strengthening
- Isolation and treatment of hospital staff who are source of infection
- Universal precautions at hospital
- Notification (periodic)
- Hospital auditing procedure maintenance
- Hospital infection control committee for policies.

WHO DEFINITION OF HEALTH

"Health is a state of complete physical, mental and social well being and not merely an absence of disease or infirmity".

Positive Health

Maintaining perfect functioning of the body by improving the quality of life is suggestive of positive health. Each country, each nation, each state, each family and each individual set their own standard for defining health. This varying concept has given a new idea of relative concept of health.

Health Team: Each member in a professional group has specific and recognised function in the team. It is a group of persons who share a common goal and common objectives which are determined by the needs of the community.

Health For All: It is an attainment of a level of health that will permit them to lead to a socially and economically productive life.

Primary Health Care: It is "Essential health care based on practical, scientifically sound and socially acceptable methods and technology made universally accessible to individuals and families in the community through their full participation and at a cost that the community and the country can afford to maintain at every stage of their development in the spirit of self-determination."

DISEASE

It is condition of body, organ or tissue in which functions are disrupted or deranged.

Epidemiological Triad—Apart from pathogen, host character and environment are also considered. It can be represented as a triangle.

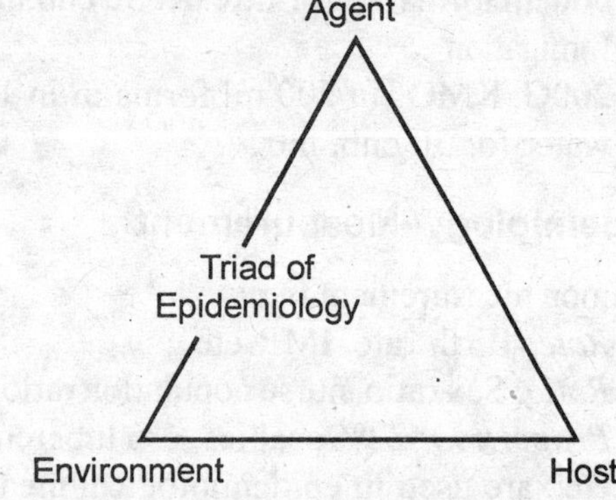

Fig. 11.5: Epidemiological triad

Community Health

It is "all the personal health and environmental services in any human community, irrespective of whether such services were public or private ones." Earlier hygiene moulded to sanitation which got changed to preventive and social medicine, the same area is now "Community Health". This is called as community medicine till today.

Prevention

Before the disease and after getting the disease body interacts to fight the disease. So nature tries to preserve and restore the health when impaired. With advance in science and technology man wants to utilize the knowledge of advancement in preventive and curative medicine to promote health. These formulations are seen with the process of prevention.

Levels of prevention are:

- *Primordial:* Prevention of development of disease by not changing the harmful life style.
- *Primary:* Action taken before disease develops to remove the possibility of getting it.
- *Secondary:* Action which halts the progress of disease.
- *Tertiary:* Action taken to reduce disability.

W.H.O. has recently recommended 2 approaches under primary prevention (first level of prevention); one is *population strategy,* which is directed at the whole population irrespective of individual risk level. Here population strategy is directed towards socioeconomic, behavioural and lifestyle changes. The other is *high risk strategy* which aims at bringing preventive care to individuals at risk through optional use of clinical methods.

Modes of Intervention

These are depicted under National history of disease which are:

- Health promotion
- Specific protection
- Early diagnosis and treatment
- Disability limitation
- Rehabilitation

Common practical activity is given in a tabular column below:

Iceberg of Disease

Like an iceberg, presymptomatic and what health professional cannot see is exceedingly high. This phenomenon is called *Iceberg of disease* (Fig. 11.6).

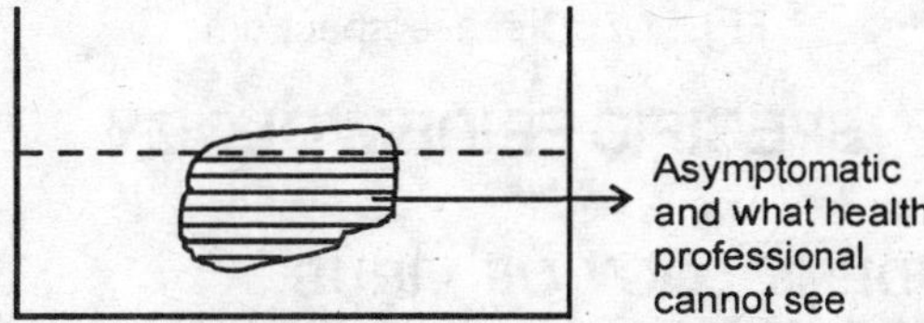

Fig. 11.6: Iceberg of disease

Disease Spectrum

Similar to light spectrum the disease gives the picture of disease at a given point of time in the community (Fig. 11.7).

Table 11.3: Examples of intervention therapy in prevention

Primary		*Secondary*		*Tertiary*
Health promotion	*Specific protection*	*Early diagnosis and treatment*	*Disability limitation*	*Rehabilitation*
• Health education	• Immunisation	• TB patient	• Physiotherapy polio case	• Artificial limb to limbless
• Life style change	• IFA prophylaxis	• Leprosy case	• IV fluid to severe dehydration	• Gardener job to leprosy cured
• Use protected water	• Chemoprophylaxis	• Hypertension case	• Bed rest, sedation to IHD	• Family restoration of TB cured
• Mosquito control	• Seat belt, helmet	• Cancer cervix case	• IV therapy in severe malaria	• Brill schooling to blind
• Food fortification	• Food safety	• Severe malnutrition	• IV therapy in Meningitis	• Reconstructive surgery to leprosy patient

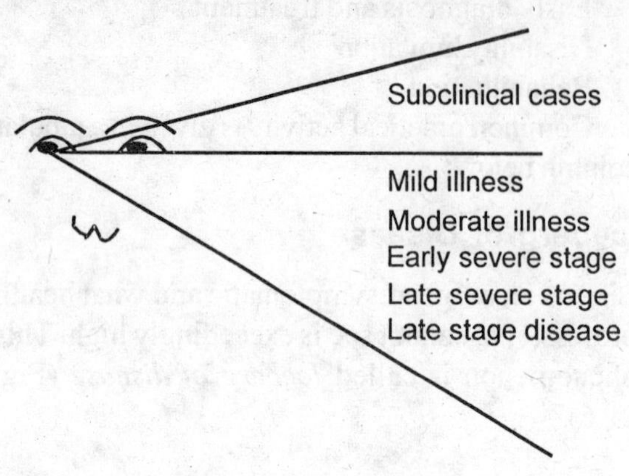

Fig.11.7: Disease spectrum

SPECIFIC EPIDEMIOLOGY

EPIDEMIOLOGY OF VIRUS INFECTIONS

CHICKENPOX

Chickenpox is a viral infection, a primary disease of children which results in a highly contagious, generalised exanthema which occurs in epidemics. It is derived from a French word to the appearance of the pox. It is endemic in developing countries. 90% of cases are below 10 years of age.

In India all population seems to have been infected once in their life time. The disease goes unnoticed because natural history of disease is 8 to 10 days and people attribute this to the curse of "Goddess *Maramma*".

Incubation period: Usually 14 to 16 days.

Mode of transmission: It is transmitted by droplet infection and by personal contact (Table 11.4).

MEASLES

It is an acute, highly contagious, vaccine preventable viral infection with a prodromal stage characterised by catarrhal symptoms and Koplik spots on buccal mucous membrane. Dusky red blotchy rash appear on the skin on 4th day affecting face and body. Leucopenia is usual. Because of red spots on the body it is called *Rubeola.*

Measles elimination strategy has following components:

i. **Catch up vaccination:** One time nationwide vaccination of children 9-12 month of age under U.I.P.
ii. **Keep up vaccination:** Vaccinating above 95% of each successive birth cohort.
iii. **Follow up vaccination:** Nationwide vaccination of all children born after catch up vaccination once in 4 years.

Mode of transmission: Person to person by droplet infection and droplet nuclei.

Incubation period is 10 days.

Clinical features: Case will have usual prodromal phase of 3 days. Catarrhal stage is characterised by upper respiratory symptoms and presence of Koplik's spots on internal buccal mucosa, which is pathognomonic of measles. The

Table 11.4: Difference between chickenpox and smallpox

		Chicken pox	*Small pox*
	Fever	*Rash develop at the same time as fever*	*Fever appears 2-4 days before rash*
Rash	Appearance	Pleomorphic (Pocks are several stages) at a given point of time	Monomorphic (Pocks are same stage) at a given point of time
	Development	Rapid	Slow
	Distribution	Centripetal (More in centre)	Centrifugal (More in periphery)
	Palm and sole	Absent	Present
	Mortality	Nil	High

child is irritable at this stage. Later, skin rash appear and lasts for 6 days, gradually fading with staining in the pale skinned children. Generalised lymphadenopathy and diarrhoea are very common. Bacterial pneumonia is seen in 4% of the cases. Very rarely S.S.P.E. (Subacute Sclerosing Panencephalitis) may occur. It is a serious infection along with malnutrition, among children.

Complications

- Diarrhoea
- Pneumonia
- Respiratory complications
- Otitis media.

Management with Nursing Care

Only symptomatic treatment. Antibiotic should be given *only* if the child has clinical signs of pneumonia or other evidence of sepsis.

Control Measures

- Isolation of cases for 7 days from rash
- Immunisation of contacts within 2 days of exposure
- Routine immunisation
- Community measures against malnutrition.

Prevention

It is given at 9-12 months under U.I.P. 0.5 ml subcutaneous single dose is given. Except fever no other side reactions are observed in every day practice. It should, theoretically, give 95% immunity for life. Pregnancy is a contraindication

Measles vaccination combined with Mumps and rubella as M.M.R. is also made available on public demand.

GERMAN MEASLES

It is worldwide in distribution. Epidemics occur in early spring. Epidemics once in 10 years and major epidemic once in 30 years are reported in global epidemiology. In 1941 Sir Norman Gregg recognised the association between Rubella and congenital abnormalities.

Occasional deafness is observed in infection at the 5th month of pregnancy.

Incubation period – 2 to 3 weeks.

Mode of transmission: By droplet infection and by person to person contact.

Congenital Rubella Syndrome

Rubella infection in pregnant woman inhibits cell division of embryo and hence congenital defects like deafness, cardiac anomalies and congenital cataract are seen; microcephalus and retinopathy have also been reported. 85 to 95% of defects occur during first 2 months of gestation.

Control and Prevention

First	• Women of child bearing age (15 to 39) are immunised.
Second	• All children 1-14 years age are immunised.
Third	• All children at 1 year age are immunised.

In India it has not been possible to affect the above strategy. It is given on voluntary request since UIP load under national programme for 6 preventable diseases is high and since detection of risk population has been cumbersome.

In mega cities, MMR (Measles, Mumps and Rubella) is available and is found equally effective weapon against German measles.

MUMPS

Mumps primarily infects 5 to 9 years old children. In developing countries like India where there is no programmed vaccination, older teenagers are also affected. Infection is by droplet or direct salivary spread and initial infection is though URI.

Incubation Period: 16-18 days.

Period of infectivity: 1 week.

Clinical Picture

Fever and malaise are the beginning symptoms and they are prodromal symptoms. This is followed by either unilateral or bilateral parotid swelling. In 10% of cases other salivary glands may also be infected. Oophoritis and orchitis are complications in post puberty period manifested with abdominal pain or testicular pain. Sterility and meningitis are observed complications of mumps. Transient hearing loss, labyrinthitis and measurable deafness have been recorded. During pregnancy abortion is observed.

Case Management

Most of the cases are treated with symptomatic treatment. In case of discomfort by orchitis or oophoritis (only when diagnosed) require 40 mg prednisolone orally for 4 days.

Control Measures

There is no specific control measure advisable for mumps control. Selective isolation, proper disinfection of articles used by the patient and surveillance of contacts are useful tools for control of mumps.

Prevention

i. Mumps immunoglobulin (MIG) is available, but not found satisfactory in protective action.
ii. Live attenuated mumps vaccine I.M. 0.5ml as single dose gives good detectable antibodies in 90% of cases.
iii. MMR (Measles—Mumps—Rubella) a combined vaccine is also found equally effective in the prevention of mumps.

INFLUENZA

Influenza is a specific acute illness caused by a group of myxoviruses-2. Common strain are $A(H_1N_1)$, $A(H_3N_2)$ and B. Recently $A(H_5N_1)$ strain has been isolated.

Man is the reservoir and source of infection are discharges from mouth and nose of infected persons. It is transmitted through droplet infection and air borne.

Incubation period is 24-72 hours. The patient will be infectious from pre-clinical phase to 1 week after clinical onset.

Influenza A is subjected to antigenic variation both major and minor. When there is sudden complete major change it is called a *shift*. When the antigenic change is gradual over a period of time it is called a *drift*.

It is common in winter and rainy seasons. Overcrowding enhances transmission. It is high in close population group like school, ship etc.

Case Management with Nursing Care

Bed rest is advocated until fever subsides. Paracetamol 0.5 to 1.0 gram 6 hourly can relieve headache and generalised pains. Amantadine and Rimantidine 100 mg BD for 3 days is found effective. Pholcodine 10 mg every 6 hours may be given to suppress cough. Specific treatment for pneumonia may be necessary.

Control Measures

i. Good ventilation, avoiding overcrowding, encouraging patients to cover while sneezing or coughing
ii. Vaccines.

International Measures

- Prompt notification to W.H.O.
- Identification of virus type and reporting
- Continued epidemiological studies and exchange of information
- Continuing attempt to mobilise development and production facilities to permit rapid shipment and use of an appropriate vaccine when a new strain appears or when it threatens to become pandemic.

POLIOMYELITIS

Poliomyelitis is a disease of early life in indigenous population in tropics, originally called *infantile paralysis*. Gentle passive movement of limbs will differentiate polio as it is the only condition in which pain is not aggravated and may even be relieved. Bulbar paralysis by polio is usually fatal.

Mode of transmission is faecal oral route.

Prevention by Vaccine

Two types of vaccine are available and in India oral (Sabin) polio vaccine is used in eradication strategy (Table 11.5).

Table 11.5: Difference between O.P.V. and I.P.V.

O.P.V. (Oral)	*I.P.V. (Injectable)*
Live attenuated	Killed formalised
Oral	I. M. or S.C.
Humoral and intestinal immunity is got	Only humoral
Prevents reinfection	Do not prevent reinfection
Useful in epidemic	Not useful
Cheap	Costly
Cold chain required	Not stringent

OPV

OPV contain live attenuated type I, II and III type virus grown in monkey kidney or human diploid cell cultures.

Under UIP programme OPV is given as per schedule under primary course of immunisation. The dose is 3 drops per dose. WHO recommends a dropper for proper use. Tilt the child's back and gently squeeze the cheeks or pinch the nose to make the mouth of the infant to open. Let the polio drop fall from dropper onto the child's tongue. It has to be repeated if the child spits out the vaccine.

For passive immunity in acute infection, human normal immunoglobulin is used at 0.3 ml per kg body weight. But it must be used along with active immunisation.

Epidemiological Basis of Polio Eradication

1. Man is the only host to get polio.
2. There is no chronic carrier state.
3. In the sewage, virus has 48 hours half life, and it spreads during this period of half life if at all it is spreading.
4. OPV multiplies in intestine and interrupts the transmission of wild polio virus.
5. OPV oral administration is easy for coverage.
6. OPV is cheap and hence is cost benefit as well as cost effective.

Based on the above 6 noted phenomena, public health personal ventured for simultaneous administration of OPV within a short period of time by mass immunisation. OPV will interrupt the transmission of wild polio virus by displacing it from intestine where the wild polio virus is expected to multiply.

Epidemiological Investigation of Polio Case in the Community

Even a single case of polio should prompt immediate active search for other cases. Now polio epidemic is defined as "Two or more local polio cases caused by same strain of virus within 1 month duration".

Line listing of cases is done by visiting the children in the community.

Operational Terminologies

i. **Mopping up:** Involves door to door OPV to below 5 years children in the village or a settlement where a case of polio was detected. This operational procedure is done in active stage as well as in final stage of polio eradication.

ii. **Ring immunisation:** Is a mopping up operation in cities where door to door OPV to below 5 year children is done covering an area with a radius of 3 kms.

iii. **Pulse immunisation:** OPV is given to all 0-5 years children in a country on a single day regardless of previous immunisation. This is maintained as an annual event. Hence the name pulse.

Polio Eradication Programme

Since 1992 all polio and non polio-flaccid paralysis were included under active surveillance activity.

National polio eradication strategy included the following:

1. Pulse polio immunisation is done every year till it is eradicated.
2. Along with pulse polio, high level of routine immunisation coverage is sustained.
3. Monitoring of OPV coverage is done at all levels.
4. Improve the surveillance capable of detecting all AFP due to polio and non-polio.
5. Rapid case investigation, stool sample collection is ensured.
6. All cases are followed for 60 days to check residual paralysis.
7. To stop transmission, conduct outbreak control for cases confirmed.

IPPI (Intensive Pulse Polio Immunisation)

Polio eradication programme was called PPI (Pulse polio immunisation) from 1995 to 1999. Later with intensification, it becomes IPPI from 2000 onwards. It is defined as sudden, simultaneous, mass administration of extra 2 doses of OPV on a single day before the transmission season which is usually January-February of every year, to children below 5 years of age.

VVM (Vaccine Vial Monitor) is made of heat sensitive material which change colour if the vaccine vial is exposed to high temperature than recommended.

AFP Surveillance (Acute Flaccid Paralysis)

The eradication of polio is based on our knowledge about polio, effective vaccine and effective surveillance.

We have achieved highest vaccination coverage. We have successfully implemented nationwide mass immunisation. Now, we have to strengthen the surveillance of Acute Flaccid Paralysis so that all cases are detected, investigated and controlled.

HEPATITIS

Hepatitis includes a range of viral pathogens. They are:

1. Hepatitis A (HAV) RNA enterovirus.
2. Hepatitis B (HBV) DNA hepadna.
3. Hepatitis C (HCV) RNA flavivirus.
4. Hepatitis D (HDV) RNA incomplete virus.
5. Hepatitis E (HEV) RNA calicivirus.
6. Hepatitis G (HGV) RNA flavivirus.

Hepatitis A (Infectious Hepatitis, Epidemic Jaundice)

Poor personal hygiene and poor environmental hygiene are facilitators of the illness. Nearly 30% of hepatitis are caused by HAV infection. India has experienced many epidemics in many cities, colonies and in camps.

Incubation period: 15 to 45 days.

Mode of transmission: Faecal oral route.

Clinical Picture

Chills, headache, malaise are succeeded by jaundice. Prominent G.I. symptoms are anorexia, nausea, vomiting and diarrhoea.

Diagnosis

i. Liver function tests (LFT).
ii. Anti HAV of IgM type (Immuno assay) is diagnostic of acute infection.

Investigation	*Reference Range*
Total Protein	6.0–7.5 G%
Albumin	3.5–5.3 G %
Globulin	2.0–2.5 G %
A:G ratio	2:1
Serum Bilirubin	0.1 to 1.0 mg %
Direct Bilirubin	0.0 to 0.35 mg %
Indirect Bilirubin	0.1 to 0.65 mg %
SGOT	0 to 40 I.U./Lt
SGPT	0 to 38 I.U./Lt
Serum Alkaline Phosphate	100 to 290 I.U./Lt
GGT	5 to 38 u/Lt (male) 5 to 29 u/Lt (female)

Common lab. tests for hepatitis infections

Case Management and Nursing Care

Acute cases (severe) need hospitalisation for required nursing care to allow early detection of acute hepatic failure. Reassurance is needed for post hepatitis syndrome. Balanced diet should provide 2000 to 3000 calories per day which should have light diet supplemented by fruit drinks and glucose. The diet should be as per wish of patient for taste. This should take care of high protein intake. IV fluid and glucose may be needed in some of the patients.

Control and Prevention

i. Case finding, notification, disinfection of stool with 0.5% sodium hypochlorite is recommended.
ii. Personal hygiene, environmental hygiene reduces the incidence of HAV infection.
iii. Passive immunity by human immunoglobulin (0.2 ml/kg) is advocated for contacts.
iv. Hepatitis A vaccine 2 doses are given at 6 months interval.

Hepatitis B (Serum Hepatitis)

Hepatitis B is transmitted by parenteral route and is an acute viral infection of liver parenchyma. In 5% of cases they become carriers. Liver cancer is associated with HBV infection.

Incubation period: 45 to 180 days.

Mode of transmission: Essentially it is blood borne infection, though other routes are demonstrated.

Case Management and Nursing Care

Nursing care should focus attention on monitoring acute liver failure. There is no specific treatment. Interferon 5 Mu daily for patients with high serum transaminase is advocated.

Interferon is found useful and helpful in HBV infection to maintain high level concentration of serum transaminase.

Prevention of HBV Infection

i. *Hepatitis B vaccine:* It is formalin inactivated sub unit viral vaccine for I.M. at 1.0 ml dose in 3 doses (0 month, 1 month and 3rd month).

Hepatitis C (HCV)

W.H.O estimate show the HCV infection as 2 to 3 percent of world population. Humans are sole source of infection. Mode of transmissions is through blood and saliva. HCV infection produces chronic infection. Incubation period is 4 to 20 weeks.

Hepatitis D (HDV) (Delta Hepatitis)

This does not have an independent existence. This requires HBV infection for its replication.

Mode of Transmission

Through blood, sexual and vertical transmission. Prevention is by effectively preventing hepatitis B viral infection.

Hepatitis E (HEV)

It spreads through faecal oral route. It is associated with water pollution to spread as waterborne epidemic. Clinically it mimics HAV infection. Recovery is usually 100 percent.

Hepatitis G (HGV)

It is caused by flavivirus through blood. Blood transfusion is blamed for its spread.

RABIES

Rabies attack all warm blooded animals; particularly fox, jackal, wolves, dog and bat population. Incidence of rabies in a country is related with its National Rabies Control Programme. Global epidemiologists have recorded high incidence of 3.3 per 100,000 population both in India and Mexico.

Rabies infects CNS and salivary glands of mammals. It is transmitted through saliva by bite or lick on aberrations. Humans are normally infected from dogs.

Incubation period is 4 to 8 weeks, but it ranges from 9 days to many months. Severe bite on head or neck is associated with shorter I.P.

Clinical Picture

Attempt to drink water provokes violent contractions of inspiratory muscles and diaphragm, making the person "fear of water". Hence the name "Hydrophobia" which is synonym with rabies. Delusion, hallucination, spitting, biting and mania are manifested with rabies patient.

Case Management and Nursing Care

As soon as a case of a dog bite by an infected dog is received, steps are taken to assure patient and his family to overcome unnecessary anxiety state. At the earliest post exposure prophylaxis with ARV is the need of the hour. In all cases post exposure prophylaxis must be started before 5 days from the day of bite to save the life of patient.

Class I	–	Licks, suspected unboiled milk consumption, scratches
Class II	–	Fresh cut, oozing blood, minor wound
Class III	–	Wound on neck, face, palm, lacerated wound

Dose of BPL inactivated vaccine schedule (Pasteur Institute Coonoor):

Wound	*Adult*	*Child*	*Duration*
I	2 ml	1 ml	7 days
II	3 ml	3 ml	10 days
III	5 ml	3 ml	10 days

Vaccination of Persons Bitten by Infected Dog (Post Exposure Prophylaxis)

a. Initially local treatment of wound by cleaning with water and soap–Alcohol or povidone iodine is preferred–Wound suturing should be avoided–Local application of ARS is advocated–Meanwhile antibiotics are started–If possible bitten dog is observed for 10 days.
b. ARS (Anti Rabies Serum)
   Horse ARS 40 i.u./kg on day zero.
   Human ARIG (Human Rabies Immunoglobulin).
   20 i.u./kg (½ I.M. ½ local site)
c. Cell culture vaccine and duck embryo vaccine WHO Intra Muscular regimen is as under:
   6 doses on 0, 3, 7, 14, 28 days and a booster on 90th day is recommended by I.M. to Deltoid muscle.

Other alternate methods are advocated for cell culture vaccine, for better immunogenic property. They are:

* *Reduced multi-site I.M. regimen.*

Rabies in Dogs

Clinically rabies is manifested in 2 forms among dogs:

i. Furious type with behavioural change like running amuck, voice paralysis etc.
ii. Dumb type with quite and spending all the time in sleep state.

Suspected died dog's head can be sent to laboratory, packing in ice in air tight container. If brain is sent, it should be immersed in 50% glycerol saline.

Dog Vaccine

- *BPL vaccine:* Single dose 5 ml for dogs, 3 ml for cats. Booster dose at 6th month is advocated. Later once in a year they are revaccinated.
- *Chick embryo vaccine:* 3 ml by single injection given once in 3 years.

Public Health Measures for Dog Menace

- Elimination of stray dogs
- Registration, licensing of domestic dogs
- Destruction of animals bitten by infected dogs
- 6 months quarantine for imported dogs
- Health awareness on Rabies in the community.

AIDS (ACQUIRED IMMUNO DEFICIENCY SYNDROME)

AIDS is caused by human Immuno Deficiency Virus (HIV). It is a serious disorder of the body immune system in which the body normal defences against infection break down, leaving the body vulnerable to a host of life threatening infections and life threatening conditions including unusual malignancies.

Indian Picture

Since the detection of HIV in Tamil Nadu in 1986, there has been a steady increase in HIV/AIDS seeking treatment in hospitals.

Agent

It is a virus (lentivirus) one of the subfamily of retroviruses. Its enzyme copies viral RNA to DNA which eventually integrates to host cell. Hence eradication of HIV/AIDS is not found possible. HIV-1 and HIV-2 are common types of infective agent.

Reservoirs of infection are men suffering from disease. Source of infection are infected blood, semen and vaginal fluids. Infected breast milk may be source of infection from mother to child.

Saliva and Tears are not source of infection.

Host Factors

Young people 20-30 years age in both sexes are found infected with HIV/AIDS. Certain group of people show higher risk of infection. They are:

- Person suffering from RTI/STD
- Frequency of exposure of unprotected sex
- Mixing pattern of population
- Drug users
- Sex workers
- Profound lymphopenia.

Socioeconomic Factors

Following socioeconomic factors influence the occurrence of HIV/AIDS:

i. Low literacy.
ii. Urbanization.
iii. Imprisonment.
iv. High mobility.
v. Migration and separation from family.
vi. Drug use.
vii. Alcohol use.

Mode of Transmission

- Intercourse with infected person
- Blood transfusion by infected blood
- Drug users by common syringe use (Includes mother to child transmission).

Natural History of HIV/AIDS

Stage 1

Infection with HIV results in rapid proliferation of the virus in blood and lymph nodes. The infected person may experience a seroconversion illness, which usually resolves within weeks. The CD_4 cell count declines rapidly before virus is controlled by the immune system, whereupon the count returns to near normal.

Stage 2

During stage 2, the immune system has controlled the virus, which is largely restricted to lymphoid tissue. In this the damage inflicted by the virus is limited to the regenerative capacity of the immune system and people with HIV are usually without symptoms. CD_4 count will be above 500/ml in this stage.

Stage 3

In this stage viral replication is very high and CD_4 cell turnover is rapid. Subtle signs and symptoms indicating compromise of immune system begin to appear. CD_4 cell count will be 200-500/ml.

Stage 4

The virus which proliferate throughout the body, overcomes the immune system.

National Guidelines for HIV Testing

1. Surveillance to monitor trend.
2. Transfusion safety.
3. Voluntary testing purpose.
4. Research.

Case Management and Nursing Care

Drug:

1. Nucleoside analogue
   Zidovudine (AZT) (Retrovir)
   500-600 mg orally daily in 3 divided doses
2. Protease inhibitor
   Saquinavir (invirase)
   600 mg orally 3 times daily
3. Non-nucleoside reverse transcriptase inhibitor
   Nevirapine (viramune)–200 mg orally daily for 2 weeks, then 200 mg orally twice daily.

Counselling

Nurse in her counselling, with the help of medical social worker, will listen, understands client's dignity and uses good communication skill and non-judgemental attitude. Pre-test counselling is done before HIV test and post test counselling is done after HIV testing.

Blood Transfusion

Promotion of voluntary blood donation should get top priority.

AIDS Education

Health education on AIDS enables people to make life saving choices.

Health Care

Primary health care for HIV/AIDS with an integration of R.C.H., F.W.P. and health education.

Nursing Management of Needle Stick Injury

Being risk group, nursing professionals have to deal with anticipated accidental exposures to HIV. Average risk is 1 in 300 (0.3%) and prevention is the main strategy to avoid occupational exposure to HIV.

Use of protective barrier

- Latex or vinyl gloves
- Heavy duty rubber glove at cleaning
- Gloves and apron at surgery
- Protective eye wear
- Safe handling of sharps.

If injury (after exposure)

- Wash the injury with soap and water
- Splash to the nose, mouth, skin should be flushed with water
- Eyes are irrigated with clean water
- Don't put prinked finger into mouth
- Report to authorities
- Post exposure prophylaxis (PEP) may be recommended.

National AIDS Control Programme

This was launched in 1987. Main aim is to reduce the spread and strengthen India's capacity in terms of production and economics.

The programme includes:

a. Blood safety programme.
b. Policy on HIV testing.
c. STD control programme.
d. Condom promotion.
e. HIV surveillance.
f. HIV sentinal surveillance.
g. IEC activities.
h. Social mobilisation.
i. Family health awareness campaign.
j. Prevention of mother to child transmission

BACTERIAL INFECTIONS

DIPHTHERIA

It is an acute bacterial infection of tonsil, pharynx, larynx and nasal mucous membrane caused by C.diptheriae. The known reservoir is man. It spreads from person to person. From case or carrier the disease spreads both by droplet infection and contact. Milk contamination can cause epidemics.

Powerful exotoxin causes:

- False membrane
- Lymphadenopathy
- Toxaemia

Case fatality rate is 10% which is reduced to 5% among treated cases.

Incubation period–2-6 days.

Clinical Feature

"Wash leather" elevated greyish green membrane on the tonsils is a diagnostic feature. The membrane has well defined edge, firm, adherent and surrounded by inflammatory zone. Bull neck and tender enlarged lymph node predominate.

In untreated case circulatory failure occurs within 10 days.

Complications

- Laryngeal obstruction, paralysis
- Myocarditis
- Peripheral neuropathy.

Schick Test

It is done to find out susceptibility to infection and success of immunisation. 0.2 ml of Schick test toxin intradermally with control is tested.

Vaccines

Absorbed DPT (Triple antigen) is available from Kasauli and Glaxo.

DPT is stored at 4-8°C. Immunisation is followed as per UIP schedule (discussed under general epidemiology). Primary immunisation is started at 6 week after birth. Three doses with 1 month interval is optimal for effective immunisation. It is given deep IM Very mild reaction like fever may follow which is ignorable. No severe complications are seen in routine immunisation. But possibility of 1 in a million, convulsion, encephalitis, Reye's syndrome should be kept in mind.

There is no contraindication for DPT. Only acutely ill hospitalized child is excluded.

In case of children above 12 years, DT (Paediatrics double antigen) is given 2 doses at 1 month interval and a booster at 12 months after second dose. For adults dT (adult double antigen) is used in the same manner.

III Antisera : Diphtheria Anti Toxin

It is passive agent 500 to 2000 units by IM as a prophylaxis. For therapy high dose is used 30,000 unit IM may be needed.

WHOOPING COUGH

Whooping cough is caused by *Bordetella pertussis.*

In unimmunised children cough, whoop and vomiting are characteristic signs. Young infants do not whoop, although the cough is still spasmodic and is followed by vomiting.

Incubation period 7-4 days.

The clinical course has a catarrhal stage lasting for 10 days, paroxysmal stage lasting for 20 days and a convalescent stage lasting for 2 weeks.

Control of Whooping Cough

Cases are diagnosed, isolated and treated. Erythromycin 50 mg/kg body weight in 4 divided doses for 10 days is recommended. Alternatively ampicillin, cotriamaxzole or tetracycline as suggested by M.O.H. Epidemic Disease Hospital or an attending paediatrician should be considered.

The problem of cases and contacts do not occur if primary immunisation under U.I.P. is done with high coverage in the community.

Vaccines

i. D.P.T. is used in active immunisation as per U.I.P. schedule.

TUBERCULOSIS

Tuberculosis is a chronic bacterial disease caused by Mycobacterium tuberculosis and an important cause of death in most parts of the world.

In developed countries added reasons are immigration from high prevalence area, social deprivation and rising life expectancy.

Problem–World

Every year 8 million new cases are occurring and is killing 2.9 million people each year.

Problem—India

Every year 2 million people are developing tuberculosis and nearly 500,000 die from it – more than 1000 per day.

Common Terms in Tuberculosis

i. *New case :* Sputum +ve pulmonary TB who has never taken treatment.
ii. *Failure case:* Sputum +ve case, after 5 months treatment, still show +ve.
iii. *Relapse:* Sputum +ve case declared cured show again sputum +ve.
iv. *Defaulter:* One who left the treatment in between.
v. *Cured:* Sputum + case after treatment show sputum –ve on at least 2 occasion.

Natural History of Tuberculosis

Nearly 80% of population must have had their exposure one day or the other to tuberculosis. Many develop sero conversion and thus a few develop different adult variants of tuberculosis.

As Sequelae of Bronchial Complications

This lead to bronchial obstruction, bronchiectasis and fibrosis.

Latent period between primary infection and the development of pulmonary tuberculosis in adult life is longer in European countries and shorter in Asia and African countries.

Tuberculin Test

It is a skin test developed to find out the evidence of past or present infection with M. tuberculosis. Mantoux test is done by 0.5 ml P.P.D. (1 T.U.) intradermally on flexor surface of forearm. It is read after 72 hours. Result will be positive if 10 mm of induration is observed.

Incubation period: 3 to 6 weeks will be the duration for infection to tuberculin +ve stage. For disease development the period is uncertain.

Mode of transmission: Droplet infection and droplet nuclei.

Community Parameters

a. Prevalence of infection–Tuberculin +ve = 30%

b. Incidence of infection–Newly infected (TB conversion index) = 2%
c. Prevalence of disease = AFB +ve = 0.4%
d. Prevalence of X-ray suspect = 2%
e. Prevalence of drug resistant = 10%
f. Mortality rate = 60 per 100,000.

Control of Tuberculosis

Tuberculosis control is said to be achieved when the prevalence of natural infection in 0-14 year children is 1%. Control is by (a) Curative by case finding and prompt treatment (b) Preventive by B.C.G. vaccination.

Case Finding Tools: Any case who show (a) Persistent cough of 1 month duration (b) Continuous evening rise of temperature (c) Chest pain and (d) Haemoptysis are subjected for sputum examination for A.F.B.

For chemotherapy we have major bactericidal and bacteriostatic drugs.

Bactericidal

i. *Streptomycin :* It acts on rapidly multiplying A.F.B. Daily dose is 0.75 to 1.0 gram in single injection. Vestibular damage and nystagmus are drug side effects.
ii. *I.N.H.:* It is the most powerful drug. It acts on bacilli. It is given as a single dose 4-5 mg/kg body weight (max. 300 mg). For intermittent therapy 700 mg twice a week is given.
Gastric irritation, neuropathy, liver damage are side reactions.
iii. *Pyrazinamide:* Acts on slow multiplying intra cellular A.F.B. Dose is 30 mg/kg body weight divided into 3 doses per day. Side reactions are liver damage and hyperuricaemia.
iv. *Rifampicin:* It permeates all tissue membranes and kill bacilli. Even extensive tuberculosis is curable with rifampicin. Dose is 10-12 mg/kg body weight taken 1 hour before or 2 hours after food. Daily convenient dose is 450-600 mg. For intermittent therapy 900 mg is given. Side reactions noticed are gastritis, thrombocytopenia and nephrotoxicity.

Bacteriostatic

i. *Ethambutol:* It is used in combination to control drug resistance. Dose is 15 mg/kg body weight given in 3 doses.
ii. *Thioacetazone:*
In combination with I.N.H., it is used. Dose is 2 mg/kg body weight. Side effects are nausea, vomiting, blurring of vision and urticaria.
iii. Other bacteriostatic drugs are ethionamide, PAS, cycloserine, kanamycin and viomycin.

Earlier regimen was domiciliary or ambulatory treatment under (a) Daily regimen and (b) Biweekly regimen. But it is now totally replaced with short course therapy under R.N.T.C.P.

D.T.C. is reference centre for diagnosis and treatment in the district. It is also responsible for training and supervision.

R.N.T.C.P.

R.N.T.C.P. Case Detection

- Spot, early morning, spot—3 sputum exam of patients with cough of 3 weeks.
- Health awareness by H.E. on Respiratory symptoms.
- Contact exam of AFB +ve children.
- Evaluation of chest X-ray.

RNTCP Treatment Regimens

Diagnosis is done as per flow chart shown as: (a) Pulmonary +ve (b) Pulmonary –ve and (c) extrapulmonary cases.

Treatment is instituted as per R.N.T.C.P. treatment regimen.

Category I : Initial phase extended by 1 month of smear if +ve after 2 months.

Category II : Re-treatment cases. Initial phase extended by 1 month if smear is positive after 3 months.

Category III : If smear is +ve at 2 months categorised as failure case and treated afresh.

DOTS Chemotherapy (Directly Observe Treatment, Short Course)

DOTS is a strategy to ensure that by providing most effective drug and confirming that the drug is taken (Fig. 11.8).

Fig. 11.8: The DOTS Strategy

It is the only documented effective programme in the world. The DOTS strategy are:

- Political commitment
- Diagnosis by microscopy
- Adequate supply of right drugs
- Directly observed treatment
- Accountability.

B.C.G. Vaccine (Bacilli Calmette Guerin)

0.1 mg in 0.1 ml (For new born 0.05 ml). It is given intra-dermally with B.C.G. syringe (Omega Microstat syringe with 1 cm sted 26 gauge needle). It is either given at birth (Hospital deliveries) or at 6th week under primary immunisation. BCG has protective value of 20 years and it prevents nonpulmonary serious complications of tuberculosis. B.C.G. is not given for cases with eczema, hypogammaglobulinaemia.

Revised National T.B. Control Programme

Details of National TB Control Programme is dealt in Chapter 17 page 255. Government of India along with World Bank revised the National TB control programme in 1992. The main strategies under revised N.T.P. are:

- Achievement of not less than 85% cure rate among infectious cases of tuberculosis through short term chemotherapy involving peripheral health functionary.
- Detecting 70% of estimated cases through quality sputum microscopy.
- Involvement of NGO's.
- Direct observed therapy short term (DOTS) as community based TB treatment and care strategy.

Tuberculosis and HIV

It is a lethal combination that accelerates tuberculosis progress from harmless infection to life threatening condition. Tuberculosis is an opportunistic infection that kills HIV +ve people. Tuberculosis with HIV can be treated effectively if early diagnosis is made.

MENINGOCOCCAL MENINGITIS

Meningitis is known as "Cerebrospinal fever" and is referred to meningococcal meningitis caused by menigococci organism.

Acute infection of meningitis is characterised by pyrexia, headache and meningism. This is associated with neck stiffness and meningeal irritation, which is demonstrated by:

India–Problem

Sporadic meningitis are being reported. Annual case is about 7 to 8 thousand and annual death is about 8 to 9 hundred.

Incubation period—3-4 days.

Mode of transmission is by droplet infection.

Clinical Feature

Headache, drowsiness, fever, neck stiffness, signs of cerebral oedema due to endotoxin/cytokine release, purpuric skin rash and circulatory failure.

Investigation—Lumbar puncture (L.P.).

Case Management and Nursing Care

Benzylpenicillin 2.4 G. I.V. 6 hourly even before hospital admission is advocated. Hospitalisations, regular nursing care, C.S.F. analysis for any treatment regimen change, are advocated. Steroid therapy is useful in paediatric patients.

Control Measures

i. **Case management:** Life saving penicillin is given as suggested under case management. Isolation has limited use.
ii. **Carrier management:** Rifampicin or more powerful antibiotics are advocated to eradicate organisms in carriers.
iii. **Contact management:** They need chemoprophylaxis. Rifampicin 600 mg BD for 2 days for adults is given.
iv. **Mass management:** In international religious congregations (e.g. Mecca), medically supervised chemoprophylaxis is undertaken.
v. **Vaccination:** Monovalent or polyvalent vaccine are administered to risk group or visiting group which gives 3 years immunity. It is not recommended to below 2 year children.
vi. **Prevention of** overcrowding and improved housing along with health awareness campaign is very helpful.

CHOLERA

Cholera is one of the International Quarantine disease caused by V. cholerae.

Man is the only known natural host of cholera. Transmission is through ingestion of contaminated food and water. Incubation is from few hours to 5 days.

- Classical cholera (Vibro cholera) known even early to 1817.
- El Tor cholera (Eltor vibrio) was found in 1961.
- 0139 strain cholera (cholera of new era) was found in 1992.
- Water transmission followed by person transmission are source of infection.
- Absolute differences between classical type and El Tor type are recorded.
- All 3 strains classical, El Tor and 0139 are causing epidemics, deaths and acute public health problem.

Clinical Features

Sudden onset of severe diarrhoea without pain, colic and is succeeded by vomiting. Clear fluid and flecks of mucus characterise diarrhoea as "Rice water" stools. Classical type produces severe dehydration by loss of fluid and electrolytes and lead to muscular cramps. Oliguria shock develops with good mental clarity. Acute circulatory failure causes death. El Tor and 0139 type manifest in mild form but are acute in children.

Community Diagnosis of Cholera

In 100 cases of diarrhoea due to cholera, 70% show rapid dehydration that requires hospitalisation. 15 to 20% die due to cholera if early action in case management is not taken (Tables 11.6 and 11.7).

Table 11.6: Differentials in cholera types in the community

Vibrio Classical	*Vibrio El Tor and 0139*
Severe cases are more	Mild cases are more
Secondary cases are less	Secondary cases are more
Not resistant to environment	More resistant to environment
No carrier stage	Carrier stage present

Table 11.7: Laboratory differentials

Classical		*El Tor*
RBC (Chicken, sheep)		
Agglutination	No	Yes
Phage IV resistance	No	Yes
Polymyxin B resistance	No	Yes
V P reaction	+ve	-ve

Stool sample collection in isolation wards:

- Fresh sample must be collected
- Should be collected before giving antibiotic.

i. *Rectal swab:* 20 cm. long wooden stick with one end wrapped with absorbent cotton, sterilised by autoclaving, is dipped into holding medium before introducing into rectum. This is placed in a sterile plastic bag, sealed and sent to laboratory with details.

ii. *Rubber catheter:* No.26-28 soft rubber catheter is sterilised by boiling. It is lubricated with liquid paraffin. This is introduced to rectum for a 4 cm length. The stool is collected to VR medium and sent to laboratory with details.

Case Management

For severe cases I.V. Ringer Lactate is best fluid. When vomiting stops, oral fluid is started. This may be 5 litres per day in humid climate.

3 days treatment with tetracycline 250 mg 6th hourly is recommended. To make bacterial load to minimum, a single dose of 300 mg doxycycline or 1 gram of ciprofloxacin is highly recommended. Children (paediatric ward) nursing care should include to check hypoglycaemia and careful attention to fluid balance.

Cholera Control

As per WHO guidelines following steps are recommended for cholera control:

a. Confirmation of cholera
b. Notification to local, national and to WHO
c. Early diagnosis and prompt treatment
d. Rehydration by:
   - Oral rehydration
   - I.V. rehydration
   - Maintenance therapy
e. Chemotherapy
f. Epidemiological investigation
g. Environmental sanitation
h. Vaccination
i. Health education.
   a. Confirmation of case of diarrhoea, due to cholera is first task before taking public health measures. Laboratory service is essential.
   b. It is internationally quarantinable and notifiable. Notification to local authorities is done who in turn do the further needful.
   c. Early diagnosis reduces mortality and early treatment reduces both mortality and morbidity. Isolation hospital, epidemic disease hospital and treatment centres take care of these as special measures.
   d. *Rehydration:*
      i. *Assessment of dehydration:* During nursing care, check the following at your assessment of dehydration:

– Blood in the stool	– Fever
– Spleen palpable	– Unconsciousness
– Convulsion	– Difficult, fast, deep breathing
– PEM in children	

ii. *Oral fluids:*

O.R.S. (Oral Rehydration Solution):

Sodium Chloride (Table Salt)—3.5 G
Sodium Bicarbonate 2.5 G
(Baking soda)
Potassium chloride 1.5 G
Glucose (dextrose) 20.0 G

Home made solution: (for emergency)

Table salt—Thumb and 2 finger pinch
Water
Or
Orange juice ½ litre
Or
Tea

iii. *Sustenance takes care of the following:* (a) Serious problems that cause or complicate dehydration (b) Maintaining rehydration and (c) Helps in nutritional rehabilitation. During this period *nursing care* should check:

- Pneumonia
- Otitis media
- Tonsillitis
- Skin infection
- Deep sighing breathing
- Malaria
- Unconsciousness
- Convulsions
- High fever.

iv. *Prevention*

- Educating mother
- Solving problem of water supply
- Solving problem of sanitation.

Making Oral Fluid in Nursing Care: One litre glucose salt solution should contain:

Sodium chloride	3.5 G
Sodium bicarbonate	2.5 G
Potassium chloride	1.5 G
Glucose	20.0 G

For clinics, hospitals, bags or bottles containing 10 times this amount for dissolving in 10 litres of water is more practical.

Standard measure is used at dispensing. Once prepared, the O.R.S. should be used within 24 hours. Every 24 hours, fresh solution is prepared. It should not be boiled.

Nutritional care during diarrhoea: Breast milk is best food for infants and should be continued in diarrhoea also.

Earlier it was believed that undernutrition is due to inadequate food consumption alone. But the role of diarrhoea and other infections in causing undernutrition is now well-recognised.

During diarrhoea, following nutritional advice is of paramount importance:

- Soft, easily digestible food which will be almost totally absorbed even if diarrhoea is present.
- Small frequent meals instead of a single large dish.
- Energy dense food like, oil, ghee or sugar which in small quantity provide more energy and reduce the bulk in food.

v. *Chemotherapy:*

- Tetracycline
  12.5 mg/kg for children — 4 times a day for 3 days
  500 mg for adults
- Doxycycline
  300 mg adults
- Trimethroprim
  5 mg/kg — Children
- Sulfamethoxazole — twice daily
  25 mg/kg — 3 days

vi. Epidemiological investigation considers source detection, sanitary survey and contact tracing.

vii. Under environmental sanitation water control, excreta disposal, food sanitation and proper disinfection of patients' secretion and excretion are advocated.

viii. *Vaccination:* Cholera vaccine is killed vaccine preserved in phenol. Two doses 0.5 ml subcutaneously each at 6 weeks interval give protection for 3-6 months.
ix. Health education on reporting, food hygiene, vaccination, breastfeeding in diarrhoea phase and nutritional care during diarrhoea are advocated.

Cholera Control Programme

It is now under Diarrhoeal Disease Control programme. (C.D.D. programme = Control of Diarrhoeal Diseases Programme).

TYPHOID

Typhoid and paratyphoid are common causes of fever in developing countries. They are rare in developed countries.

Mode of Transmission: Faecal oral route or urine oral route. Directly by ingestion of contaminated water, food or flies and indirectly by contaminated hands.

Clinical Features

During first week of infection, fever, headache, myalgia, relative bradycardia, constipation (Diarrhoea and vomiting in young patients) are common.

During second week of infection, rose spots on trunk, splenomegaly, cough, abdominal distension and diarrhoea are common.

During third week, in untreated cases delirium, complications, coma and death are noticed.

In case of paratyphoid, symptoms are milder, onset is abrupt with acute enteritis, rashes will be abundant and complications are rare.

Complications

- Perforation and haemorrhage of intestine
- Septicaemic foci cause bone infection, joint infection, meningitis and cholecystitis
- Toxic pneumonia
- Myocarditis
- Nephritis

Investigations

- W.B.C. count for leucopenia
- Blood culture in first week
- Stool culture in second week
- Widal test in second week.

Case Management and Nursing Care

i. Ciprofloxacin 500 mg 12 hourly
ii. Cotrimoxazole 2 tablet 12 hourly
iii. Amoxicillin 750 mg 6 hourly
iv. Chloramphenicol 500 mg 6 hourly.

In resistance case, third generation antibiotics like Cephalosporins, Ceftriaxone and Cefotaxime are used with caution.

The treatment is continued for 14 days. Pyrexia persists for 5 days with treatment. Chronic carriers are treated with ciprofloxacin for 4 weeks. In some cases of carrier's stage, cholecystectomy may be needed.

Control of Typhoid

i. Case management by early diagnosis.
ii. Carriers are given one course of drugs
iii. *Sanitation:*
   - Water purification
   - Food hygiene
   - Environmental hygiene
iv. *Immunisation:*

Monovalent, bivalent and trivalent vaccines are available.

Oral vaccine is available (Typhoral): It contains Ty21 strain. It is available in enteric coated capsule form. One capsule on 1st, 3rd and 5th day one hour before meal in tepid water; gives protection from 15th day to 3 years.

Prevention

Improved sanitation and improved living condition reduces the incidence. Travellers visiting endemic area are immunised to overcome the infection.

LEPROSY

Leprosy is a chronic bacterial infection caused by *Mycobacterium leprae*. Common organs involved are nerve, skin, eye, bone and internal organs. Two major entities are clinically recognised. They are:

a. Infectious type (Lepromatous) (LL).
b. Non-infectious type (Tuberculoid) (TT).

For the purpose of treatment and prognosis, leprosy is classified according to bacterial presence. They are:

a. *Multibacillary:* This contains LL, BL and BB.
b. *Paucibacillary:* This contains indeterminate (I), TT and BT.

Problem–India

- Prevalence rate 3.8 per 10,000
- Single skin lesion among new cases 4.1%
- Proportion of multibacillary and paucibacillary type:
  MB = 49.2% PB 50.8%
- New case rate is 55 per 100,000
  Mode of transmission: Droplet and contact
  Incubation period: 3-5 years.

Clinical Features

Hypopigmented anaesthetic patches and thickened nerves are markedly seen. Nodules are seen on skin, face, ears.

In late phase of leprosy, loss of fingers, nasal depression, foot drop, claw toes, plantar ulcers are seen.

Lepromin Test

It is an useful tool in case evaluation on immune status, for classification and to estimate prognosis. 0.1 ml of lepromin intradermally to inner aspect of forearm is given. The reaction is read at 48 hours and on 21st day.

a. If induration and redness is more than 10 mm at 48 hours, it is +ve and is called early reaction (Fernandez reaction).
b. On 21st day a nodule of more than 5 mm is positive. This is late reaction (Mitsuda reaction).

Leprosy Reactions

There are 2 types of leprosy reactions:

A. Reversal Type–1 Reaction:
This is cell mediated hypersensitivity and is called Arthus Phenomenon. Clinically it shows painful tender nerves, loss of function, swollen skin lesions, new skin lesions and rarely fever. Loss of nerve function is sudden, with foot drop by overnight. Recovery is good with M.D.T. regimen.

B. Erythema Nodosum Leprosum
Type–2 Reaction: This is due to immune complex deposition. Clinically it shows tender nodules and papules. They may ulcerate. Painful tender nerve, loss of function, iritis, orchitis, myositis, lymphadenitis, fever and oedema are other reactions.

Treatment of Leprosy Reaction

Arthus Phenomenon

a. Aspirin 600 mg 6th hourly
b. Prednisolone 40-80 mg tapered in 9 months.

Erythema Nodosum Leprosum

a. Aspirin 600 mg 6th hourly
b. Prednisolone 20-40 mg tapered in 6 months
c. Local treatment for eye involvement.

National Leprosy Elimination Campaign

N.L.E.C. has the following objectives:

a. To carry out intensive awareness campaign about leprosy involving the community in the campaign.
b. To give 1 day training to MOH, HS, MPW (M) and (F), VHG, AWW etc., to appraise them about the case detection procedure is adopted.

c. To give 3 days training to PHC staff who have joined the service recently.
d. To give I.E.C. training to Media officers, B.E.E., H.E. and H.S.
e. To detect hidden leprosy cases by active house to house search for 6 days or at fixed voluntary reporting centres on 2 previously fixed dates.
f. To confirm and treat all the detected cases with M.D.T.

L.E.C.: Leprosy Elimination Campaign is an initiative to detect leprosy that remained undetected and to cure them. Elements involved in L.E.C. are:

i. Capacity building measures for local health workers to improve M.D.T.
ii. Increasing community participation; and
iii. Diagnosis and curing leprosy patients.

S.A.P.E.L.: Special action projects for elimination of leprosy is an initiative aimed at providing M.D.T. services to patients living in "special difficult to access areas" or situation or to those belonging to "neglected population groups."

WHO "MDT" Regimen:

A. **Clinical grouping:**

Lesion	*PB Single skin lesion (Patch)*	*PB Paucibacillary*	*MB Multi-bacillary*
1. Skin lesion	1	2-5	6 and above
2. Nerve involvement	No	only one	More than one
3. Skin smear	-ve	-ve	+ve

B. **Treatment:**

	Drug	*Dose*	*Frequency*	*Criteria for cure*
M.B.	Rifampicin	600 mg	Once monthly	Completion of
	Dapsone	100 mg	Daily	12 monthly
	Clofazimine	300 mg	Once monthly	Pulses
		50 mg	Daily	Within 18 months
P.B.	Rifampicin	600 mg	Once monthly	Completion of 6
	Dapsone	100 mg	Daily	monthly Pulses Within 9 months
Single Skin Lesion	Rifampicin Ofloxacin Minocycline	600 mg 400 mg 100 mg	Single dose	Single dose treatment

Under N.L.E.P., Leprosy control units and SET centres play vital role. Major points are tabulated as under :

L.C.U. (Leprosy control treatment unit)		*S.E.T. (Survey education unit)*
800	Number	6000
1%	Prevalence	0.5 to 1.0%
A control unit	Status	a sub-centre
1 M O 12 Para-medical workers	Staff	1 non medical Supervisor 5 PM worker
150,000 population	Coverage	10,000 population

In India NLCP was started in 1955. Later in 1983 Government of India declared to eradicate leprosy by 2000. Now the goal is to reduce 1 per 10,000 population by 2005.

TETANUS

Tetanus is caused by clostridium tetani bacteria which is an ubiquitous organism in soil. Tetanus is of public health importance because of N.N.T. (Neonatal Tetanus) causing Neonatal mortality in developing countries. Generalised tetanus from infected umbilical stump is characteristic of neonatal tetanus. The main causes of death are pneumonia, respiratory failure, circulatory failure, haemorrhage and septicaemia; even sudden death by severe spasm is recorded.

In India, tetanus, being still a public health problem made the administration to gear up priority work. This gave rise to district grouping according to risk of N.N.T.

Tetanus is an occupational hazard among agricultural workers. Soil, agriculture, animal husbandry compounded by social factors will influence the occurrence of tetanus in the community. It is also associated with unhygienic delivery practices; custom and habit of applying *Bhasmum* or cow dung on the stump; use of unsterilised instrument to cut the cord is illustrations of tetanus being a social disease.

Incubation period: 6-10 days.

Types of clinical tetanus according to its source are:

1. Traumatic
2. Puerperal
3. Otogenic
4. Neonatal
5. Idiopathic.

Case Management and Nursing Care

Neutralise toxin by :

By I.V. injection 3000 I.U. human tetanus antitoxin.

Prevent further toxin by:

- By debridement of wound
- Benzylpencillin 600 mg 1 V 6 hourly (metronidazole as alternative).

Control the Spasm by

- Nursing in a quiet room.
- Avoid noise, light and other stimuli
- I.V. diazepam for spasms.

General nursing by:

- Hydration
- Nutrition (tube feeding)
- Treating secondary infections.

Wound treatment strategy in hospital:

Vaccine

1. D.P.T. as suggested under U.I.P.
2. D.T. or dT as suggested under diphtheria management.
3. TT 2 doses of 0.5 ml each IM at 1 month interval, Third dose is given at 1 year, Fourth dose after 5 years of primary dose. Immunologists and surgeons are of the opinion that frequent booster dose is useless and must be avoided.
4. Human tetanus hyper immunoglobulin is best prophylaxis. Dose is 250 I.U.

ACUTE RESPIRATORY INFECTION (ARI)

It is a common cause of morbidity among elderly and common cause for mortality among young children. Depending on the site of infection, upper and lower respiratory tract infections are classified.

Clinically the entities are grouped under (a) Very severe (b) Severe (c) Pneumonia and (d) No pneumonia for the case management. Common sequelae are: (a) Ear problems and (b) sore throat.

Problem–India

A.R.I. is one of the major cause of I.M.R. in India. Hospital data show that about 13 to 14 percent of paediatric outpatient load is by acute respiratory infections. Two problems are encountered with respect to the case management. They are:

Common causative agents of A.R.I. are as under (Table 11.8):

Table 11.8: Common pathogens causing A.R.I.

Virus	*Bacteria*	*Others*
Adenovirus type 2 and 5	Bordetella	Chlamydia Type B
Influenza B	Klebsiella	Mycoplasma
Measles	Streptococci	
Respiratory syncytial		
Corona		

Mode of transmission: It is airborne and by person to person contact.

Management of the child with cough or difficult breathing

ASSESS

ASK

- How old is the child ?
- Is the child coughing ? For how long?
- Age 2 months upto 5 years: Is the child able to drink ?
  Age less than 2 months: Has the young infant stopped feeding well ?
- Has the child had fever ? For how long ?
- Has the child had convulsions ?

LOOK, LISTEN

(Child must be calm)

* Count the breaths in one minute.
* Look for chestin drawing.
* Look and listen for stridor.
* Look and listen for wheeze. Is it recurrent?
* See if the child is abnormally sleepy or difficult to wake.
* Feel for fever; or low body temperature (or measure temperature).
* Look for severe malnutiriton.

CLASSIFY THE ILLNESS

	THE YOUNG INFANT AGE LESS THAN 2 MONTHS	
Signs	* Stopped feeding well * Convulsions * Abnormally sleepy or difficult to wake * Stridor in calm child * Wheezing or * Fever or low body temperature	
Classify as	VERY SEVERE DISEASE	
Treatment	‣ Refer urgently to hospital ‣ Keep young infant warm ‣ Give first dose of an antibiotic	
Signs	* Severe chest indrawing Or * Fast breathing (60 per minute or more)	* No severe chest indrawing and * No fast breathing (Less than 60 per minute)
Classify as	SEVERE PNEUMONIA	NO PNEUMONIA : COUGH OR COLD
Treatment	* Refer urgently to hospital * Keep young infant warm * Give first dose of an antibiotic (If referral is not feasible: treat with an antibiotic and follow closely)	* Advise mother to give the following home care * Keep young infant warm * Breastfeeding frequently * Clear nose if it interferes with feeding * Return quickly if: * Breathing becomes difficult * Breathing becomes fast * Feeding becomes a problem * The young infant becomes sicker

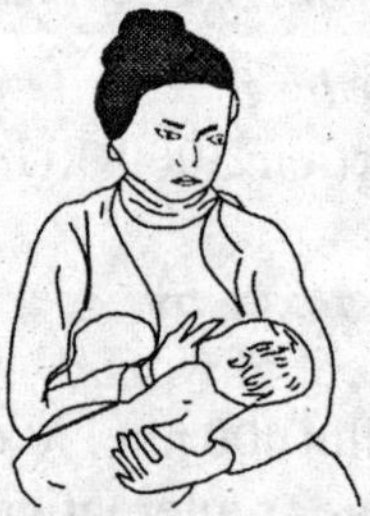

THE CHILD AGE 2 MONTHS UPTO 5 YEARS

Does child have danger signs ?		
	SIGNS	* Not able to drink * Convulsions * Abnormally sleepy or difficult to wake * Stridor in calm child or * Severe malnutrition
	CLASSIFY BY	VERY SEVERE DISEASE
	TREATMENT	‣ Refer URGENTLY to hospital ‣ Give first dose of an antibiotic ‣ Treat fever, if present ‣ Treat wheezing, if present ‣ If cerebral malaria is possible, give an antimalarial

Does child have pneumonia ?				
	SIGNS	* Chest indrawing Or (If also recurrent go directly to ‣ **Treat Wheezing**	* No chest indrawing and * Fast breathing (50 per minute or more if child 2 months upto 12 months ; 40 per minute or more if child 12 months up to 5 years	* No chest indrawing and * No fast breathing (Less than 50 per minute if child 2 months upto 12 months; Less than 40 per minute if child 12 months upto 5 years)
	CLASSIFY AS	SEVERE PNEUMONIA	PNEUMONIA	NO PNEUMONIA COUGH OR COLD
	TREATMENT	* Refer URGENTLY to hospital * Give first dose of an antibiotic * Treat fever if present * Treat wheezing, if present (If referral is not feasible, treat with an antibiotic and follow closely)	* Advise mother to give home care * Give an antibiotic * Treat fever if present * Treat wheezing, if present * Advise mother to return with child in 2 days for reassessment, or earlier if the child is getting worse	* If coughing more than 30 days refer for assessment * Assess and treat ear problem if present (see chart) * Assess and treat other problems * Advise mother to give home care * Treat fever, if present * Treat wheezing, if present

	Reassess in 2 days a child who is takin an antibiotic for pneumonia		
SIGNS	WORSE * Not able to drink * Has chest indrawing * Has other danger signs	THE SAME	IMPROVING * Breathing slower * Less fever * Eating better
TREATMENT	* Refer URGENTLY to hospital	Change antibiotic or refer :	Finish 5 days of antibioutic

Advise Mother to Give Home Care (For the child age 2 months upto 5 years)*

- **Feed the child**
  - Feed the child during illness
  - Increase feeding after illness
  - **Clear the nose if it interferes with feeding**
- **Increase fluids**
  - Offer the child extra to drink
  - Increase breastfeeding
- **Soothe the throat and relieve the cough with a safe remedy**
- **Most important: In the child classified as having No pneumonia: Cough or Cold, watch for the following signs and return quickly if they occur:**
  - Breathing become difficult
  - Breathing becomes fast
  - Child is not able to drink
  - Child becomes sicker

  } This child may have pneumonia

* See section on young infant for home care instructions for that age group

A.R.I. Control Programme

It was initiated in 1990. When C.S.S.M. programme was launched in 1992, the ARI control programme became the part and parcel of CSSM. Since 1997 it is part of RCH programme at national level.

Training of health workers to recognise and treat at first contact, distribution of cotrimoxazole supplied to RCH drug kit is main activity under ARI control programme.

Home Care Instructions for Mother

i. *Infant below 2 months*
- Keep infant warm
- Breast feed frequently
- Clear nose if it interferes with feeding
- Take the child to doctor if
  a. Breathing becomes difficult
  b. Breathing becomes faster
  c. Feeding is not possible
  d. Infant seems to be really sick

ii. *Infant from 2 months to 5 years.*

Figure 11.9 gives specific idea for home care of children from 2 months to 5 years. Mother or patients must take precaution to:

a. Feed the child.
b. Fluid intake is maintained by extra drink and breastfeeding.
c. Safe remedy for cough and throat irritation is given; and
d. Watch for warning signs and to take the child to doctor, if they occur.

DIARRHOEA

Diarrhoea is a predominant symptom which signifies passage of loose, liquid or watery stools usually more than 3 times a day.

According to WHO, acute diarrhoea is an attack of sudden onset diarrhoea, lasting to 3-7 days or even upto 10-14 days, which is also called "G.E.". Common organisms causing acute watery diarrhoea are:

- Rotavirus
- Salmonellosis
- E. coli
- Cholera.

In case of acute bloody diarrhoea, following pathogens are commonly found in the diagnosis:

- Shigella (Bacillary dysentery)
- Giardiasis.

Nowadays new entry "Travellers diarrhoea" has emerged which is self limiting with oral fluid and salt replacement.

Epidemiological importance of community history directs to the aetiology of diarrhoea.

i. Fever, bloody diarrhoea suggests invasive dysenteric process.
ii. Incubation of below 18 hours suggests food poisoning.

Feed the child
* Feed the child during illness
* Increase feeding after illness
* Clear the nose if it interferes with feeding

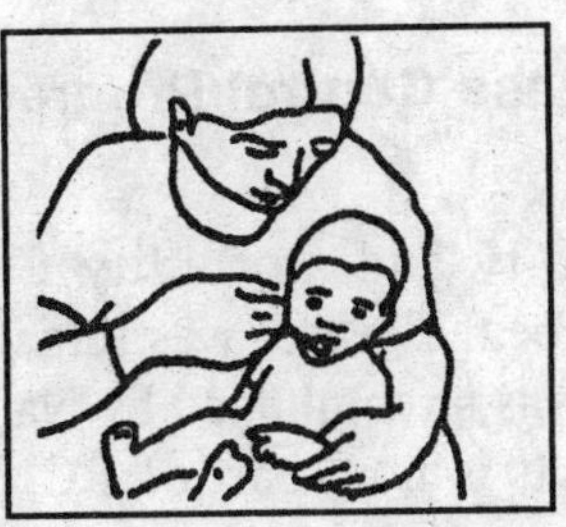

Increase Fluids
* Offer the child extra to drink
* Increase the breast feeding

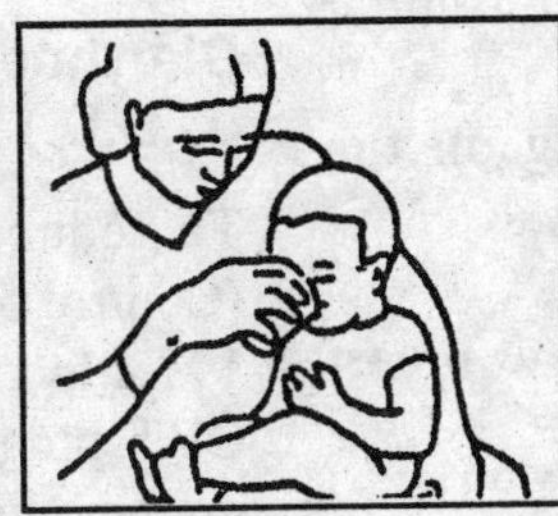

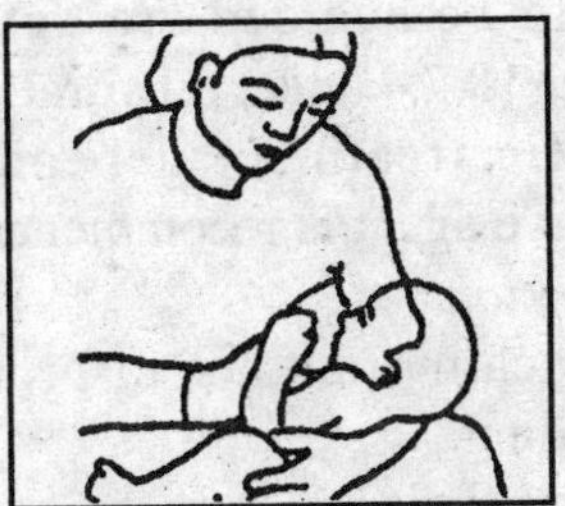

Soothe the throat and relieve the cough with a safe remedy

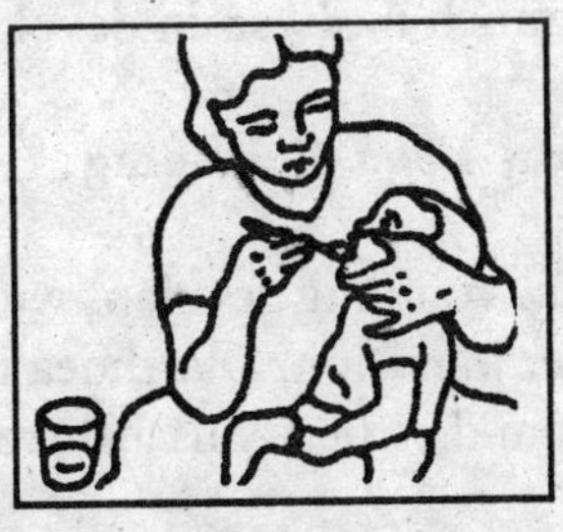

Most Important :
Watch for the following signs and return quickly if they occur:

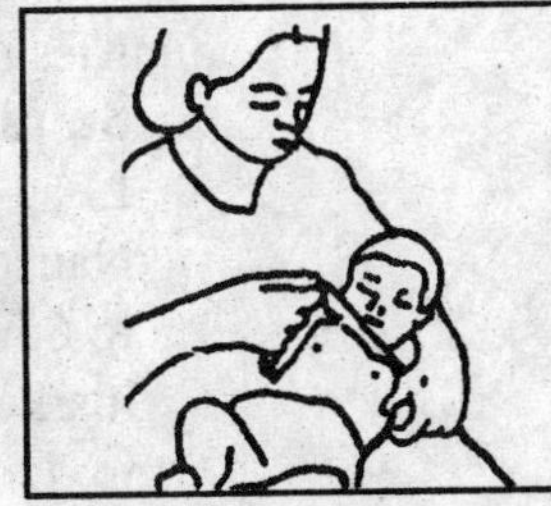

* Breathing becomes difficult
* Breathing becomes fast
* Child is not able to drink
* Child becomes sicker

This child may have pneumonia

Fig. 11.9: Home care instructions for children aged 2 months upto 5 years with acute respiratory infections

iii. Incubation above 4-5 days suggests protozoal or helminthic.

Problem–India

Diarrhoea is a major public health problem causing morbidity and mortality.

Mode of Transmission–Faecal Oral Route

Control and Prevention of Diarrhoea

i. *Confirmation of cause of diarrhoea:* With available laboratory facility, cause is ascertained for case management and for public health measures.

ii. *Notification:*
Depending on local health authorities, the given cause of diarrhoea has to be notified.

iii. *Early diagnosis and prompt treatment:*
Assessment of dehydration, special check during assessment, rehydration, oral fluids, sustenance of O.R.S. and medicines that need to be avoided are detailed under chapter 18.7.4 under rehydration.
Specific treatment depending on the causative agent is recommended.

iv. *Prevention:*
- Educating mother to promote breast feeding
- Food hygiene
- Improved water supply
- Provision of sanitary latrine.

v. *Making of ORS* (Fig. 11.10 and Table 11.9)

Fig. 11.10: Requirement of HAF, ORS and I.V. fluid

- In 100 cases of diarrhoea 90 cases may show no sign of dehydration

REQUIRING HAF
- 10 cases may show some sign of dehydration

REQUIRING ORS
- 1 case may develop severe dehydration

Requiring Hospitalisation for I.V./ORS

(Home available fluid, oral rehydration solution and intravenous fluid)

Table 11.9: Minerals and calories in ORS

	Na	*K*	*Cl*	*Calorie*
WHO	90	20	80	160
Orange juice	0.2	49	-	440
Breast milk	22	36	28	670

vi. Source detection, sanitary survey and contact tracing are done through epidemiological investigation.

vii. Health education on safe water, excreta disposal by sanitary way, food sanitation and concurrent disinfection of patient are undertaken.

Diarrhoeal Disease Control Programme (C.D.D.)

To reduce mortality and morbidity C.D.D. (Control of Diarrhoeal disease) was initiated in 1978. In 1985, it was strengthened by National ORT programme. It is now part of RCH programme in the country.

FOOD POISONING

Food poisoning is acute gastroenteritis by bacterial toxin, chemical toxin, plant toxin or by animal toxins. It is characterised by a common source, many will have same symptoms at one time.

Food poisoning is still a public health problem in the world. It is much more so in developing countries like India.

i. **Staphylococcal Food Poisoning:**
I.P. 1-6 hours
Nausea, profuse vomiting develops within 1 to 6 hours after ingestion. Diarrhoea is not marked. It is intra-dietetic toxins that produce toxic effect.
Antiemetic, fluid replacement is advocated. Suspected food is sent for laboratory examination. If food vending is involved, public health authorities are informed.

ii. **Bacillus cereas:**
Preformed toxin of *B.cereas* produces rapid onset of vomiting within 1 hour of food consumption.
Rapid and judicious fluid replacement and appropriate notification are mandatory.

iii. **Clostridium perfringens:**
This is common by contaminated meat, or incompletely cooked meat and when stored in anaerobic condition.

iv. **Cl. Botulism:**
It is due to neurotoxin of *Cl.botulinum* which is manifested in paralysis and neurological dysfunction. It is common in canned meat and preserved vegetables.

v. **Salmonella poisoning:**
S. Typhimurium from contaminated meat, milk and milk products produce symptoms with an I.P. of 12 to 24 hours. Fever, nausea, vomiting and watery diarrhoea are common. Reservoirs are poultry and farm animals.

Investigation of an Epidemic of G.E.

i. List of people involved is done.
ii. They are subjected for laboratory tests
iii. Survey of eating places; kitchen and food, handlers are done.
iv. Data is analysed for time, place and person distribution.
v. In all epidemics of acute G.E, cholera is ruled out at investigation. Differences between cholera and food poisoning are as under (Table 11.10):

Table 11.10: Differences between food poisoning and cholera

	Cholera	*Food poisoning*
History of common meal	No	Yes
Incubation period	5 days	1 day
Onset	Diarrhoea	Vomiting
Nausea	Absent	Present
Stool	Rice watery	Offensive mucus and blood
Dehydration	Marked	Not marked
Muscle cramp	Severe	Less
Fever	No	Yes
Urine	Suppressed	Not suppressed
Differential WBC count	Leucocytosis	Normal

Control and Prevention of Food Poisoning

i. Food sanitation includes meat hygiene, milk hygiene, food hygiene, sanitary method of preservation and food handling techniques. Health education on personal hygiene is essential.
ii. *Refrigeration:* Keeping food in cold storage (below 4°C) prevent bacterial growth and toxin liberation.
iii. *Food surveillance:* Periodic and suspected food analysis helps in preventing food poisoning.

SEXUALLY TRANSMITTED DISEASES (STDs)

They are contagious bacterial, viral, protozoal, fungal and ectoparasite infections of man whose principle mode of transmission is by intimate sexual contact. Earlier five classical venereal diseases viz., syphilis, gonorrhoea, chancroid, lymphogranuloma venerium and granuloma inguinale are added with many more sexually transmitted diseases which formed a giant group called STD's. They are enumerated in the Table 11.11.

Table 11.11: Sexually transmitted diseases

First generation STD:
1. Syphilis
2. Gonorrhoea
3. Chancroid
4. LGV (Lympho granuloma venerium)
5. GI (Granuloma inguinale)

Second generation STD:
1. Trichomonos vaginalis
2. Scabies genitalia
3. Thrush
4. Herpes simplex
5. Warts of genitalia

Third generation STD:
1. HIV/AIDS

Syphilis

Syphilis is caused by *Treponema pallidum* (a spirochaete) and is sexually acquired with the entry of treponemes through abrasions in skin and mucous membranes. Clinically it is manifested in primary, secondary and tertiary forms.

Primary syphilis: The incubation period is 9-90 days. Chancre at the site of genital area develops which gets eroded to form an indurate ulcer.

Secondary syphilis: After 2 months of development of chancre multisystem disease is noted.

Tertiary syphilis: This stage develops after 3-10 years of infection.

Congenital syphilis can lead to stillbirth, syphilitic baby, early congenital syphilis and late congenital syphilis.

Laboratory test commonly done is VDRL.

Procaine benzyl penicillin G 6 lakh units I.M. daily for 17 days or Benzathine penicillin G 2.4 million units I.M. weekly for 3 doses are recommended. Doxycycline 100 mg 12 hourly for 14 days and Erythromycin 500 mg 6 hourly for 14 days are alternatives.

During nursing care Anaphylaxis, Jarish Herxheimer reaction (malaise, headache, myalgia, optic neuritis etc.) and procaine reactions are to be attended as per hospital procedures.

Gonorrhoea

It is caused by *Neisseria gonorrhoea* and clinically Urethritis, Cervicitis, Epididymitis salpingitis, PID and neonatal conjuctivitis are manifested. It is the common STD causing genital discharge. I.P. is 2-10 days. Gram negative intracellular diplococci under microscopy are diagnostic. Untreated cases go for complications like Prostatitis, Epididymoorchitis, Bartholin abscess, PID and Opthalmia neonatorum.

Ciprofloxacin 500 mg stat or ofloxacin 400 mg orally stat or Ampicillin 3 G with Probenecid 1.0 Gram orally stat, are recommended specific treatments.

Chancroid

Chancroid, a soft sore is a disease causing genital ulceration caused by *Haemophilus ducreyi* (Gram –ve bacteria). It is highly prevalent among prostitutes. Single or multiple painful ulcers with ragged undermined edges are seen. Inguinal nodes are enlarged. I.P. is 3-10 days. Microscopy and culture of scraping of ulcer gives diagnosis.

Treatment choices are:

1. Azithromycin 1 gram orally once.
2. Ceftriaxone 250 mg I.M. once.
3. Ciprofloxacin 500 mg 12th hourly orally for 3 days.
4. Erythromycin 500 mg 6th hourly orally for 7 days.

L.G.V.

It is caused by *Chlamydia Trachomatis* I.P. is 3 to 30 days. Genital lesion is small, transient, painless ulcer. Vesicle and papule often are unnoticed. Inguinal nodes are enlarged and tender. Serological tests are diagnostic. Case is managed with Doxycycline Hydrate 12 hourly orally for 21 days or Erythromycin 500 mg 6 hourly orally for 21 days.

Granuloma Inguinale (G.I.)

The disease is strongly associated with low socio economic state and prostitution. It is common in south India. It is caused by *Klebsiella Granulomatis* (Donovan bodies) and has an I.P. of 3-40 days. Hypertrophic granulomatous painless ulcers on genitals are common findings.

Inguinal Lymph node enlargement, abscess and ulceration follow at a later stage. Identification of Donovan bodies is specific and diagnostic tool. Case is managed with Azithromycin 1 G. weekly orally or 500 mg daily orally is suggested. Alternatively Doxycycline Hydrate 100 mg 12 hourly is recommended.

T.V. Infection

Trichomonas vaginalis is a pathogenic protozoan in lower female genitourinary tract. It is world wide in distribution, both in rural and urban situation. High prevalence is in high level sexual activities. It is a common cause of nongonococcal urethritis. Microscopical examination for T.V. and specific treatment with Metronidazole 400 mg orally 12 hourly for 5 days are measures for effective control of T.V.

Scabies of Genitalia

This is attributed to sexually transmitted disease. Poor personal hygiene and prostitution are contributing factors. Its diagnosis and case management are discussed in the Chapter 5 page 80 and Chapter 11 page 99.

Thrush

Vulvovaginal condition or balanitis condition is fungal (candidiasis) infection contracted through sexual activity. Cardinal clinical features are pruritus vulvae and vaginal discharge (curd like plaques adherent to vaginal wall. Case is managed with:

i. Clotrimaxazole 500 mg pessary once at night
ii. Clotrimaxazole cream 12 hourly
iii. Econazole pessary 150 mg for 3 nights
iv. Fluconazole 150 mg orally stat.

Herpes Simplex

Herpes (genital) by HSV-1 or HSV-2 are known, asymptomatic primary course followed by asymptomatic general viral infections are recorded. Irritable vesicles rupture and ulcerate on genitalia. Fever, malaise, headache are common clinical features of herpes. Tissue culture and typing are diagnostic of herpes simplex infection.

The treatment will be

i. Aciclovir 200 mg 5 times a day
ii. Famciclovir 250 mg 8 hourly
iii. Valaciclovir 500 mg 12 hourly.

S.T.D. Control in the Community

Case detection is done by screening, contact tracing and cluster testing. After confirmation, case is held for complete course of treatment. All contacts must be tested and positive are treated (epidemiological treatment). Health education of the community for personal prophylaxis is undertaken.

STD clinics are established which is found useful to maintain confidentiality, free treatment, counselling and integrated essential care services.

Lab facilities like VDRL, serological examination, smear examination and microscopic facilities are requirement in case finding activities.

STD activities are integrated with primary health care through VHG, MPW at subcentre and PHC, help in overcoming social stigma attached in hiding the disease.

Surveillance of STD

"Surveillance is the continuous scrutinising of factors involved in the distribution and trends of STD through systematic collection, consolidation and evaluation of mortality and other relevant data. This is linked to a system of feedback and action."

STD surveillance is collection of information on STD for community action. Surveillance systems are of 2 types:

1. **Routine reporting:** S.T.D. case detection and reporting by health personnel include routine report and sentinel report.
2. **Sentinel reporting:** It is the selection of a few reporting units to participate in the process of surveillance.

Syndrome Approach

Syndrome approach is a method of management and control of STD's where diagnosis and treatment is based on a group of symptoms and signs. Treatment is targeted towards all diseases that could cause that syndrome. It allows diagnosis without extensive laboratory tests and treatment within a single visit. This approach is relevant in the context of Indian condition where laboratory facilities for diagnosis is limited. Syndrome approach for "5 field-approach" are given in appendix for the following areas (Appendix VII):

- Genital ulcers
- Vaginal discharge (no speculum examination)
- Vaginal discharge (with speculum examination)
- Urethral discharge
- Lower abdominal pain in the female (PID).

National STD Control Programme

It is linked with HIV/AIDS and is ongoing since 1946. Diagnosis and treatment, condom promotion, STD surveillance, IEC activities and family health awareness campaign are detailed under National Health Programmes Chapter 17 page 253.

MALARIA

There are 4 species of plasmodium that produce malaria. They are:

1. P. vivax
2. P. malaria
3. P. ovale
4. P. falciparum.

Global Malaria Problem

Almost all countries have malaria cases. About 3 million are dying every year of whom 1 million are children under five years (Table 11.12).

Table 11.12: Endemicity of malaria

Spleen rate or Parasite rate	*Endemicity*
0-10%	Hypoendemic
10-50%	Mesoendemic
50-75%	Hyperendemic
75% above	Holoendemic

Vector Bionomics

Urban area	*Anopheles stephensai*, which breed in used well overhead tank, transmits malaria.
Rural area	*A. culicifacies*, which breeds in stagnant or slow running water, transmit malaria.
Hilly area	*A. fluviatilis* which breeds in slow running water, transmits malaria.
Sea coastal area	*A. sundaicus* which breeds in salt water, transmits malaria.
Tea plantation area	*A. minimus* which breeds in slow running water, transmits malaria.
Waterlogging area	*A. philippensis* which breeds in high level subsoil water, transmits malaria.

Malaria Problem in India

Upto 1976 there was a good improvement in malaria situation. But after 1977 resurgence of malaria is a common feature. Since 1977 till 2003 we are getting higher API, ABER, SPR, and SFR which hallmark alarming situation (Annual Parasite Incidence, Annual Blood Examination Rate, Slide Positive Rate and Slide Falciparum Rate). Severe malaria due to P.falciparum is also increasing.

P. vivax – Benign tertian malaria
P. malariae – Quartan malaria
P. ovale – Ovale tertian malaria
P. falciparum – Malignant tertian malaria

Incubation period is 15 days in P.vivax, 15 days in P. ovale, 12 days in P. faliciparum and 30 days in P. malariae.

Clinical Features

Vivax and Ovale Malaria

Illness starts several days of continued fever before classical fever on alternate days. Fever starts with rigor. Patient feels very cold but body temperature rises to 40°C. Hot phase is followed after 30 minutes of temperature. 4-6 hours later profuse perspiration and fall in temperature. Splenomegaly and hepatomegaly which show tenderness are later manifestations. Slowly anaemia develops. In 20% of cases development of herpes simplex is seen. Relapse is common even after 2 years in case of vivax and ovale malariae.

Malariae Malaria

It produces mild symptoms. Fever appears every third day. Even a symptomatic case with MP smear +ve is known. Among children malariae is known to cause nephrotic syndrome and glomerulonephritis.

Falciparum Malaria

This produces severe malaria. Onset is slow with malaise, headache, vomiting and often mistaken for influenza, mild diarrhoea and cough are seen in most of the patients. Fever does not follow a specific pattern. Because of liver dysfunction and haemolysis, clinical jaundice appears early. Splenomegaly and hepatomegaly are common and they are tender. Very rapid, development of anaemia is seen with falciparum malaria. A patient with severe falciparum malaria present with confusion, drowsiness, extreme weakness, prostration. The following clinical entities are noticed with severe malaria which needs special nursing care in day-to-day practice.

Cerebral malaria, defined as unarousable coma not attributable to any other cause in patient with falciparum malaria.

Malaria Measurement in the Community

i. **Spleen rate:** Percentage of children 2-10 years who show splenomegaly.
ii. **Parasite rate:** Percentage of children 2-10 years who shown M.P. smear +ve.
iii. **Infant parasite rate:** Percentage of infants (0-1) who show M.P. smear +ve.
iv. **Proportional case rate:** It is number of malaria cases out of 100 attending hospital patients

Parasitological indicators of malaria in a community.

i. $\text{A.P.I.} = \dfrac{\text{Confirmed cases during 1 year}}{\text{Population under surveillance}} \times 1000$

(Annual Parasite Incidence)

ii. $\text{A.B.E.R.} = \dfrac{\text{No. of slides examined}}{\text{Population}} \times 100$

(Annual Blood Examination Rate)

iii. A.F.I. (Annual Falciparum Incidence)
iv. S.P.R. (Slide Positive Rate)
v. S.F.R. (Slide Falciparum Rate)

Case Management and Nursing Care

P.vivax, P.ovale, P.malariae infections should be treated with chloroquine 600 mg base followed by 300 mg base in 6 hours, Later 150 mg base 12 hourly for 2 more days. Relapse is overcome by antimalarial drugs in suppressive doses. Primaquin 15 mg daily for 14 days will destroy hypnozoits phase in liver. Haemolysis and cyanosis are common but not dangerous.

P.falciparum is best treated with quinine 10mg/kg body weight 8 hourly by mouth till clinical improvement and till M.P. smear is –ve. This is followed by single dose of sulfadoxine 1.5 G combined with pyrimethamine 75 mg. In pregnancy 7 days Quinine is given. Alternatively Atovaquone 250 mg + Proguanil 100 mg 4 tablets once daily for 3 days is given.

Special Nursing Care in Severe Malaria of a Child

Nursing care should include all well established principles of the care of unconscious child. Every 2 hours frequent turning of the child, careful attention to airways, eyes, mucosae, skin and fluid requirements. The child should be nursed in the lateral or semi-prone position.

Special paediatric nursing care should include:

- Insert nasogastric tube to minimise risk of aspiration pneumonia
- Correct hypoglycaemia
- Restore circulating volume

National Level Malaria Control Programmes

Malaria Effective Control

a. Case Management:

Case detection: All fever cases are subjected to M.P. smear examination (under surveillance).

Active surveillance: Fortnightly visit by health worker who detects fever, collects blood smear for M.P.

Passive surveillance: All health care institutions detect fever cases, collect blood smear for M.P.

Treatment

i. Presumptive treatment with chloroquine in low risk areas:

Age	*Chloroquine*	*Remarks*
Below 1 year	75 mg (½ Tab)	– Blood smear taken to all
1-4 years	150 mg (1 Tab)	
4-8 years	300 mg (2 Tab)	
8-14 years	450 mg (3 Tab)	– P. T. given after food
Above 14	600 mg (4 Tab)	

ii. Radical treatment for vivax, malariae, ovale

Age	*Chloroquine (mg)*	*Primaquine (mg)*	*Remarks*
Below 1 year	75	—	
1-4 years	150	2.5	– No primaquine for pregnant and infant
4-8 years	300	5	
8-14 years	450	10	
above 14 years	600	15	

iii. Radical Treatment for Faliciparum and Malaria :

Age (years)	*Chloroquine (mg) (days)*			*Primaquine (mg)*	*Remarks*
	I	*II*	*III*	*1 day*	
Below 1	75	75	37.5	–	No primaquine for pregnant and infant
1-4	150	150	75	7.5	
4-8	300	300	150	15	
8-14	450	450	225	30	
Above 14	600	600	300	45	

Malaria Chemoprophylaxis

Person should take any one of the following till he moves in endemic areas:

i. Chloroquine–500 mg weekly
ii. Chloroquine–300 mg weekly + proguanil – 200 mg daily
iii. Chloroquine–300 mg weekly + pyramithamine – 500 mg daily

b. Public Health Measures:

Area with A.P.I. Above 2

- Spraying 2 rounds D.D.T./3 rounds H.C.H.
- Entomological assessment
- Surveillance
- Case management.

Area with A.P.I. Below 2

- Focal spraying
- Surveillance
- Case management
- Follow up
- Epidemiological investigation.

c. Integrated Vector Control:

Following are the major measures through integrated vector control:

- Residual spray
- Antilarval measures
- Personal protection
- Control of breeding places by intermittent irrigation and source reduction.

AMOEBIASIS

Intestinal amoebiasis is very common and ubiquitous in distribution, extra intestinal amoebiasis is seen in tropics and subtropics as minor entity.

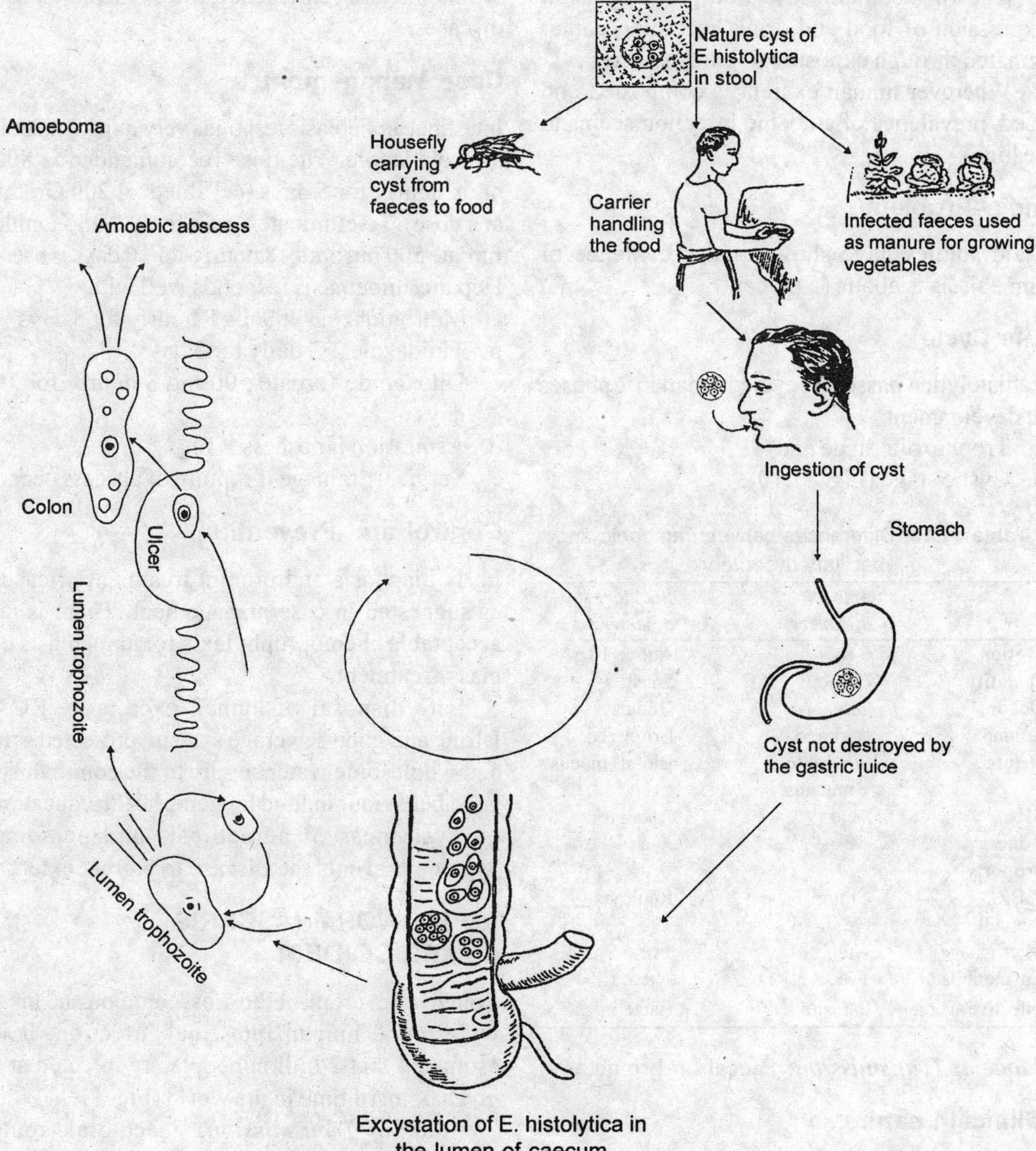

Fig.11.10: Life cycle of E. histolytica

W.H.O. has defined this as a clinical condition which harbour entamoeba histolytica irrespective of whether the case is symptomatic or asymptomatic.

Known faeco-oral infection probably is an expression of food and drink becoming contaminated through exposure to human excreta.

Wherever human excreta is composted and used, prevalence of amoebic infection seems to be high.

India–Problem

Field studies have shown that prevalence of amoebiasis is about 15 percent.

Life Cycle

E. histolytica passes its cycle in man in 2 phases of development:

a. Trophozoite stage and
b. Cystic stage (Fig. 11.10).

Table 11.13: Differences between amoebic and bacillary dysentery

	Amoebic dysentery	*Bacillary dysentery*
Motion	6-8	Above 10
Quantity	Copious	Small
Odour	Offensive	Odourless
Colour	Dark red	Bright red
Nature	Stool+blood + mucous	Blood+mucus
pH	Acid	Alkaline
Adherent property	-ve	+ve
R.B.C.	Clump	Rouleaux
Pus cell	-ve	+ve
Microphage	-ve	+ve
Eosinophils	+ve	-ve
Infective agent	Parasite	Bacteria

Mode of Transmission: Faecal oral route.

Clinical Feature

Incubation period is 15 days to few years. Grumbling abdominal pain, 6-8 motions a day, alternating diarrhoea and constipation are features. Stools are characteristics and diagnostic (Table 11.13) patient may present acute bowel symptoms, as an emergency, in a small proportion of cases.

Case Management

Intestinal amoebiasis responds very quickly to oral Metronidazole. The dose recommended is 800 mg 8 hourly for 5 days (4 Tablets of 200 Grams at a dose). To eliminate cystic forms, Diloxanide furoate 500 mg orally 8 hourly for 10 days is used. Hepatic amoebiasis responds well with:

a. Metronidazole 800 mg 8 hourly for 5 days
b. Tinidazole 2 G daily for 3 days
c. Diloxanide furoate 500 mg 8 hourly for 10 days
d. Aspiration if abscess is big
e. Surgical drainage if rupture of abscess occur.

Control and Prevention

Early diagnosis and prompt treatment of cases as suggested in case management. There is no acceptable chemoprophylaxis for amoebiasis or mass treatment.

Safe disposal of human excreta by RCA latrine and good sewerage system, protected safe and wholesome water supply to the community, good behaviour in food hygiene, health education on awareness of amoebiasis and personal hygiene prevents the disease to a great extent.

ROUNDWORM (ASCARIS LUMBRICOIDES)

Roundworm is one of the most common and most widespread human intestinal infection. It is estimated that 2 billion people are infected at a given point of time in the world (Fig. 11.11).

Mode of Transmission: Faeco-oral route when the infective eggs are swallowed with food. Raw foods convey infection readily. Water pollution also makes infection vulnerable.

Incubation period is about 50 days. Course of larvae in man is showed in diagram.

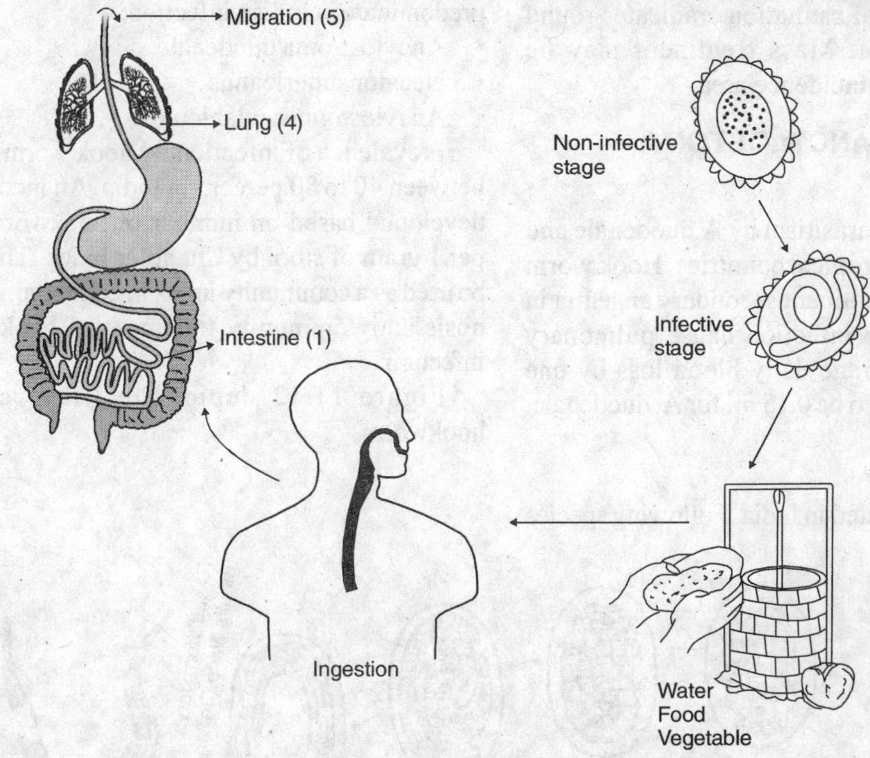

Fig.11.11: Life cycle of roundworm

Clinical Features

Mainly gastrointestinal manifestations in the form of vague abdominal pain form the main symptom. Extreme cases manifest as malnutrition. Migrating larvae produce (Ascaris pneumonia) fever, cough, dyspnoea, Sputum examination show larvae. In 25% of cases urticarial rash and eosinophilia are seen. Due to circulating larvae, functional disorders of brain, heart and kidney are unusual manifestations.

Adult worm destroy nutrients and consume calories leading to subnutrition and malnutrition. Even Vitamin A deficiency can also be seen. Ascarin in the body can also lead to oedema of the face, conjunctivitis, urticaria and other toxic manifestations. Rarely, intussusceptions, obstruction and peritonitis (penetration through ulcers) are reported. Ectopic ascarisis can cause vomiting, suffocation, appendicitis, obstructive jaundice, pancreatitis and liver abscess.

Laboratory diagnosis is examination of ova by direct examination under microscope and concentration by floatation method. History of passing adult worms in the stool or vomitus and X-ray by barium examination is added pathognomonic investigations.

Specific Treatment

a. Mebendazole 100 mg 12th hourly for 3 days
b. Albendazole 400 mg as single dose
c. Piperzine citrate 4 G as a single dose
d. Pyrentol 10 mg/kg body weight (IG. adult).

Surgical obstruction may need nasogastric suction for worms.

Improvement of sanitation eradicates round worm infestation. Mass treatment may be advocated in high incidence area.

HOOKWORM (ANCYLOSTOMA DUODENALE)

It is an intestinal parasitism by A.duodenale and N. americanus in tropical countries. Hook worm anaemia is a predominant secondary anaemia in the world. Heavy infection cause pulmonary eosinophilia. Average daily blood loss by one worm is estimated to be 0.15 ml for A. duodenale.

Problem–India

It is widely distributed in India. Following species predominate in Indian infection:

- Ancylostroma duodenale
- Necator americanus
- Ancylostoma ceylanicum.

Prevalence of infection by hook worm range between 40 to 80 percent in India. An index was developed based on number of hookworm egg per 1 gram of stool by Chandler index. This can be used as a community index in community diagnosis and community treatment of hookworm infection.

Figure 11.12 depict the life cycle of hookworm.

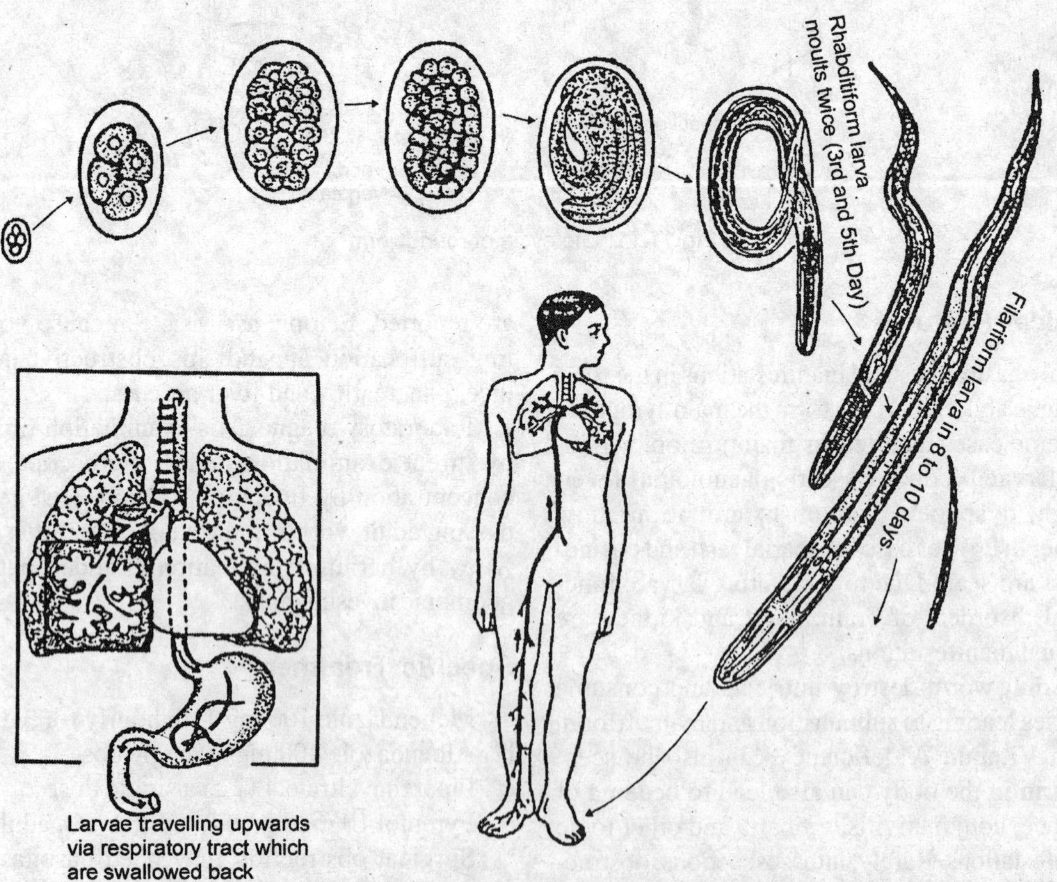

Fig. 11.12: Life cycle of hookworm

Mode of Transmission: Infective stage larva enter through skin.

Incubation period: It ranges from few weeks to few months.

Clinical Feature: Ground Itch is common in early infection. Patient may come with presentation of dermatitis. Migration through lung is manifested with cough with blood stained sputum. Clinically there may be patchy consolidation. Vomiting and epigastric pain are common in intestinal habitat phase. Loose motion may be subjective manifestations in some of the cases. Signs and symptoms of iron deficiency anaemia is very common in late phase of intestinal parasitism. Among undernutrition population, protein loosing enteropathy and hypoproteinaemia are observed. Iron deficiency anaemia can cause high output cardiac failure. Among children it effects growth and development. Creeping eruption by migrating larvae, bronchitis and bronchopneumonia produce specific clinical manifestations of respiratory systems.

Case Management

a. Mebendazole 100 mg 12 hrly for 3 days.
b. Albendazole 400 mg single dose.
c. Oral iron preparation for anaemia.
d. Severe anaemia need blood transfusion.

Community Management

a. Sanitary disposal of human excreta by RCA latrine.
b. Treatment and early diagnosis of hookworm infection.
c. Nutrition correction and anaemia treatment.
d. Health education on use of *chappal* and not to walk barefoot in open field defecation area.
e. Integrated approach of above (a) to (d).

MYIASIS

Myiasis is a clinical condition caused by the attack of larvae of common housefly. They attack tissues, intestine or bladder. When maggots cause furuncle, attack and multiply in wound they cause creeping eruption. When they enter through natural orifice the manifestation depends on the body cavity attacked. If accidentally ingested, it can enter intestine.

Wound Myiasis

Wound of a person which could be a chronic ulcer, a post operative wound or very commonly advanced cancer wound are produced by facultative parasite of Musca domestica (housefly) larva.

Control and Prevention

Personal hygiene and environmental sanitation are best suited answers for the control and prevention of Myiasis due to housefly larva.

SCABIES

Morphology, life cycle and other details are highlighted under Chapter 5.

Itch mite which is also called as scabies mite (Sarcoptes scabiei) causes human scabies.

It is transmitted by person to person contact, through bedding and through clothing. The infective agent is fertilized female. The itch mite female makes a permanent burrow in the horny layers of the skin.

Case Management and Nursing Care

All the members of the family of case are given simultaneous treatment. 20% emulsion of benzyl benzoate is applied from neck down after a bath and allowed to dry and clothing is put. The next day second bath and clothing wash are a must. The treatment is repeated on 6th day.

Secondary infection is treated by penicillin one course for 5 days.

Other alternative drugs are:

a. NBIN emulsion (1:15 water before use)
   Benzyl benzoate 68%

DDT	6%
Benzocaine	12%
Polysorbate	14%

b. BHC–Malathion lotion

Malathion	0.5%
BHC	1%

c. Crotamiton daily application for 5 days. It is suitable for infants since it is antipruritic.
d. Tetmasol 5% solution.

Control and Prevention

Personal hygiene and environmental sanitation can control and prevent scabies.

CHAPTER TWELVE

Occupational Health

IMPORTANCE

Industrial revolution and progress in science and technology has brought in changes in the occupational status. Gradually, for the past 50 years, these changes have become cognizant of the benefit of nurse's professional skills in safeguarding health status of workers.

DEFINITION

According to I.L.O., it is defined as "Occupational health is the field of science which aims at the promotion and maintenance of the highest degree of physical, mental and social well-being of workers in all occupations, at prevention of departures from health at work place.

Ergonomics

It is derived from Greek meaning work + Law. It is a recognised discipline for developing efficiency of man and machine.

OCCUPATIONAL ENVIRONMENT

It is the sum of external conditions that influence health status of workers. It can be represented by a diagram (Fig. 12.1).

Agents mentioned above may be adverse to the health of a person in a working condition. Accidents due to fatigue, muscle and joint impairment are common occurrence. Human relation with co-workers decides good working atmosphere.

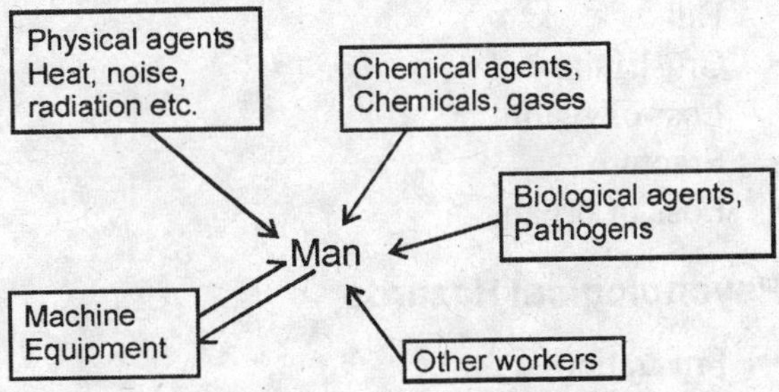

Fig 12.1: Man in his working environment

HAZARDS IN OCCUPATION

Physical Hazards

Heat	:	Burns, heat exhaustion, heat stroke, heat cramps, fatigue
Cold	:	Chilblains, erythrocyanosis, immersion foot, frostbite
Light	:	Eye strain, headache, eye fatigue, miner's nystagmus
Noise	:	Hearing loss, nervousness, annoyance
Vibration	:	White fingers by spasm, joint injury
U.V. Rays	:	Welder's flash, conjunctivitis
Radiation	:	Cancer, depilation, sterility.

Chemical Hazards

Local – Dermatitis

Gases – Inhalation and lung change, poisons

Dust – Fibrosis of lung, malignancy

Biological Hazards

- Anthrax
- Brucellosis
- Encephalitis
- Fungal infections
- Hydatid disease
- Leptospirosis
- Psittacosis
- Tetanus.

Mechanical Hazards

- Fall
- Crush injury
- Loss of vision
- Fracture
- Loss of organ.

Psychological Hazards

- Frustration
- Lack of job satisfaction
- Emotional tension
- Depression
- Alcoholism
- Psychosomatic like headache, peptic ulcer.

PNEUMOCONIOSIS

Organic or inorganic chemical dusts (of size 0.5 to 3 micron in size) when inhaled over a period of time cause lung changes by with or without infection leading to reduced ventilatory capacity called "Pneumoconiosis".

Common types of pneumoconiosis are described in the following section:

Inorganic Dust Induced Pneumoconiosis

Anthracosis

Coal dust inhalation over a period of 12 years causes simple pneumoconiosis. Later with the development of progressive massive fibrosis (PMF) severe respiratory disability and premature death occurs. It is a notifiable disease.

Asbestosis

A silicate of magnesium is a fibrous material, which when inhaled gives rise to Asbestosis. Sputum examination showing "Asbestos bodies" and X-ray showing ground glass appearance are established criteria of diagnosis. It is associated with a serious cancer called Mesothelioma of pleura which kills the worker within 3 months.

Siderosis

Lead is common metal used in many industries like, battery, glass, ship building, printing, potteries, rubber etc., There are non-occupational sources like gasoline use, lead paint on toys, water running through lead pipes etc.

Silicosis

Inhalation of silica in mining, ceramic industry, metal grinding, construction work, iron and steel industry cause premature death.

It produces nodular fibrosis, poor ventilatory capacity, X-ray shows snow storm appearance and found, on most of the occasions, with tuberculosis.

Organic Dust Induced Pneumoconiosis

Bagassosis

Inhalation of cane bagasse dust produces bagassosis. Industry like paper, cardboard and rayon show a fungal growth (actinomyces) on kernel of sugarcane which causes bronchiolitis changes. Reduced pulmonary ventilatory capacity, fibrosis, emphysema and bronchiectasis are common.

Dust control, personal protection and sprinkling 2% propionic acid on kernel prevents bagassosis.

Byssinosis

Inhalation of cotton fibre produces byssinosis. Cotton industry show, among its workers chronic cough, progressive dyspnoea, chronic bronchitis and emphysema.

Containment of cotton dust and periodic examination of workers help in the control of byssinosis.

Farmer's Lung

It is also called Hay fever since grain dust is inhaled which produces lung change causing fibrosis and corpulmonale. Fungal infection causes lung changes. In the beginning it manifests as allergic disorder and later as infective disorder.

Personal protection and health awareness help in the control of farmer's lung.

Tobacossis

Nicotine in tobacco when inhaled constantly produces lung changes causing bronchitis and emphysema. It is associated with bronchogenic carcinoma.

Personal protection and periodic examination help in the control of tobacossis.

CANCER AND OCCUPATION

Certain occupations are found associated with specific cancers. They are:

Blood cancer: Work with X-ray, work with Isotopes, Exposure to Benzol may lead to blood cancer (Fig. 12.2).

Lung cancer: Industries handling nickel, Chromium, arsenic, uranium, asbestos, tobacco are associated with lung cancers in their workers.

Skin cancer: Workers at X-ray, oil, dyes, gas works, tar distillery and chimney sweeping are found to get skin cancer.

Urinary bladder cancer: Industries handling rubber, aromatic amines, dyeing industry, electric cable, magenta and aniline affect this organ to develop cancer changes.

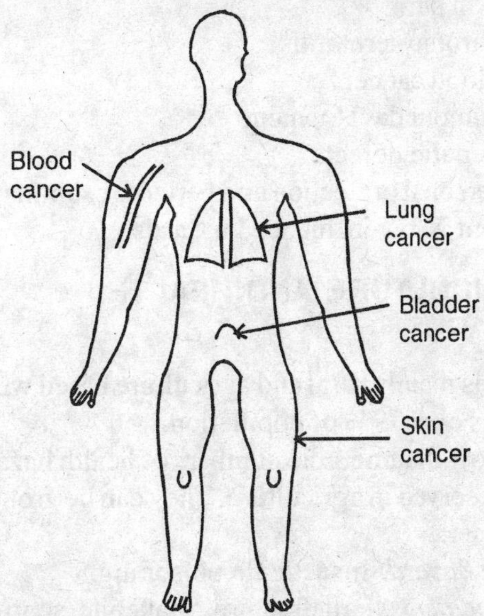

Fig. 12.2: Common occupational cancers

SKIN AND OCCUPATION

Dermatitis is known in almost all working placements where physical agents like heat, cold, moisture, friction, pressure, X-ray, chemical agents like acid, alkali, dye, solvents, phenols, biological agents like bacteria, parasite and plant products like dust of flower and vegetable dust come in constant contact with skin.

Occupational dermatitis can be prevented by following measures:

- Preplacement examination
- Skin protection
- Personal hygiene.

X-RAY INFLUENCED HAZARDS

Occupations like radiology, radiodiagnosis, Radiotherapy, watch industry, radioactive ore, arc welding, foundry work etc. have effects of radiation which can cause following health hazards:

- Skin burn
- Chronic dermatitis
- Blood cancer
- Tumour development
- Genetic defects

Personal protection and periodic examination prevent X-ray influenced hazards.

AGRICULTURE AND HEALTH HAZARDS

India is mainly rural and agriculture based which covers over 79% of population.

Now innumerable numbers of health hazards are observed in agriculture. They can be grouped as under:

Toxic hazard: Insecticide poisoning.

Accidents: Fall, fracture, Snakebite, scorpion bite.

Zoonotic disease: Man may get diseases of lower animals like anthrax, brucellosis, tuberculosis.

Soil contamination: Tetanus.

Physical environment: Rain, hot sun.

Respiratory diseases: Organic dust.

ACCIDENT AND OCCUPATION

Accidents are causes of production loss, human suffering and loss of worker's day in occupation. Human and environmental factors play a vital role in occupational accidents.

Human factors: Incapability of worker, vision impairment, hearing impairment, immature mind, fatigue, carelessness, emotion.

Environmental factor: Poor light, unsafe machines, high temperature.

DIAGNOSIS OF ABSENTEEISM (SICKNESS ABSENTEEISM)

It is defined as absence from work attributed to sickness or injury and accepted as such by the employer or the social security system.

Gross absence rate should be below 5%; if it is 10% it is serious as per standards.

Sickness absence rate if high and is above 4%, this indicates a high degree of morbidity in working class and this points out to a medical rather than a managerial problem.

Unauthorized absence rate of spells more than 14, require special attention as per standard.

Incidence: India is showing 15 to 20% sickness absenteeism as per findings from the National Productivity Council (NPC).

Causes of Sickness Absence

- As a privilege for benefit, workers are entitled for pay during sick period which is used by them for financial benefit and at the same time working to earn elsewhere.
- Wedding, festival, property acquisition and other social and family obligation make the worker to get absented.
- Social disorders like alcoholism, drug addiction, horse race, *Matka* are found to be responsible for absence.
- Medical illness of genuine nature form 8 to 10 percent of days lost in occupation.

Prevention of Sickness Absence

- Provision of health services and medical facilities.
- Ergonomics
- Good worker relations
- Pre employment examinations
- Periodic screening
- Good Occupational Management Techniques.

HEALTH PROBLEMS IN OCCUPATION

In all, occupations are means of economic and social revolution; they carry associated health hazards. Be it an industry, a hospital, a rehabilitation centre, it takes a role of an organisation to face inevitable health upsets during the course of its working culture.

Main problems are enumerated below:

Housing	– Shelter problem is increasing in vertically grown cities.
Water	– Scarcity, pollution leading to water borne diseases.
Air	– Toxic gases, dusts pollute the air causing allergy, asthma, chronic bronchitis.
Sewage	– Poor sewage system leads to soil pollution, high parasitic and helminthic infestations.
Diseases	– Tuberculosis, STD and Malaria are raging due to overcrowding of cities.
Food	– Typhoid, Hepatitis are becoming more conspicuous due to poor food sanitation.
Mental health	– Psychoneurosis, behaviour disorders, delinquency are increasing due to altered, and urbanized ways of life.
Accidents	– Congestion and vehicular traffic is leading to many highway traffic accidents leading to mortality and morbidity.
Social problems	– Alcoholism, drug addiction gambling, prostitution, divorce, crime have increased in densely populated industrialised areas.

SPECIFIC PROTECTION OF HEALTH OF WORKERS IN OCCUPATION

International Labour Organisation, through its subsidiary National Labour Organisations, is trying to uphold health protection measures as its aim in promotion and maintenance of the highest degree of physical, mental and social well-being of workers in all occupations. They are summarized as under:

i. *Health education:* Health awareness for personal hygiene, personal protection, good and healthy atmosphere of working condition are the need of the day.

ii. *Mental health:* Workers in any occupation require love, affection, recognition, job satisfaction; rewards and discipline, nursing profession being highly skilled occupation requires utmost attention in this regard.

iii. *Nutrition:* Balanced diet at reasonable rate to workers of an organisation is a must. This is compulsory as per legislative standards when the number of employees exceeds 250.

iv. *Medical care:* Facility for diagnosis, treatment, hospitalization of affected workers is obligatory on the part of the employer.

v. *Environmental sanitation:* Any factory, industry or organisation require facilities under this, which are the prime requisite for health of workers. They are:
   - Protected water supply
   - Hygienic food
   - Separate toilet for male and female
   - One Latrine for every 25 workers
   - General cleanliness of industry, factory, Hospital, Nursing home or organisation
   - Floor space of 500 cub.ft per worker
   - Good lighting
   - Good cross ventilation
   - Anti fire measures
   - Good dust containment measures.

vi. *Special care of women:*
   - Maternity leave to expectant mothers
   - M.C.H. services
   - Crèche in factories, industries or organisation if more than 30 women are working which can take care of their children.

vii. Welfare schemes for small family norm.

PREVENTION OF OCCUPATIONAL DISEASES

They are grouped under 3 heads:

1. Medical
2. Engineering
3. Legislation.

Medical Measures

a. *Medical examination before appointment:* This is called preplacement examination. The purpose is to place proper person in a given work placement, depending upon his ability and capacity.
b. *Periodic examination:*Normally annual examination is recommended. In case of occupations, where radium, dyes, lead are used; it will be every month. In case of irritant chemicals, ionising radiation, High dose cobalt therapy, Investigations with radioactive isotopes-daily examination at the end of shift is advocated.
c. *E.S.I. hospitals:*In case of factories, industries and organisations, facility for medical check up, treatment and investigations are made available to workers.
d. *Notifications:* Notification of cases and suspected cases in occupational diseases are mandatory as per legal standards.
e. *Supervision of working environment:* Physician and nurse should enlist the cooperation of safety engineers, psychologists and industrial hygienists for the health and welfare of workers in an occupation.
f. *Occupational records:*Records on worker's health, disability or absence help in improving the best device for good working condition.
g. *Use of protective devices:*Mask, glove, helmet, apron, shoes, lead or cloth working white coat help in personal protection in occupation.

Universal precaution is a typical example of personal protection of nursing profession from infectious diseases.

Special protective devices in AIDS cases, SARS cases are other examples.

Engineering Devices

a. Design of factory, industry, hospital, health centre should start from blue print stage.
b. *Good house keeping:* It includes general cleanliness, lighting, ventilation to eliminate occupational hazards.
   Hospital waste management is an example of good house keeping in Nursing Care services.
c. *Containment:* To collect all dust and eliminate from working area is called containment of dust or agents
d. *Dilution:* Developing green belt around factory, industry, hospital or organisation maintain air purity and hazards due to atmospheric pollution can be reduced.
e. Engineering devices for personal protection are well-known. Apron, glove, mask, helmet, sterile suit are examples.
f. *Monitoring:* Environmental monitoring for permissible limits and statistical monitoring for health criteria are required for positive occupational health.
g. *Research:* It is a podium for better understanding of health problem in occupational health.

Legislation

To govern the condition of a factory, an industry, a hospital, a nursing home or an organisation and to safeguard the health and welfare of the worker, laws are framed at national level and are amended from time to time.

The Factory Act 1948

Since 1881 earlier rules and regulations were in force till the Act was promulgated.

Many revisions took place and latest revision (amendment) was in 1987.

Scope: Any organisation which appoints 20 workers comes into its preview. (It is 10 when power is not used which is becoming rare). It includes contract labour also.

Health, safety, welfare, provision of working environment, medical and nursing facility, provision of waste disposal etc., are included in the provision. Agewise, sexwise limit is prescribed for effecting work in an occupation. "Safety Officers" for every 1000 workers is made mandatory. It describes special welfare measures like washing, first aid, lunchroom and crèches. A canteen for every 250 workers, a crèche for every 30 women workers and a welfare officer for every 500 workers are recommended.

Child labour: Prohibits employment of children below 14 years of age.

Shift basis: It prescribes 48 hours of work per week which should be 8 to 9 hours per day.

Leave with pay: 1 day for every 20 days is advocated.

It is obligatory to notify specified occupational disease. Hazardous process should be viewed for service condition of employees.

E.S.I.S., 1948

Employees' State Insurance Act, 1948 was amended recently in 1989.

Scope: It covers all establishments where 20 or more people are working. It includes shops, hotels, cinemas, transport service and newspaper establishments. In the year 1997 it included clerks, supervisors and technical workers drawing salary upto 7500 per month. The limit was proposed as Rs. 10,000 by Employees State Insurance Corporation (ESIC) in June 2006 which came to effect from 1-10-2006.

Benefits

Medical benefit: Investigation, treatment, hospitalization, individual health care and family care of employee is taken care under this. ESI dispensaries are set up where more than 1000 workers are employed, a part time ESI dispensary where 750 workers are employed and through General Practitioners in other situations.

Sickness benefit: The benefit of 91 days wage per year is allowed. It pays 7/12 of wage of employee; certain long term illness are considered for allowing 309 days since chronic course of disease need long time. They are:

Maternity benefit: Twelve weeks for confinement, 6 weeks for miscarriage are allowed.

Disablement benefit: 72% of wage for temporary disability and life pension (72%) for permanent disability.

Dependent benefit: Dependents get 40% of standard benefit rate periodically.

Funeral benefit: This is an amount of Rs. 1000 towards funeral expense. Expense of not exceeding 2500/- is available.

Rehabilitation allowance: At insurance of Rs. 10 per month by worker, medical treatment of disabled and members of family till life.

Other Acts

The Mines Act, The Plantation Act, The Minimum Wages Act, The Maternity Benefit Act, etc.

OCCUPATIONAL HEALTH NURSE

In early days home nursing service for workers was given by industrial nurses. Nursing care at hospital, nursing homes, health centres, physician or dentists office and nursing education are predominant areas of placement of nurses. Now new area of interest for nursing care services are:

- School health
- Occupational health.

In developed countries nurses are employed in factories. This requires specialized knowledge and skill with proper training. U.K. and Canada are imparting advanced courses in occupational health nursing. Standing committees are giving service activities which are now under the banner of American Association of Occupational Health Nurses (AAOHN).

Apart from general nursing, special nurse management in performing lung function tests, audiograms, vision tests are the needs of nursing care.

Job description of occupation health nurse:

- Assist rehabilitation of employee at plant site.
- Conduct walk through inspection of plant from health point of view.
- Treating, educating employee.
- Attend safety meetings.
- Assist occupational physician in clinical examination.
- Maintaining records.
- Act as a liaison.
- Check over hazard data sheets.

CHAPTER THIRTEEN

Mental Health, Mental Health Nursing, Community Psychiatry

IMPORTANCE

In nursing care, a nurse has a duty of very many complicated issues which include:

- Mental illness of patient depicting many mental disorders.
- Working of a good practice in nursing care where psychology of nurse works a lot.
- Understanding of hospital and community where, role, status, morale, leadership work upon her.

INTRODUCTION

Concept of Normalcy, Abnormalcy

Mental health is poorly understood with regard to a person's normal and abnormal behaviour and prescribes the word mad or not mad. If a person is not found adjustable then he is termed mad, which is not the case. Degree of mental health varies and no one is hundred percent healthy; varying degrees of adjustments, understanding and ability to cope with emotional problems make a person normal or abnormal.

Criteria of Abnormal Behaviour

- Always worrying.
- Unable to concentrate.
- Unhappy without justified cause.
- Very often and very easily loose tempe-rament.
- Regular insomnia.
- Depression which makes incapacitated to fight.
- Routine life is not normal.
- Unnecessarily getting frightened.
- Total disparity with always right and always wrong.
- Somatic incurable pains and aches.

Defence Mechanism

This defence mechanism is automatic uncons-cious response that helps a person reduce painful feelings associated problems. It helps in the following manner:

- Protects from anxiety.
- Insult is protected by self esteem
- Done or occurred at unconscious stage; it is a natural protective phenomenon.
- It acts by denying mistakes, denying true motives and denying actions or impulses.

Common Defence Mechanisms are:

Repression: Forgetting unacceptable idea.

E.g., Under fits patient urinates which he can not recollect a month later.

Sub-limitation: Diverting unacceptable feeling.

E.g., Unmarried is dedicated to career.

Reaction formation: Unconscious dealing for unacceptable desire.

E.g., Afraid of surgery, patient jokes at it.

Dissociation: Unconscious removal of pain-ful experience.

E.g., Parents are charred to death in front of child and child cannot recollect it.

Conversion: Change feelings to emotions.

E.g., Man does not want to marry gets fits (Common in hysteria).

Rationalisation: Give excuses (Unconsciously).

E.g., A girl always seen semi-nude, when asked says that she can never find anything else to wear.

Projection: Shift the blame to others.

E.g., Poor dancer blames floor level.

Regression: Childish behaviour.

E.g., Anxious husband become completely dependant on wife, refusing to do even smallest thing for himself.

Problem of Mental Disorder

General behaviour is changed–loss of appetite, refusal of food, hostile, angry, give up a job, restless, irrelevant and incoherent talk and obsession.

Perception change: Illusion, hallucination.

Memory change: Amnesia.

Altered consciousness: Disorientation.

Emotional disturbance: Mood change, depression.

Motor activity change: Stupor, pathological imitations (ecopraxia), immobile positions (catalepsy).

Classification of Mental Disorders

I. Schizophrenia (Split Personality)

1. Schizophrenia (Simple)
   a. with +ve symptoms
   b with –ve symptoms
2. Paranoid schizophrenia (Delusion + Jealousy)
3. Hebephrenic schizophrenia (Disorganised)
4. Catatonic schizophrenia (Stupor or rigid)
5. Residual schizophrenia (Eccentric)
6. Undifferentiated schizophrenia.

II. Maniac Depressive Psychosis (Excitement or depression)

1. Hypomania
2. Manic excitement.

III. Paranoia

1. Psychoneurosis
2. Character disorders.

Therapeutic Nurse-Patient Relationship

Therapeutic relation starts with giving little possible attention "Talking of nursing the whole patient" which refers to body and mind is key to success for physical and emotional difficulties. Patient's new social attachment to ward may not be overlooked.

There is a need to perform many treatments in private in order to spare sensitive patients the distress of watching and being observed.

Nursing staff creates the feeling of relaxation (Optimism). Strain (or pessimism) is also possible in her nursing role.

In recent years the atmosphere in paediatric ward and geriatric ward are receiving much attention. The pathetic loneliness of the aged when they are in bed is a handicap to recovery. Deafness, short-sightedness and inhibited movements make it too difficult to bridge the conventional distance of beds. Playrooms are used for each child patient which is an advantage in case of paediatric ward.

In Mental hospitals the therapeutic effect of group treatment where, use of patients' ability to help each other has been found immensely helpful.

The term "Therapeutic Community" was originally coined to describe how in a particular hospital for psychopathic, a community spirit developed which helped many patients to gain self-respect, to cultivate their assets to the fullest degree and to gain control over their antisocial and aggressive tendencies.

Understanding of stages of motivation helps the approach in such important matters as toilet training, weaning, feeding, play, education etc., among child patients.

THE INDIVIDUAL WITH FUNCTIONAL PSYCHOTIC DISORDERS

Schizophrenia

It is a functional psychosis characterised by disturbances in thinking, emotion, violation and perception. Finally it leads to personality deterioration. Nearly 50% of mentally ill are Schizophrenic. It could be due to imbalance between interacting biological, psychological and social factors. Genetic basis is thought to be around 0.8%. Diagnosis is based on eliciting positive symptoms like Delusion, Hallucination, Aggression, Suspicion and Conceptual Disorganization: negative symptoms like apathy, social withdrawal, artificial gestures and lack of spontaneity.

Treatment method include anti-psychotic drugs, ECT, psychotherapy and health education.

The nursing management needs may vary from defining reality, handling patient control; strengthening the patient's self-image and strengthening inter-personal relationships. The chronic patients need stimulation, occupational and recreation therapies.

Mood Disorder

Mood disorder (affective disorder) is an emotional state characterised by an excessive swing of mood. Manic depressive psychosis (now called Bipolar disorder) is common manifestation of mood disorder. In India 1-6 percent of population suffer from mood disorder. Apart from heredity, imbalance of biogenic amines in the brain can cause depression. This may be associated with alcohol. Suicide is common among these patients. Management include hospitalization, drug therapy (Anti-depressant) ECT and psychotherapy.

Nursing care is required for good sleep, food intake, drug intake, safety measures and health education.

THE INDIVIDUAL WITH ORGANIC DISORDERS

Mental illness resulting from transient or permanent CNS dysfunction caused by brain pathology which may be acute or chronic (delirium or dementia) constitute organic mental disorders.

Differences between acute and chronic organic mental disorders are:

Acute (Delirium)	*Chronic (Dementia)*
Disorientation, anxiety	Disturbed memory
Drowsy	Alert
Illusion, hallucination common	Cerebral function is lost
Variable clinical course	Progressive
Reversible	Irreversible

Common Causes of Delirium

Infection of brain, head injury, uraemia, pellagra, drug toxicity due to atropine, cocaine and bromide.

Common Causes of Dementia

- Degeneration of nerve (Alzheimer's)
- Infection (Syphilis, AIDS, Multiple sclerosis
- Toxic (alcohol, carbon monoxide and heavy metal poisoning)
- Metabolic (Hypothyroidism, chronic uraemia, pellagra)
- Tumours (Meningioma, hydrocephalus)
- Trauma (Head injury).

Management of Organic Mental Disorders

Treatment of delirium	*Treatment of dementia*
Diagnosis, treatment	Drug treatment (Papaverine), piracetam lecithin
Sedation	Psychosocial management
Diet	Patients' safety
Rest	Restraint violent cases
Reassurance	Reassurance
Support	Educate for no bed wetting
	Education of relatives

Toxin and poison need specific treatment by stopping drug, using antidote and reassurance.

Epilepsy

Sudden loss of consciousness which is often accompanied by repeated jerky movements called convulsions (Fits or Seizures). It may be primary or secondary epilepsy. In primary epilepsy cause is not known. Secondary epilepsy is caused by tumour, brain haemorrhage, electrolytic imbalance and alcohol withdrawal. Grand Mal is major epilepsy characterised by aura, tonic phase, clonic phase and recovery phase; other types are focal epilepsy which show jerky movement of one part of body. One of the complications of epilepsy is status epilepticus which is an emergency. Diagnosis is done by history, investigation of blood for VDRL, calcium and sugar, X-ray, EEG and CT scan of brain.

Management of epilepsy include drug treatment by phenytion sodium, carbamazepine, sodium valproate, diazepam, pheonbarbitone. Nursing care during attack include maintaining calmness, clear the area, actions to prevent aspiration pneumonia and allowing for full rest. Status epilepticus need 10 mg slow IV diazepam.

Nursing care after attacks include health education, guidance and counselling.

THE INDIVIDUAL WITH PSYCHO NEUROTIC DISORDERS

They are less severe form of psychological disorder where patients show either excessive or prolonged emotional reaction to any given stress. Symptoms are anxiety, fear, sadness, vague aches, pains and other bodily symptoms. Nearly 10% of population suffer from psychoneurotic disorders.

Anxiety

We are in the "era of anxiety", current conflict of civilization and rapid changes in urbanised life. It is an unpleasant emotion when a man seeks urgent relief. They are classified into 4 groups:

1. Generalised anxiety disorder
2. Panic disorder
3. Phobic disorder
4. Obsessive compulsive disorder.

Dissociative Disorders (Hysteria)

Hysteria, a common type of neurosis cause hysterical personality which may be dissociative disorder or conversion disorder. In dissociate disorder he separates from original self and acts in a new manner. In conversion hysteria pain, paralysis, fits and aphonia are common which is due to increased stress, repeated ideas and maladaptive coping methods.

Multiple personality: The existence within individual of two or more distinct personalities, one of which is dominant at a particular time. The original personality is not aware of this. It is associated with psychological stress and tends to become chronic.

Nursing Care in Psychoneurotic Disorders

i. *Anxiety disorders:*
   - Health education on psychological problems.

- Simple relaxation exercises
- Encourage to take care of ones own activities
- Comfort and safety

ii. *Hysteria:*
- Problem identification
- Assurance of relatives
- Attention and sympathy
- Encourage independence

iii. *Dissociative disorder:*
- Reassurance
- Avoid exposing patient to memory recollection
- Expose patient to stimuli that represent pleasant experience.

The Individual with Psycho Physiological Disorders (Psycho Somatic)

They are group of disorders in which emotional factors have a demonstrable role in the aetiology.

Common Disorders Seen are

- High B.P.
- Asthma
- Peptic ulcer
- Ulcerative colitis
- Irritable bowel syndrome
- Arthritis
- Headache
- Eczema
- Diabetes
- Anorexia nervosa
- Obesity
- Psychogenic pain.

Common causes could be response to emotion, personality traits, family pattern and prolonged stress.

Management include symptomatic treatment. Nursing care includes:

- Good therapeutic relationship
- Encourage patient to discuss his problem
- Create a feeling of acceptance
- Encourage family participation in therapy
- Teach relaxation exercises.

THE INDIVIDUAL WITH CHARACTERISTICS DISORDERS

Sexual Disorders

It is difficult to define it because the disorder is decided by social norms and customs which vary in different countries and cultures. We have certain normal sexual behaviour.

Psycho sexual disorders can be:

i. Sexual dysfunction
ii. Gender identity disorder (Trans-sexualism)
iii. Perversions like Fetichism (Sexual gratification by objects), Transvestism (Cross dressing), Paedophilia (child-sex), Sexual sadism (inflicting pain), Sexual masochism (seek beaten), Exhibitionism (body exposure) voyeurism (peep undressing).

Alcohol and Substance Dependence

Alcohol withdrawal delirium occurs in 5% of alcoholics who stop alcohol. Corrections of dehydration, electrolytic imbalance, control of fits are to be attended along with careful monitoring of vital signs.

Opioids, antipsychotic drugs show involuntary muscle contractions ending with stiff neck, stiff mouth, elevated eyeball.

Care has to be managed as inpatient along with the special nursing care of psychiatric emergencies.

Sociopath Reaction

Antisocial, cruel minded personality needs attention of safety, security and its management is similar to psychiatric emergency.

CHILDHOOD DISORDERS

Proportion of childhood mental disorders can be gauged by the fact that they constitute 38 to 40%

of our population which comes to about 390 million at present as per 2001 census.

Common causes of disorders are Biological cause (hereditary, illness), Psychological cause (broken homes) and Social cause (poverty).

Common illness are:
- Mental retardation
- Autism (driven to fantasy)
- Conduct disorders
- Specific developmental disorders
- Personality developmental disorders
- Hyperkinetic disorders
- Tics
- Mannerism.

Basic responsibility of nurse should be based on recognising child on following features:
- Child behaviour not appropriate to age.
- Child behaviour leads to disability.
- It is against social expectation.

Apart from carrying out instructions for therapy, a nurse should:
- Obtain detail of problem
- Explain parents
- Assurance to parents
- Play therapy.

MODERN THERAPY

In mentally ill health person treatment is not specific since it varies from person to person. Nurse being closer with patient, has important role in therapy. Her action, attitude and skills to help patient to deal with his problems are themselves an essential part of his treatment.

a. *Physical therapy:* It includes drug treatment, ECT, psychosurgery.
b. *Psycho pharmacology:* This includes psychotherapy of individual, group, family.
c. *Hypnosis:* By altered state of consciousness induced by conditioning and skilled use of suggestions.
d. *Play therapy:* Very helpful for young and the old. Diversion by play can get over tension and anxiety.
e. *Activity therapy:* There are specific therapy like occupational, music, dance, psychodrama, recreation and psychosocial therapies.

CRISIS SITUATION

It is also called crisis intervention which is a type of brief psychological method of treatment for the person who is in an emotional crisis. Crisis is a sudden event in one's life that disturbs the mental equilibrium during which the usual coping mechanisms fail.

Grief is a crisis which normally does not require intervention. Reassurance, suggestion and environmental manipulation are found sufficient. In some cases it may require psychotropic medication.

Suicide is an emergency crisis which needs one or two sessions of treatment. If necessary hospitalization may be necessary. It is possible to prevent suicide by behavioural therapy and relaxation therapy.

LEGAL ASPECT OF MENTAL HEALTH NURSING

Law is involved in many situations which compel us to focus our attention on this aspect. Legal aspects of mental health are:

Civil Responsibility

Mentally ill person cannot make will (Testamentary incapacity). Marriage with mentally ill is declared null and void.

Mentally ill person cannot give witness and cannot (a) Transfer or sell property (b) Stand for election (c) Enter into business.

Criminal Responsibility

According to section 84 of IPC.

"Nothing is an offence which is done by a person, who at the time of doing it, by reason of unsoundness of mind, is incapable of knowing the nature of act, or that he is doing what is either wrong or contrary to law".

Mentally ill is exempted from punishment for a crime.

The Indian Lunacy Act, 1912

It has been the governing Act for many years in India. It is being replaced by original Mental Health Act for the reason of incorporation of human rights of the mentally ill.

The Mental Health Act 1987

In India, it governs the welfare of mentally ill. It controls the treatment procedure of mentally ill. It takes care of human right aspect and property also. The lunatic is replaced with mentally ill and asylum is replaced by psychiatric hospital.

Community Psychiatry

It is a branch of psychiatry that develops and maintains organised programmes for the prevention, promotion and rehabilitation of mentally ill person.

In a defined population, care given through health workers and community health guide for a continuous care and integrated with regular health service is called community mental health care.

Primary Prevention

- Elimination of causative agent.
- Reducing risk factors.
- Enhancing man's resistance.
- Reducing stress.
- Counselling (Student, marriage, sex and genetic).
- Mental health education.

Secondary Prevention

- Population screening.
- Crisis intervention service centres are established.
- Health awareness for early diagnosis.

Tertiary Prevention

- Rehabilitation after defects noticed.

The Nurse in Mental Health Nursing

It is now a well-established fact that it is not just diagnosis and treatment, but requires promotion and preservation of good mental health. There are many areas where mental health nursing play vital role. They are:

- Early diagnosis, prompt treatment
- Rehabilitation
- Group psychotherapy
- Individual psychotherapy
- Mental health education
- Use of psychoactive drugs
- Follow-up services.

National Mental Health Programme

Government of India has launched National Mental Health Programme during VII five year plan with the objectives of:

- Ensuring availability of service.
- Make mental health service accessible.
- Its application in general health care.
- To promote community participation.
- To help for self help.

Now, it is under the shade of comprehensive mental health programme where mentally ill is treated with common man in community health activity.

CHAPTER FOURTEEN

Health Education and Communication (IEC)

HEALTH EDUCATION

INTRODUCTION

Health Education is an essential tool of community health. Every branch of community health has health educational aspects in the end. Health education brings scientific knowledge to the people so that they can use such knowledge for betterment of their own health and of their community in which they live.

Aims and Objectives

1. To ensure that health is valued as an asset in the community.
2. To equip people with skills, knowledge and attitudes to enable themselves to solve their health problems by their own actions and efforts.
3. To promote the developmental and proper use of health services and improving their sense of responsibilities for their own health.

Definition

According to the National conference on Preventive Medicine in U.S.A. the definition of Health Education is:

"A process that informs, motivates and helps people to adopt and maintain healthy practices and lifestyles, advocates environmental changes as needed to facilitate this goal and conducts professional training and research to the same end."

PURPOSE OF HEALTH EDUCATION

Help people to become self relevant, not dependent on others, to be central actors and not spectators.

Democracy and Health Education go hand in hand in a community.

Creates will power, develops personality, and make them to work voluntarily.

Encourage people to adopt and sustain health promoting lifestyles and practices.

Promote the proper use of health services available to them.

Provide knowledge to develop positive attitude and to practice on rational decisions to solve their problems.

Stimulate self-reliance and community participation for achieving health development.

In reality health education gives an opportunity to make realistic improvements in the quality of life.

Scope

We have many situations in day-to-day life and day-to-day activities. Main situations have been home, school and community.

Home

- Hygienic habits and practices of adults and guidance to children
- Positive attitude towards prevention of illness
- Family budgeting for priority expenses

- Sanitation of home
- Preparation, serving and preservation of food
- Selection of entertainment in the family
- Molding in religious and cultural behaviour of the family.

School

- Cleanliness of environment and facilities
- Good feeding practice or midday school meal
- Participation in community project
- Teacher's health behaviour to become example for children.

Community

- Service and advice from health personnel
- Participation in health programmes
- Observing ceremonies
- Leisure time activities.

APPROACHES TO HEALTH EDUCATION

a. **Regulation:** By Government Acts, Amendments and Rules the behaviour of man can be managed hence it is called regulatory approach.
   E.g.,
   Compulsory helmet wearing by two wheelers users.
   Child Marriage Restraint Act.
   Regulatory approach is not appropriate because health education do not carry force or law.
b. **Service:** By giving service, people can be made to inculcate the habit of changing their behaviour.
   E.g.,
   - Free health care to mothers and children to make them to accept small family norm.
   - Sanitary latrine is provided free of cost under basic health service to reduce faecal borne disease.

   Here the drawback is that people do not accept or use unless they feel that there is a felt need of the situation.
c. **Education:** New attitude and new habit for healthy life by creating health awareness is a task which takes longer time to achieve. It depends on mass media and social organisation. Stopping smoking, using filtered water or planning one child for their family etc., need an autonomy of person on their lives. Planned learning experience and motivation by satisfied people can take us a long way under this approach.
d. **Primary health care:** Active involvement and community participation, a new approach of first contact care by the people is taking a boost as a good approach in health education.

Table 14.1: Difference between health education and health propaganda

	Health education	*Health propaganda*
Knowledge	Acquired	Instilled
Skill	Acquired	Instilled
Animal instinct	Taken away	Put to action
Action	Think and act	By reflex act
Emotion	No	Yes
Reasoning	Yes	No
Attitude	Positive	Negative

PRINCIPLES OF HEALTH EDUCATION

i. Trustworthy and credible message must be given
ii. It should be related to the interest of the people
iii. People's participation should be encouraged
iv. Use of motivation is a requisite
v. Health education must be given in an understandable language and to the level of I.Q. of people
vi. Repeated efforts are needed
vii. Learning by doing encourage positive outlook
viii. Awareness must be from known to unknown at health education
ix. Good human relation is mandatory
x. The person giving H E should be a model

xi. Command and respect help health education. Leaders of village, religion, politics etc. can help us in conveying health message.

METHODS OF HEALTH EDUCATION

I. Individual
- Contact
- Home visiting
- Postal

II. Group
- Lecture
- Demonstration
- Group discussion
- Panel
- Symposia
- Workshop
- Conference
- Seminar
- Role play

III. Mass
- Museum
- Poster
- Newspaper
- Radio
- T.V.
- Folk method
- Internet.

Individual Method

When a nurse individually contacts a patient in ward and/or in home visiting, she will be in a position to discuss, argue and persuade the patient to change his/her behaviour in the interest of patient's health status. However there is limitation in the above method since the size of the population needing counselling being such that they cannot be reached individually by the nursing community.

Group Methods

Lecture

It must be combined with AV aids like flip chart, Flannel graph, model, specimen and charts. 20 minutes talk followed by discussion is preferred.

Demonstration

It is of great value in environmental sanitation like hand pump, sanitary latrine, ORS packet use etc. It arouses interest and makes "seeing is believing".

Group Discussion

It is face to face interaction of a small group on health education. A group leader has to lead this. A well-conducted discussion is found effective; however one person may dominate as there may be a shy group. Deviation causes the group discussion irrelevant. OTC (Orientation training camp) of village leaders is example.

Panel Discussion

A given topic discussed by 4 to 8 members who are experts in the field.

Symposium

It is a series of speeches on a selected topic by experts.

Workshop

Series of meeting about 3-4 with emphasis on individual work. Here resource persons help in conducting workshop.

Conference

It is held at District, State, National or International level, for a given duration making use of group method of education using media.

Seminar

Seminar contain large component of material for a day or two on a given topic or on selected group of topics. Report prepared is also circulated later as material of reference and awareness.

Role Play

Sociodrama like mono acting on family planning, street play on HIV/AIDS etc., getting popular methods of propagating the messages.

Mass Media

T.V. radio, newspaper, internet, printed material, posters, health exhibition and folk media like *Harikatha, Yakshagana*, puppet show, drama etc., are made use of in creating health awareness through mass media. All these are called media of health education.

Planning and Management of Health Education

Since health education has to be carried out within the context of socio-cultural, political and socio-economic conditions, planner should take care in:

- Programming
- Planning
- Implementation
- Evaluation
- and its administration.

Step in Organisation of Health Education

1. Information on health problem is collected
2. Problem is properly identified
3. Priorities in the process are decided
4. Goals and objectives are set
5. Resources are mobilised
6. Possible solution to the problem are kept ready
7. Plan of action as to who is giving HE? On what aspect is giving? And when is that done?
8. Actual HE session
9. Monitoring and evaluating
10. Reorganising by noted flaws.

ADMINISTRATION

SEARB – South East Asia Regional Bureau
CHEB – Central Health Education Bureau
SHEB – State Health Education Bureau
DHEB – District Health Education Bureau
DAVP – Directorate of Advertising and Visual Publicity
PIB – Press Information Bureau
AIR – All India Radio.

Content of Nursing Health Education

- Human biology
- Better nutrition
- Personal hygiene
- Family health
- Mental health
- Health programmes
- Disease control
- Others (relevant to local area).

Ultimate Aims of Health Education

Every individual is made physically fit, mentally alert, bodily vigorous, socially responsible, culturally cooperative, emotionally stable, ethically sound, professionally competent, psychologically unworried.

SPECIAL AREAS

There are 4 areas which have widened their coverage, need special mention. They are:

a. AIDS education
b. Cancer education
c. Nutrition education
d. Population education.

AIDS Education

An educational programme which provide a study of AIDS situation for a better development of responsible attitude towards HIV/AIDS.

Content

- Making life-saving choices.
- Guidelines for prevention of AIDS.
- Nature of AIDS.
- Transmission of AIDS.
- Risk factors in AIDS.
- National AIDS situation.

There is a requirement of high political commitment for AIDS control. Educational goals for AIDS control should be self-awareness on benefits of living in simple and self-cultured to be disseminated. Available treatment for AIDS facilities and clinics are explained.

Cancer Education

An educational programme which provide a study of cancer situation for a better development of responsible attitude towards cancer control.

Content

- Warning signs of cancer
- Risk factors
- National cancer situation
- Political commitment for cancer centres
- Educational goal of cancer centres
- Benefits of simple living
- Economics of smoking
- Economics of alcoholism
- Occupational aspects of cancer
- Carcinogens in atmosphere
- Cancer screening programmes
- Available treatment for cancer.

Nutrition Education

This is aimed at providing a study of nutritional situation for a better development of responsible attitude towards better nutrition and better health.

Contents

- Malnutrition
- National nutritional status
- Political commitment for better nutrition
- Food hygiene
- Special group requirement
- PFA Acts
- National programme on nutrition
- Balanced diet
- Nutritional assessment
- Nutrition and health.

Population Education (Extension Education)

An educational programme which provides a situation for a better development of responsible attitude towards population growth.

Content

- National demographic situation
- National political commitment to population growth
- Educational goal for population growth
- Benefits of small family norm
- Economics of population growth
- Sociology of population growth
- Statistics of population growth
- Levels of living by population growth
- Effects of population explosion.

COMMUNICATION

INTRODUCTION

In recent years, communication is one of the crucial elements in administrative behaviour. The art of communication is greatly complicated by the deficient language. Most of the communications are verbal.

Communication is the process of giving message to people either through talk or through written message. Communication is essential to minimize conflict, confusion and chaos. It eliminates friction, frustration and help in motivating the man; and thus becomes dynamic interaction process of connecting people.

"It is a two-way process of exchanging and shaping ideas, feelings and message."

Communication can be for:

- Acquiring knowledge
- Learning skills
- Develop good attitude.

Definition

Communication is the broad field of human understanding and interchange of facts and opinions and not the technologist of telephone, telegraph or radio.

It can also be the sum of all the things one person does when he wants to create understanding in the minds of another man. Thus it forms the bridge of meaning.

Components

Communication is very important to the smooth functioning and very survival of an organization; forming the foundation of cooperative group activities. Moreover planning requires perfect understanding.

Components of communication are represented as under (Figs 14.1 and 14.2):

Communication Barriers

1. Physiological – Difficulty in hearing
2. Psychological – Emotional disturbance
3. Environmental – Loud noise.
4. Cultural – Urban: Rural
   – Foreign: Local (National).
   – Positive: Negative attitude.

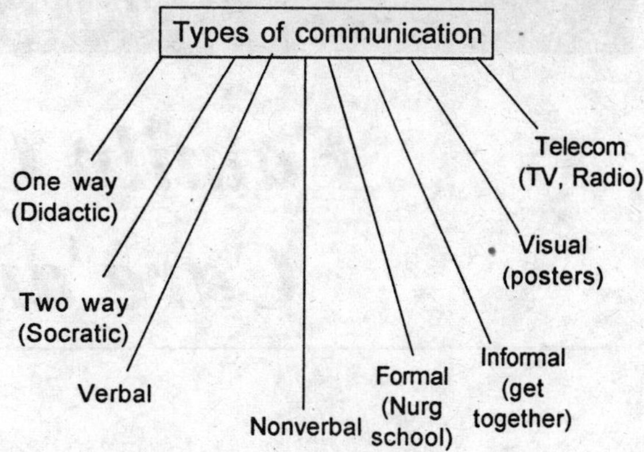

Fig. 14.2: Types of communication

Need of Communication

- To inform other
- To educate the group (formal and non-formal)
- To motivate people
- To persuade people
- To give counselling
- To raise morales of a group
- For health development
- To organise a programme.

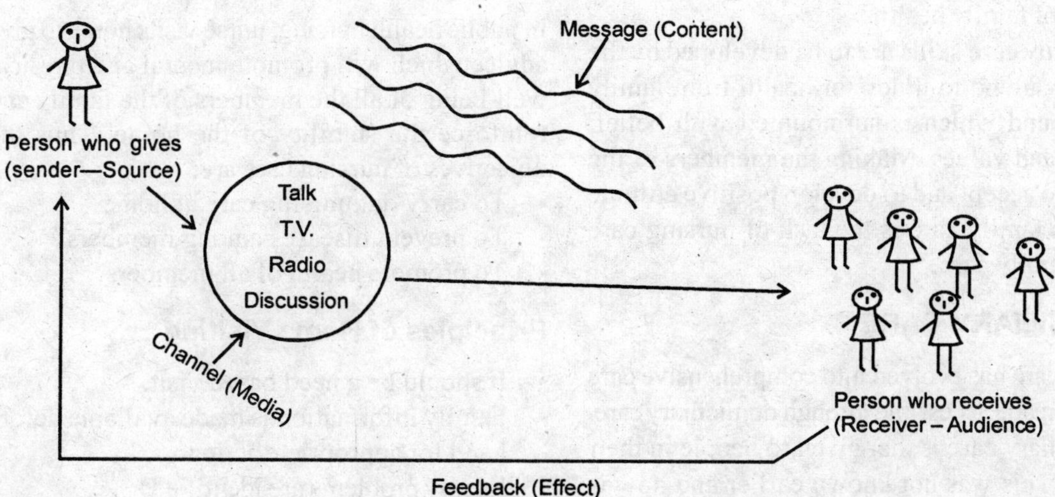

Fig. 14.1: Components of communication

CHAPTER FIFTEEN

Family Care, Domiciliary Care and Home Visiting

FAMILY CARE

Family is the unit of society or community and here maximum interaction occurs within the family and outside the family. Studying individual or a patient from his family background, managing the case at family within available resources make an effective care called Family Care.

Family care needs a good nurse-family relationship. Nurse needs her public health training to treat common illness at family. Integration of Indian systems of medicine, if requested by the family, is to be considered as priority based health care. Family care involves recording system of family composition, size and type of family and pattern of family health.

Family care skills are to be developed by the nurse to attend to illness or health from family background which is surmounted with belief, culture and values. Making the members of the family to accept and to develop positive attitude towards family care is the task of nursing care under family care.

DOMICILIARY CARE

Family care has evolved into comprehensive care and it is made accessible through domiciliary care. Domiciliary care is that given to people in their homes. This was not known earlier and now is an organised controlled practice in health care services.

Domiciliary care was (earlier) the responsibility of churches. Florence Nightingale revolutionized and took the nursing task to people in their living atmosphere (to their doorstep). As a friend and advisor, nurse gives domiciliary care in the following specific situations:

- Mother craft
- Pregnancy, delivery, childcare
- Tuberculosis treatment
- Leprosy nursing
- Mental illness
- S.T.D. care
- Malaria surveillance and treatment.

HOME VISITING

In public health nursing, nurse visits home to give advice which will promote mental and physical well-being of all the members of the family and reinforce the stability of the home. Thus the objectives of nursing care are:

- To carry out nursing care at home
- To prevent diseases among members
- To promote health of all members.

Principles of Home Visiting

- It should be a need based visit.
- Family information is made available before hand for appropriate action.
- Family problems are identified.
- Technical skill learnt and nursing procedure known is to be put into action.

- Make sure of scientific base in creating health awareness among members at home.
- Nursing approach should build a sense of confidence.
- Kind and courteous at care.

Home Visit Planning

This is to be planned with available resources and on the available information on families. Map of the area, approaching roads, family folders if available, individual health cards will help in initiating home visit.

Needs are identified for home visit. They include pregnant woman, lactating mothers, a child, a sick or a family problem.

During initial home visits, introducing her, building up confidence and clarification of their doubts mark the success of home visiting.

Nursing bag is carried for primary care and treatment of minor illness. There are two nursing bags one for delivery and the other for general nursing. The content of delivery kit and nursing bag are given in the appendix.

Home visit will be incomplete without follow-up of cases. Achievement of home visiting can be assessed by many available methods.

Bag Technique

Canvas, leather or light metal bag is used. This is stitched in such a way that it can be carried either by hand or over shoulders. It should have an outer packet to keep a note book, measuring tape, newspaper sheet, towel, soap and a nail brush.

Bag Usage Technique

Since the bag is used for many home visiting, it must be kept clean. When a home visit is made the bag is placed over a newspaper, hands are washed before opening the bag, only required are removed for the given nursing procedure, used ones are washed and carried in an other bag for future sterilisation. After nursing care, soiled dressings are burnt; newspaper is folded with used side inside and kept in outer packet of bag.

Content of Nursing Bag

- Clinical thermometer
- Rectal thermometer
- Scissors
- Dressing forceps
- Artery forceps
- Kidney tray small and medium
- Sterilised dressing set
- Foetoscope
- Sterilised swabs
- Rubber gloves
- Common and essential drugs (Paracetamol Tab, BB emulsion, Boric acid or Zinc boric, APC, Chloroquine, ORS, Spirit, KMNO4 cristal, Belladona tab, Phenobarbitone tab, Antacid tab, Vit A solution, 2% Gentian Violet, Vasaline, Antepar tab, Alcopar tab, Calamine lotion, Tr. Benzoin, Tr. Iodine
- Cord dressings
- Perineal dressings,
- Cord ligatures
- Detergent soap
- Towel
- Nailbrush
- Enema set
- Female catheter (urinary)
- Measuring tape
- Spring balance
- Mucus catheter
- Eye drops and ear drops
- Urine test set
- Big newspaper to spread and keep nursing bag and contents at home visit
- Small cut pieces of paper for tablet dispensing
- Extra bag that can carry used material after home visit
- Umbilical cotton (0.3 × 25 cm)
- Blade with holder
- Sanitary pad

- Dusting powder
- Antiseptic lotion
- Roller bandage
- Triangular bandage
- Adhesive plaster
- Exercise book and pencil
- Routine health education charts.

Care of Nursing Equipments

- Bag—Metal bag to be washed with soap and water canvas bag to be washed and dried.
- Rubber goods—Sterilised by boiling for 10 minutes; but disposal gloves are disposed by sanitary method.
- Thermometer—Soaked in antiseptic lotion.
- Glass bottles—Sterilised in boiled water.
- Enamel or steel items—20 minutes boiling.
- Cord ligature—Pre-sterilised pack is available; otherwise thread is boiled for 20 minutes. It is handled with sterile forceps and scrubbed hands.
- Eye drops—Opened ones are used within 10 days; later to be discarded and a new one is to be procured.
- Dry dressing and swabs—Autoclaved material is carried and used ones are disposed by burning.
- Instruments—Sterilisation procedure learnt is followed.
- Weighing machine, B.P. apparatus and Foetoscope or stethoscope are handled properly.

Precautions in Bag Technique

- No personal material are kept in the nursing bag
- No meddling of the content without hand wash
- Open only when required
- Used items are not put into nursing bag
- It is kept on a stool or box or a paper at home visiting.

Referral at Home Visiting

Cases are categorized into:

- Fatal condition
- Serious condition
- Minor condition.

One has to think and take decision in fatal case because if the same cannot be saved even with treatment with referral, it may be a waste of energy and sometimes may be against the will of members of the family. Serious condition may be serviced with first aid and immediate referral by transport. The attempt may be life saving. Minor ailments can allow delay in referral.

A referral card should have following information:

- Name, address of patient
- Complaint
- Treatment given
- Name and designation of persons referring
- To where reference made
- Date and time of referral.

Recording System

In public health practice recording system is to be updated at health centre after each home visiting. Records help in early action, minimize repetition, help in follow-up or progress.

Type of records may be:

- Village record
- Family folders
- Individual health records
- MCH (RCH) cards
- Immunisation card
- Growth chart
- TB treatment card
- Leprosy treatment card
- School health record
- Records of vital events (Birth, Death, Marriage)
- OPD record
- IPD discharge slip

- Daily log book
- Monthly reports.

Recording system should have data in complete form. It is preferred to be in structured format (which minimize clerical work). They are kept confidential.

Recording system may have following types:

- Folder type
- File type
- Envelop type
- Card type
- Book type.

Health Education at Home Visits

Nurse play greater role in educating, informing and motivating the members of the family at home visit. Selection of appropriate content, use of appropriate method is required for an effective health education.

EXTENSION OF HOME VISITING—A NEW CONCEPT OF PUBLIC HEALTH NURSING

Home Care

Nurse acts as nurse practitioner in giving primary health care, required nursing care or home care services.

Nursing (Homes)

Recent upsurge of nursing homes expect over 60 percent of health care activities by a trained nurse. The nursing component of a nursing home is catered at all levels viz., reception, advice, counselling, ward duty, follow-up of instructions, case preparation, O.T. assistance, dressing, maintenance of ICU, ICCU etc.

R.C.H. Nursing

The nursing component includes conducting home deliveries and after nursing care. It includes newborn care also.

School Health Nursing

It includes health check-up, health teaching, dental health, first aid, recording system and referral care.

Public Health Nursing

Public health in health and FW service has these designated posts and it includes family care at health and in sickness. R.C.H. care, immunisation, psychosocial counselling and carrying out P.H.C. function in the service area.

Industrial Nursing

As highlighted earlier, nursing care is a requisite in factories where more than 500 workers are employed. In the background of industrial setup care of sick, injured, first aid, safety, crèche, rehabilitation and nursing administration are the main nursing care activities.

Rehabilitation Centres

Nursing component in diagnosis, surgical correction, prosthesis provision, orthopaedic appliances are demanding nursing care services in rehabilitation centres.

Mental Health Nursing

Community psychiatry and community mental health demand the services of nursing profession. Nursing component in diagnosis, Drug administration, guidance, counselling, body care, personal hygiene of mentally ill demands the call for nursing care without which there cannot be comprehensive mental health care.

Geriatric Nursing

It is in hospital, health centre, old age home or elderly in their home call for nursing care which itself is 90% of total health care of the elderly. Along with clinical rehabilitation staff home visiting is demanded by the community.

THE HOME HELP SERVICE

With widening of dimension of nursing component through midwifery, home nursing and health visiting, adequate domestic help in the home is a created demand of urban family life. Nursing component is accepting shopping, cooking, washing and keeping house clean apart from regular nursing care on mutually agreeable terms.

Hospital deliveries, hospital admission in chronically ill, post operative cases of spouse are demanding home-help services.

The aim in providing all these facilities is to ensure sufficient support so that medical and nursing care in the home is a practical possibility.

CHAPTER SIXTEEN

Community Health Nursing

COMMUNITY HEALTH NURSING

Definition

A public health nurse is professionally equipped with additional qualification to serve the community. WHO has defined public health nursing as under:

"Public health nursing combines the skills of nursing, public health and some phases of social assistance and functions as a part of the total public health programme for the promotion of health, the improvement of conditions in the social and physical environment, the prevention of illness and disability and rehabilitation. It is concerned for the most part with the care of healthy families and with non-hospitalized sick persons and their families, with groups of people and with health problems that affect the community as a whole."

History and development of nursing in India is highlighted in Chapter 1.

Principles

The nurse who is engaged to serve the community has to follow the following nursing principles:

i. **Appraisal of community health:** Already existing base line data of the community under a primary health centre will give background picture of the community. It reflects Demographic, Socioeconomic, Morbidity and Mortality characteristics of the community. Nurse has to establish contact with the community through village leaders to appraise health status of members of the family. Family being the unit of observation, the problem study, centres round the family.

ii. **Identification of health problem:** Survey, surveillance and screening help to identify health problem in the community, survey information, PHC records individual health assessment of the family, mortality data, fertility data give clues to identify existing problem. The problem can be sickness, deaths, poverty, malnutrition or social problems.

iii. **Identification of cause of health problem:** This is a community assessment to find out the cause of problem. Individual health examination, social interaction with members of the family give the clue to the source of infection, cause of poverty, cause of malnutrition or root cause of social problems.

iv. **Setting priority for public health intervention:** Priority is fixed based on Home visiting findings which determines:
   a. Frequency of occurrence of problem.
   b. Seriousness of problem for the individual and for the family.
   c. Urgency with which the problem is to be tackled; and
   d. Practicability or feasibility of control of the problem.

A scoring system may be used for fixing the priority.

Qualities

i. **Patient sympathy and understanding:** In order to be able to help the community in her adjustment to pain, frustrations and limitations of illness. She must exercise tact in her social interaction with the members of the family and must show tolerance towards their likes and dislikes.

ii. **Gentleness and willingness:** In carrying out of all nursing duties however trivial it may be exercising self control and remaining calm and gracious at all the time is required.

iii. **Reliability:** All instructions given by MOH to her must be carried out correctly and conscientiously. She must observe honestly in deed and word.

iv. **Resourcefulness:** So that she may act immediately in any emergency using her commonsense to protect the family from ill effects.

v. **Loyalty to the MOH:** Upholding his authority at all times and never allowing anything to be said or done that may undermine the confidence of the community and family on the health staff.

vi. **Power of observation:** So that she may report accurately any changes in the health of the community, and may also anticipate and fulfil the community requirements at her earliest.

Functions

Public health nurse has to be member of health team and should be able to make decision, have management skill to help all national health programmes. Main functions of public health nurse are:

Aspect of Community Health Nursing

Family health and personal health dealt in terms of RCH, FP and school health form main aspect of community health nursing. They are dealt in detail under chapters 7, 4 and 7 respectively.

Terms Used

Health care, nursing care are services rendered to individual, families and community by health professionals.

Health system relates to management sectors involving service givers.

Levels of health care are:

Primary—Care at first contact.

Secondary—District hospitals, Community health centres.

Tertiary—Super speciality care.

Health team: Each member in a professional group has specific and recognised function in the team. It is a group of persons who share a common goal and common objectives which are determined by the needs of the community.

Health for all: It is an attainment of a level of health that will permit them to lead to a socially and economically productive life.

Primary health care: It is "Essential health care based on practical, scientifically sound and socially acceptable methods and technology made universally accessible to individuals and families in the community through their full participation and at a cost that the community and the country can afford to maintain at every stage of their development in the spirit of self-determination."

Disease

It is condition of body, organ or tissue in which functions are disrupted or deranged.

Public Health

The organised application of local, state, national and international resources to achieve health for all i.e. real public health.

Preventive Medicine

It is a branch of medicine based on aetiology as applied to healthy people. It is timely application of all means to promote the health of people.

Community Health

It is "all the personal health and environmental services in any human community, irrespective of whether such services were public or private ones." Earlier hygiene molded to sanitation which got changed to preventive and social medicine. The same area is now "Community Health". This was called community medicine till today.

Social Medicine

It is the study of man as a social being in his total environment.

Community Medicine

It is the successor of public health, preventive medicine, preventive and social medicine. In community medicine we come across measures like community diagnosis and community treatment.

NURSING STAFF

Nursing Staff Development

It is a requisite to see that all round development of nursing staff is advocated for an effective nursing services, since nursing care has become vast, special nursing requires update of knowledge and skill. If this component is forgotten, the nursing service is downgraded and achievement of nursing care goal will be lowered.

Following staff development programmes are advocated from time to time for an effective use of nursing manpower. They are:

- In-service education
- Continued education
- Specific orientation courses
- Specific skill training.

Nursing Management of Unit/Ward/Dept

Nursing management requires certain qualities in a nurse which are time tested and remunerative from humanitarian angle. They are:

- Patience, sympathy, understanding
- Gentleness and willingness
- Reliability
- Resourcefulness
- Power of observation.

Rules to be observed in cleaning:

i. All should be cleaned before start of a nursing act
ii. Clean duster, rubber, brushes and clean water must be used
iii. Sweeping should be before dusting except in high dusting of walls
iv. A damp duster is preferred for furniture
v. Corner and edges should not be forgotten
vi. Cleaning must be done with little disturbance
vii. All rubbish collection and disposal must be done twice a day
viii. Check for forbidden articles by the patient.
ix. Tiles, floors are scrubbed with yellow soap and water
x. Everyday cleaning with dry cloth of electric lights is a requirement
xi. Metal fittings are periodically checked for proper cleaning.

i. **Treatment and preparation room:** For safe aseptic practice surgical dressings are done in an annexe, one annexe for "Clean" preparation of sterilisation procedure, another for "septic" treatment.
ii. **Ward bath and sanitary annexes:** Soap and water are used for washing. For bowl and mug hot soap water containing 1: 80 Lysol is used. The dressing piles need crude phenol (1:10).
iii. **Ward/Unit kitchen:** Basic principles of kitchen sanitation are followed.
iv. **Bedpan and urinals:** Automatic bedpan washers in which bed pans are enclosed for flushing with hot and cold water are used.

Sputum mug is boiled for 5 minutes; sodium bicarbonate solution (1:160) is added before taking sputum mug to patient.

Water closet are sprinkled with chlorinated soda and left for 30 minutes. The brush used for water closet is disinfected with Jeyes fluid (1:40).

Care of bedspreads and beddings are followed as per hospital disinfection procedure. Bed mackintoshes, air rings and beds are mopped with 1:20 phenol or 1:30 Lysol before wash.

Ward linen has to follow procedures adopted by hospital infection control committee as per guidelines for nursing procedures so that care of soiled linen is taken to prevent cross infection.

Stain Removal Procedures

- Blood—Use of peroxide of hydrogen or ammonia and rinse later.
- Ink—Rubbing a paste of salt and lemon juice and a wash.
- Ball pen ink is removed by methylated spirit.
- Tea coffee cocoa—Use of a bleaching agent and a rinse.
- Fruit stain—Rub with salt and wash.
- Rust mark—Salt and lemon juice and exposure to sun light.
- Iodine mark—Apply ammonia, rinse and wash.
- Skin ointment, paste liniment—They are resistant to removal.
- Laundries have special methods.

Duties of a Nurse

To the Patient

Apart from earlier detailing, chief factors to be looked into are:

- Rest
- Toilet
- Diet
- Excretion of waste material
- Mental outlook.

To the Doctor

Carrying out instruction and written report avoids risk of omissions:

- Temperature, pulse, respiration
- Action of bowl, nature and composition of stool
- Type, amount of urine
- Nature of sleep
- Appetite, type of food taken
- Report of any pain, relief given
- Report of vomiting, nature
- Report of cough, nature
- Medicines administered
- Chart of fluid intake and fluid output.

To Herself

Nurse has to use rules of personal hygiene to maintain her health and for service efficiency:

- Cleanliness
- Clothing
- Food
- Rest, exercise.

Concepts in Community Health Nursing

Health For All (HFA)

Member countries of WHO has defined HFA as under:

"Attainment of a level of health that will enable every individual to lead to socially and economically productive life."

India developed its policies, strategies and plan of action to launch H.F.A. under its own norms and indicators. W.H.O. has established 12 global indicators as the basic point of reference to assess the progress towards H.F.A. Two major goals that all member countries have adopted are (a) Life expectancy of 60 years and (b) IMR 50 per 1000 live births.

In India, the laid down goals for HFA are:

i. Attaining IMR below 60 per 1000 LB
ii. Rise in expectation of life to 64 years
iii. To reduce CDR to 9 per 1000 MYP
iv. To reduce CBR to 21 per 1000 MYP
v. To achieve NRR of 1
vi. To provide potable water to the entire rural population.

Primary Health Care

The Alma Ata has defined Primary Health Care as under:

"Primary health care is essential health care made universally accessible to individuals and acceptable to them, through their full participation and at a cost the community and country can afford."

Elements of Primary Health Care

i. Health education on health problems and their control
ii. Promotion of food supply and proper nutrition
iii. Safe and wholesome water and basic sanitation
iv. M.C.H. and F.P. (RCH)
v. Immunisation against major diseases (UIP)
vi. Prevention and control of locally epidemic diseases
vii. Appropriate treatment of common diseases and injuries
viii. Provision of essential drugs.

Principles of Primary Health Care are:

i. Equitable distribution
ii. Community participation
iii. Intersectoral coordination
iv. Appropriate technology.

National Health Problems

Both health status and health problems need community diagnosis for their identification. In any health planning, the requirement of health status and health problems determine action plan. Data required for the community diagnosis of health problem are morbidity, mortality, demography, environmental aspect, socioeconomic aspects, sociocultural aspects, health service available and level of community participation.

Health problem of India can be grouped under 5 categories:

1. Population problem
2. Health care system
3. Environmental sanitation problem
4. Nutritional problem
5. Communicable disease problem.

Health Team

At district level, CHC level, PHC level or sub centre level, working health group complement each other. They share a common goal. After training, all possess ability and skills to manage any community health problem.

Health teams have set objectives formulated by health and family welfare services and postulated by the felt need of the community. Health team follow certain rules, procedures and legal obligations in delivering health goods to the community.

Health teams by their organised effort; plan, implement and evaluate health activity and health programmes is based on set of objectives. Team with their mutual cooperation and with the help of community participation render care, prevention and promotion of health to the sick, disabled and handicaps.

Health team of a community centre of a primary health centre and a sub-centre are listed under rural health services.

M.O.H. of P.H.C. is the leader who supervises and administers the health activities.

District Public Health Nurse

District public health nurse will have the placement as district level nursing officer attached to district health and family welfare. All district public health nursing activities are coordinated, supervised and monitored by the public health nurse. At directorate level assistant director of health and family welfare services (nursing) will guide her from technical point of view. All P.H.C., sub centres, F.W. centres and all national health programmes in the district will come under her care.

Duties

General

- Plan, develop and direct all district community health nursing activities.
- Take part in all district level meetings.
- Will convey the district need to D.H. and F.W.O. and Z.P. in terms of general and special community nursing care services.
- Take part in district level H and F.W. planning
- Guide district manpower in training activities.

Administration

- Help in policy decision matters of the district.
- Make recommendations regarding selection, appointment, leave, transfer, continued education and promotion of nursing staff of the district
- She does the needed job of material management for the district and its related budgetary planning
- Does evaluation of activity progress of nursing staff of the district
- Submit monthly reports and annual reports of the district.

Supervisory

She does the job of supervision in district public health nursing activities; bring out modifications and alterations for an effective work output in the district.

Education

- Continued nursing education
- Orientation training programme
- Dais training programmes
- M.P.W. (F) training programme
- A.W.W. training programme
- Training of student nurse in rural field training centres.

Multi Purpose Health Workers

The committee on "MPW under H and FW" was recommended by Kartar Singh Committee 1973, that there is a need of integrated health activity by a band of multi purpose workers. Thus MPW (M) is the redesigned term for BHW, malaria surveillance worker, vaccinator, health education assistant, FP health assistants. The M.P.W. (F) is redesigned term for nurse midwives.

One M.P.W. (M) and one M.P.W. (F) are posted to sub-centres which cover a population of 5000. They are given the assistance of voluntary workers.

These MPW's are supervised by health assistant male and health assistant female (Who are redesigned as male and female health supervisors).

In spite of training and recruitment, MPW manpower is not fulfilling the norms suggested by planning commission.

MPW (F) is given 6 weeks training for the transformation of unipurpose state to multi purpose work. The new entrants of MPW (F) have to undergo 18 month training and should be a matriculate. Her job responsibility is given in appendix.

MPW (M) is given 8 weeks of training for his transformation from unipurpose job.

MPW (M) and MPW (F) form a health team of the subcentre to carry out comprehensive health care services.

Health assistant female are either recruited afresh or promoted ANMs after promotional training. Existing LHV training schools are used to give promotional training of 6 months. New entrants will have to undergo 2 years training.

Nursing Personnel

Nursing personnel are group of auxiliary health workers who go to form members of health team in sub-centre, in PHC, in community health centre, in civil hospital and in teaching hospital. Accordingly categories of nursing personnel fall under following groups:

- Nursing advisor to Central Government.
- Nursing specialist under CHS scheme.
- Nursing tutors in nursing education.
- Nursing administrators like nursing superintendent, matron, District public health nurse.
- Senior nursing staff like head nurse, health supervisor female.
- Junior nursing staff like staff nurse, ward nurse, MPW(F).
- Student trainees.

Study of the Community

Study of the community is needed for community diagnosis and community treatment.

Study of the community can be by:

- Community survey
- Community screening
- Community surveillance.

Community survey can be:

- Demographic survey
- Socioeconomic survey
- Sociocultural survey
- Morbidity survey
- Mortality survey
- Fertility survey
- Epidemiological survey for incidence, prevalence
- Research survey on a specific project
- Specific disease survey
- Environmental survey
- K.A.P. survey.

At P.H.C. basic information is available which is obtained by base line health survey done at the beginning. Annual re-survey is done to update the community information which are required for progress report and future year goal fixation.

Community survey is done by personal interview, proforma filling, structured questionnaire entry, case studies, family schedule, individual health records, MCH cards, child cards, tuberculosis treatment card, leprosy treatment card, and beneficiary enrolment survey forms.

Content of community survey:

a. Physical and geographic characteristics like boundary, road, rivers, schools, civil amenities
b. Demographic characteristics like population, age, sex, race, religion, ethnic group, language
c. Socioeconomic characteristics like occupation, income, family pattern, belongings, socioeconomic class
d. Sociocultural characteristics like culture, tradition, taboo, belief
e. K.A.P. characteristics on knowledge, attitude and practices
f. Target group survey like school age, elderly, reproductive age, lame, blind, deaf, handicapped
g. Environmental characteristics like housing, refuse disposal, sewage disposal, water supply, vectors
h. Characteristics of health service utilisation.

Data thus obtained through house to house survey, records, reports, personal enquiry is very useful in planning, implementing and evaluation of community health programmes through community diagnosis and community treatment.

HEALTH CARE

Health care is now a team work. The Team includes professional and auxiliary health personnel who are needed to give health care; nursing care is nearly 50% of health care in the context of care, control and prevention.

Health committees have reported the desired nurse population ratio of 1:5000. But national average of nurse population ratio as per estimate 2001 is 1.02 per 5000 (2,10,000 nurses for 1,027,015,247 population).

Health manpower requirement of nurse, health assistant female, MPW female and trained dais are fulcrum for the Indian health scheme.

AREA

Major area of nursing care include three areas as under:

1. *Maintaining the individuality of man:* A patient is an individual member of society who has rights, privileges and immunities which should be respected regardless of his race, creed, social or economic status and personal fears and needs which usually are exaggerated by his illness.
2. *Maintaining physiologic functions in man:* The human body requires that certain physiologic activities be maintained if the body is to function effectively.
3. *Protecting man against external causes of illness*: Appropriate precautionary measures will help or eliminate physical, chemical or biologic factors in the environment which cause disease in man.

DAILY NURSING ROUTINE

The nursing care of each patient should be planned to meet the needs of individual patient physically, mentally and spiritually in the best possible way. His likes, dislikes and habits are to be respected.

Bed making, bed pan services are privilege of the nurse. She should supervise the disinfection of body discharges which are infective in nature.

Indian habit of using water for cleansing after urination and defecation is allowed since patient is accustomed to it. A check over instructions before ward rounds is a routine. Recording of vital rates like pulse, BP, respiration are common added routines in the sick.

Ward Management

Unit of a hospital which host the sick for medical care and nursing care form a ward in the hospital.

According to WHO the hospital is "an integral part of a social and medical organisation, the function of which is to provide for the population the complete health care, both curative and preventive and whose out-patient services reach out to the family and its home workers and for bio-social research."

Expected functions of professional care are:

- Care of the sick
- Care of the injured
- Prevention of diseases
- Promotion of health
- Diagnosis
- Treatment
- Rehabilitation
- Vocational training
- Nursing education
- Research.

Nursing Management Include

- Division of work starting from nursing superintendent, matron, department sister, nurse in-charge, staff nurse, ANM, clerk, ward aides, cleaning staff.
- Division of work starting from principal senior sister tutor, junior sister tutor at nursing college level.
- Authority and responsibility in nursing duties.
- Discipline as per nursing code.
- Unity of command from one source.
- Unity of direction of work or activity.
- Subordinate coordination.
- Adequate remuneration.

Nursing Skills at Hospitals and Health Centres are

- Conceptual skills
- Human relation skill

- Technical skill.

Nursing ward management is summarized by the following diagram (Fig. 16.1):

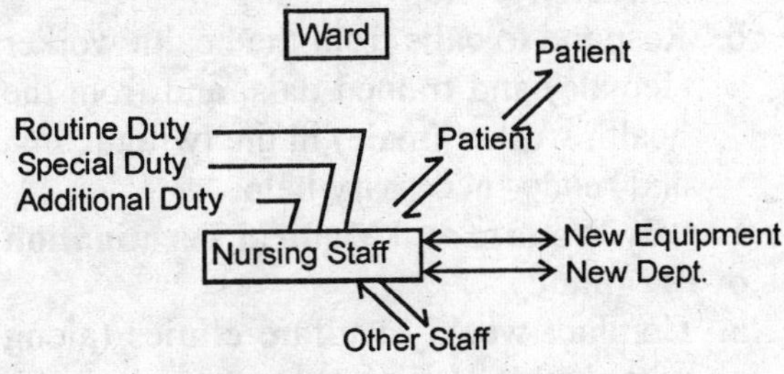

Fig. 16.1 : Ward management

SPECIAL ROUTINE

In hospital procedures following are special routines that are to be attended in nursing care services:

i. Employing techniques for infection prevention and control
ii. Using proper positioning, mobilization and transferring techniques
iii. Managing female reproductive procedures and immediate care of the newborn
iv. Managing G.I. procedure
v. Managing respiratory procedures
vi. Managing cardiovascular procedures
vii. Managing renal—Urinary procedures
viii. Managing musculoskeletal procedures
ix. Managing neurosensory procedures.

ADDITIONAL ROUTINE

- Family health counselling
- Inspection, survey of home, farm, school, industry plant, playground
- Managerial responsibilities
- Education and supervision of other workers
- Participation in research activity.

JOB RESPONSIBILITIES

Job responsibilities of nursing profession in community health nursing, which constitute comprehensive health care for the following staff, are enumerated in the following pages:

1. Health assistant female
2. MPW female
3. Health guide
4. *Dais.*

Job Responsibilities of Health Assistant (Female)

Note: Under the multipurpose workers scheme, a health assistant (female) is expected to cover a population of 20,000 in which there are four sub-centres, each with one health worker (female). However, in future she may cover one PHC with six sub-centres having 5,000 population each.

The health assistant (female) will carry out the following functions:

1. Supervision and Guidance

a. Supervise and guide the health worker (female) in the delivery of health care services to the community.
b. Strengthen the knowledge and skills of the health worker (female).
c. Help the health worker (female) in improving her skills in working in the community.
d. Help and guide the health worker (female) in planning and organising her programme of activities.
e. Visit each sub-centre at least once a week on a fixed day to observe and guide the health worker (female) in her day-to-day activities.
f. Assess periodically the progress of work of the health worker (female) and submit an assessment report to the medical officer of the primary health centre.
g. Carry out supervisory home visits in the area of the health worker (female).

2. Teamwork

a. Help the health worker to work as part of the health team.
b. Coordinate her activities with those of the health assistant (male) and other health personnel including the dais.

c. Coordinate the health activities in her area with the activities of workers of other departments and agencies, and attend meetings at block level.
d. Conduct regular staff meetings with the health workers in coordination with the health assistant (male).
e. Attend staff meetings at the primary health centre.
f. Assist the medical officers of the primary health centre in the organisation of the different health services in the area.
g. Participate as a member of the health team in mass camps and campaigns in health programmes.

3. **Supplies, Equipment and Maintenance of Sub-centre**
a. In collaboration with the health assistant (male), check at regular intervals the stores available at the sub-centre and help in the procurement of supplies and equipment.
b. Check that the drugs at the sub-centre are properly stored and that the equipment is well-maintained.
c. Ensure that the health worker (female) maintains her general kit and midwifery kit in the proper way.
d. Ensure that the sub-centre is kept clean and is properly maintained.

4. **Records and reports**
a. Scrutiny of the maintenance of records by the health worker (female) and guide her in their proper maintenance.
b. Maintain the prescribed records and prepare the necessary reports.
c. Review reports received from the health workers (female), consolidate them and submit periodical reports to the medical officer of the primary health centre.

5. **Training**
a. Organize and conduct training for dais with the assistance of the health worker (female).

6. **Maternal and child health**
a. Conduct weekly MCH clinics at each sub-centre with the assistance of the health worker (female).
b. Respond to calls from the health worker (female) and trained dais, and from the health worker (male) in the twilight area and render necessary help.

7. **Family Welfare and Medical Termination of Pregnancy**
a. Conduct weekly welfare clinics (along with the MCH clinics) at each sub-centre with the assistance of the health worker (female).
b. Personally motivate resistant cases for family planning.
c. Provide information on the availability of services for medical termination of pregnancy and refer suitable cases to the approved institutions.
d. Guide the health worker (female) in establishing female depot holders for distribution of conventional contraceptives and train the depot holders with the assistance of the health worker (female).

8. **Nutrition**
a. Identify cases of malnutrition among infants and young children (zero to five years), give the necessary treatment and advice and refer serious cases to the primary health centre.

9. **Immunization**
a. Supervise the immunization of all pregnant women, and infants (zero to one year).

10. **Primary Medical Care**
a. Provide treatment for minor ailments, provide first-aid for accidents and emergencies and refer cases beyond her competence to the primary health centre or nearest hospital.
b. Attend to cases referred by the health workers and refer cases beyond her competence to the primary health centre or nearest hospital.

11. Health Education

a. Carry out educational activities for MCH, family planning, nutrition and immunization with the assistance of the health worker (female)
b. Arrange group meetings with leaders and involve them in spreading the message for various health programmes.
c. Organize and conduct training of women leaders with the assistance of health worker (female)
d. Organize and utilize *mahila-mandals*, teachers and other women in the community in the family welfare programmes.

Job Responsibilities of Health Worker (Female)

Note: Under the multipurpose workers scheme, a health worker (female) is expected to cover a population of 5,000. (At present, however, she is expected to cover a population of 10,000 of which about 4,000 will be her intensive area, she will be responsible for all the activities listed and in the twilight area for maternal and child health activities only on request).

She will carry out the following functions:

1. Maternal and Child Health

a. Register and provide care to pregnant women throughout the period of pregnancy.
b. Test urine of pregnant women for albumin and sugar and estimate haemoglobin level during her home visits and at the clinic.
c. Refer cases of abnormal pregnancy and cases with medical and gynaecological problems to the health assistant (female) or the primary health centre.
d. Conduct about 50 per cent of total deliveries in her intensive area and whenever called in the twilight area.
e. Supervise deliveries conducted by dais and assist them whenever called in.
f. Refer cases of difficult labour and newborns with abnormalities and help them to get institutional care and provide follow-up care to patients referred to or discharged from hospital.
g. Make at least three postnatal visits for each delivery conducted in the intensive area and render advice regarding care of the mother and care and feeding of the newborn.
h. Assess the growth and development of the infant and take any necessary action.
i. Help the medical officer and health assistant (female) in conducting MCH and family planning clinics at the sub-centre.
j. Educate mothers individually and in groups for better family health including MCH family planning, nutrition, immunization, control of communicable diseases, personal and environmental hygiene and care of minor ailments.

2. Family Planning

a. Utilize the information from the Eligible Couple Register for the family planning programme.
b. Spread the message of family planning to the couples and motivate them for family planning individually and in groups.
c. Distribute conventional contraceptive to the couples, provide facilities and help the prospective acceptors in getting family planning services, if necessary by accompanying them or arranging for the dais to accompany them to hospital.
d. Provide follow-up services to family planning adopters and identify side-effects for a given treatment on the spot for side-effects and minor complaints and refer those cases that need attention by the physician to the PHC/hospital.
e. Establish female depot holders; help the health assistant (female) in training them,

and providing a continuous supply of conventional contraceptives to the depot holders.

f. Build rapport with acceptors, village leaders, dais and others and utilize them for promoting family welfare programmes.

g. Identify women leaders and help the health assistant (female) to train them.

h. Participate in *mahila-mandal*/meetings and utilize such gathering for educating women in family welfare programmes.

3. **Medical Termination of Pregnancy**

a. Identify the women requiring help for medical termination of pregnancy and refer them to the nearest approved institution.

b. Educate the community of the availability of services for medical termination of pregnancy.

4. **Nutrition**

a. Identify cases of malnutrition among infants and young children (0 to 5 years) give the necessary treatment and advice and refer serious cases to the PHC.

b. Distribute iron and folic acid tablets as prescribed to pregnant and nursing mothers, infants and young children (0 to 5 years) and family planning acceptors.

c. Administer vitamin 'A' solution as prescribed to children from 1 to 5 years.

d. Educate the community about nutritious diet for mothers and children.

5. **Communicable Disease**

a. Identify cases of notifiable diseases, i.e. cholera, plague, poliomyelitis and persons with continued fever or prolonged cough, or spitting of blood, which she comes across during her home visits and notify the health worker (male) about them.

6. **Immunization**

a. Immunize pregnant women with tetanus toxoid.

b. Administer BCG vaccination to all newborn infants, DPT vaccination, oral poliomyelitis vaccine (where available) and BCG vaccine (if not given at birth) to all infants (0 to 1 year).

7. **Dai Training**

a. List dais in the intensive and twilight areas and involve them in promoting family welfare.

b. Help the health assistant (female) in the training programme of dais.

8. **Vital Events**

a. Record births and deaths occurring in the intensive area in the births and deaths register and report them to the health worker (male).

9. **Record Keeping**

a. Register (a) pregnant women from three months of pregnancy onwards; (b) infants zero to one year of age; and (c) women aged 15 to 44 years through systematic home visits in the intensive area and at the clinic.

b. Maintain the prenatal and maternity records and child care records.

c. Assist the health worker (male) in preparing the Eligible Couple Register and maintaining it up-to-date.

d. Prepare and submit the prescribed periodical reports in time to the health assistant (female).

e. Prepare and maintain maps and charts for her area and utilize them for planning her work.

10. **Primary Medical Care**

a. Provide treatment for minor ailments, provide first-aid for accidents and emergencies and refer cases beyond her competence to the primary health centre or nearest hospital.

11. **Team Activities**

a. Attend and participate in staff meeting at primary health centre/community development block or both.

b. Coordinate her activities with the health worker (male) and other health workers including the health guides and dais.
c. Meet with the health assistant (female) each week and seek her advice and guidance whenever necessary.
d. Maintain the cleanliness of the sub-centre.
e. Participate as a member of the team in camps and campaigns.

Activities of Health Guide

Note: A health guide will be expected to cover the population of a village or, if the village is a large one, a population of about 1,000. He/she will receive technical guidance from the health worker (male/female).

After training, the health guide will be able to carry out the following activities:

1. Malaria

a. Identify fever cases
b. Make thick and thin blood films of all fever cases
c. Send the slides for laboratory examination
d. Administer presumptive treatment to fever cases
e. Keep a record of the persons given presumptive treatment
f. Inform the health worker (male) of the names and addresses of cases from whom blood slides have been taken
g. Assist health worker (male) and the spraying teams in spraying and larvicidal operations
h. Educate the community on how to prevent malaria.

2. Communicable Diseases

a. Inform the health worker (male) immediately an epidemic occurs in his/her area.
b. Take immediate precautions to limit the spread of disease.
c. Educate the community about the prevention and control of communicable diseases.

3. Environmental Sanitation and Personal Hygiene

a. Chlorinate drinking water sources at regular intervals.
b. Keep a record of the number of wells chlorinated.
c. Assist the health worker (male) in arranging for the construction of the following:
   - Soakage pits
   - Kitchen gardens
   - Compost pits
   - Sanitary latrines
   - Smokeless *chulhas.*
d. Educate the community about the following:
   - Safe drinking water
   - Hygienic methods of disposal of liquid waste
   - Hygienic methods of disposal of solid waste
   - Home sanitation
   - Kitchen gardens
   - Advantages and use of sanitary latrines
   - Advantages of smokeless chulhas
   - Food hygiene
   - Control of insects, rodents and stray dogs.
e. Educate the community about the importance of personal hygiene.

4. Immunization

a. Assist the health worker (male/female) in arranging for immunization.
b. Educate the community about immunization against diphtheria, whooping cough, tetanus, tuberculosis, poliomyelitis, measles, cholera and typhoid.

5. Family Planning

a. Spread the message of family planning to the couples in his/her area and educate them about the desirability of the small family norm.
b. Educate the people about the available methods of family planning.

c. Act as a depot holder, distribute *nirodh* to the couples and maintain the necessary records of *nirodh* distributed.
d. Inform the health worker (male/female) of those couples who are willing to accept a family planning method so that he/she can make necessary arrangements.
e. Educate the community about the availability of services for medical termination of pregnancy (MTP).

6. Maternal and Child Care

a. Advise pregnant women to consult the health worker (female) or the trained *dai* for prenatal, natal and postnatal care.
b. Advise pregnant women to get immunized against tetanus.
c. Educate the community about the availability of maternal and child care services and encourage them to utilize the facilities.
d. Educate the community about how to keep mothers and children healthy.

7. Nutrition:

a. Identify cases with signs and symptoms of malnutrition among pre-school children (one to five years) and refer them to the health worker (male/female).
b. Identify cases with signs and symptoms of anaemia in pregnant and nursing women and children and refer them to health worker (male/female) for treatment.
c. Assist health worker (male/female) in administering vitamin A solution as prescribed to children from one to five years of age (9 months to 3 years under RCH).
d. Teach families about the importance of breastfeeding and the introduction of supplementary weaning foods.
e. Educate the community about nutritious diet for mothers and children.

8. Vital Events

a. Report all births and deaths in his/her area to the health worker (male).
b. Educate the community about the importance of registering all births and deaths.

9. First-Aid in Emergencies

a. Give emergency first-aid for the following conditions, refer these cases to the primary health centre as necessary and inform the health worker (male/female):
   - Drowning
   - Electric shock
   - Heat stroke
   - Snake bite
   - Scorpion sting
   - Insect stings
   - Dog bite
   - Accidents
b. Carry out procedures in dealing with accidents.
c. Keep a record of first-aid given to each patient.

10. Treatment of Minor Ailments

a. Give simple treatment for the following signs and symptoms and refer cases beyond his/her competence to the subcentre or primary health centre:
   - Fever
   - Headache
   - Backache and pain in the joint
   - Cough and cold
   - Diarrhoea
   - Vomiting
   - Pain in the abdomen
   - Constipation
   - Toothache
   - Earache
   - Sore eyes
   - Boils, abscesses and ulcers
   - Scabies and ringworm.
b. Keep a record of the treatment given to each patient.

11. Mental Health

a. Recognise signs and symptoms of mental illness and refer these cases to health worker (male/female).
b. Give immediate assistance in emergencies associated with mental illness.
c. Educate the community about mental illness.

Activities of *DAI*

The Dai is an important person in her village. She serves as a link between the families in her village and the health worker (female)/ANM. These are some of the things she can do to improve maternal and child health in her village.

1. She should contact every pregnant woman in her area and see that she is registered at the sub-centre or primary health centre.
2. She should attend the weekly prenatal clinic and assist the health worker (female)/ANM.
3. She should try to ensure that every pregnant woman in her area attends the prenatal clinic at least three times, i.e. after the third month to confirm pregnancy, during the seventh month and during the ninth month.
4. She should try to ensure that every pregnant woman is immunized against tetanus (two doses—the last dose at least one month before the delivery and the first dose one month before the last).
5. She should try to ensure that every pregnant woman takes iron and folic acid tablets as prescribed.
6. If any abnormal pregnancy is detected she should show the case immediately to the health worker (female)/ANM or health assistant (female)/LHV or refer the case to PHC.
7. She should ensure that preparations for delivery are made either at home or at the PHC or hospital.
8. If she finds any abnormality during labour she must seek medical aid without delay.
9. When she receives a call for delivery:
   - She should take her kit with her.
   - She should watch the progress of labour carefully.
   - She should allow labour to progress normally without any unnecessary interference.
   - She should observe aseptic techniques while conducting the delivery.
10. She should see that her kit is always replenished, clean, and ready for use during a delivery.
11. She should make the mother and baby comfortable and attend to the nutrition of both.
12. She should instruct the mother and the relatives as to when she should be called immediately, e.g. in case the mother has excessive bleeding or there is bleeding from the baby's cord.
13. In the postnatal period if she finds any complications in the mother, e.g. fever or foul lochia, or in the baby, e.g. cord infection or jaundice she should immediately inform the health worker (female)/ANM or refer the mother or baby to the PHC.
14. She should try to ensure that all infants in her area are immunized with BCG, DPT, measles and poliomyelitis vaccine.
15. She should motivate the eligible couples in her area to use a contraceptive method or to undergo sterilization.
16. She should distribute *nirodh*, foam tablets, and jelly to those couples who require these contraceptives.
17. She should report all births and deaths in her area to the health worker (male) or health worker (female)/ANM.

HEALTH CARE DELIVERY IN THE FIELD OF COMMUNITY HEALTH

a. **Comprehensive health care:** It denotes provision of integrated preventive, curative and promotional health services from womb to tomb to all residing in a defined geographical area.

b. **Basic health service:** It is a network of coordinated, peripheral and intermediate health units capable of performing effectively a selected group of functions essential to the health of an area and assuring the availability of competent professional and auxiliary personnel to perform these functions. It is called total patient care under nursing component.

TEAM NURSING

Very few activities in nursing are carried out in isolation. Most of nursing works are to be done in Team Nursing. History helps to explain the elusive boundaries between various fields of medical, health and nursing practice. Centuries ago a doctor and a nurse used to be treatment givers. With the expansion of scientific knowledge, diagnostic and therapeutic approach has multiplied and specialization in nursing is seen. Thus in a team we see additional members like medical social workers, nutritionist, physical therapist, occupational therapist, clinical psychologist, rehabilitation officers, vocation officers, health educators, medical clerks, laboratory technicians, anaesthetists and many more.

In a set up of health centre nurse has to work with medical officer of health, LMO, X-ray technician, health supervisor male, health supervisor female, MPW male, MPW female, trained dais, health educator and many more.

For the total programme, team work is mandatory because Job responsibilities are laid down at hospital, at centre and at home visiting. Thus group dynamic has become a process for the spirit of team nursing.

In team nursing, quality of leadership, element of supervision and able administrative efficiency are called for.

SCIENTIFIC PRINCIPLES OF NURSING

Nursing is an art which requires a sympathetic heart and willing hands. The chief purpose of nursing today is to help the individual to attain or maintain health. Nurse has dual responsibility; one is concerned with relieving suffering in relation to caring for the sick; the other is placed upon preventive and educational aspects. Along with attendant, she is a teacher of health also.

Skills to be learnt by a nurse are:

- Skills in dealing with and influencing people
- Skills in observing
- Skill in manual dexterity needed in certain techniques
- Skill in operating different types of machines used in giving nursing care.

Scientific principles in nursing can be classified under following heads:

1. **Principles related to meeting the need of patients:**
   - Safe and comfortable environment for patient
   - Bed making
   - Admission procedures
   - Observation and charting
   - After receipt of instructions in ward rounds, sound planning of nursing care
   - Discharge procedures.
2. **Principles of daily fundamental care:**
   - Comfort position
   - Care of the skin
   - Care of nails
   - Care of hair
   - Care of mouth
   - Food requirement in terms of balanced diet or therapeutic adaptation of normal diet
   - Elimination and treatment of large intestine
   - Elimination and treatment of bladder.
3. **Principles to vital signs:**
   - Temperature recording, treatment
   - Pulse and BP recording

- Respiration and nursing treatment of respiratory tract.

4. **Principles of drug administration:**
   - Oral medicine
   - Injections
   - Infusions
   - Transfusions
   - Radiation (X-ray, Cobalt).
5. **Therapeutic measures and diagnosis test:**
   - Heat application and withdrawal
   - Treatment of vaginal canal
   - Treatment of eye
   - Treatment of ear, nose, throat
   - Treatment of stomach
   - Diagnostic tests.
6. **General principles to meet the need of special patients:**
   - Communicable diseases
   - Surgery and post surgery
   - Wound bandaging and care
   - Chronic ill patient
   - Care of dying and dead.

MAN—THE RECIPIENT OF CARE

Man is a bio psychosocial being and understanding him in his environment is utmost important for an effective treatment. Apart from health need, other aspects of needs (human needs) are to be contemplated in diagnosis, therapy and rehabilitation of a given patient. Following different situations (personalities) are encountered that need elucidation.

Infancy

He is completely a helpless patient. He has only reflex and no activity can be carried out. He is totally dependent for everything. Breastfeeding by mother is an added compliment which the nursing component should look for. Another point of consideration is to look into growth and development at hospital admission. Because the infant has no speech, no thought in terms of adult concepts, it must be assumed that her early experiences are recalled in the realm of feeling.

Early Childhood

A great deal of success in case management depends on the mother's skill in giving hand with nursing care. Again growth and development, importance, breastfeeding is to be considered in analysis of the case. Toilet training, family closeness, play therapy are to be included in the nursing component of health and nursing care.

School Age Child

School age children always want to conform. They do not know what is expected of them. They have to be informed and even if they know would have forgotten. Hence, they need to be reminded and this could help in correcting their behaviour.

Adolescence

The transformation from childhood to adulthood is the adolescence stage. There is instability and immaturity in emotional and social behaviour. They suffer from identity crisis. They are rebellious in their attitude. Nursing component has to understand and accept the above group of patients in their background. This will go a long way in offering nursing care effectively and efficiently.

Adult

It is possible to widen the scope for emotion and to feel strongly about patient's feeling and causes as well as about people.

Old Age

Eye sight and hearing loss should be remembered in this category of patient for an appropriate action through nursing component. Loneliness, worries, anxiety are to be taken note in problem evaluation. Recently geriatrics nursing is becoming a speciality.

ILLNESS AND SICK ROLE

Illness is an unwelcome intrusion: some may regard this as a challenge : many people's attitude to illness is much less constructive, and many nursing problems arise because sick people often behave not as adults but as if they were much younger. Under stress they revert to earlier pattern of behaviour (Regress). It is not uncommon for people to adopt this attitude of guilt and shame towards their own suffering. It is interesting to note that word *pain* has come from Greek word *poine* which means penalty. Some of the diseases attract negative attitude by the attending health professional. STD, HIV, AIDS, leprosy, tuberculosis are such examples.

Some patients turn to God and desire comfort from such action.

Whatever people suffer from, at treatment, patient (sick) must give up oneself and submit to the authority of nursing. In some respect sick resembles that of a child who needs attention from his/her mother.

Nursing component should visualize "attention seeking" behaviour of patient.

COPING STRATEGIES BY THE SICK

Hostility

Hostile attitude of the sick is a deterrent to all nursing care unless it is tackled in the beginning itself. Non-cooperative, non-submissive takes away nurse's energy in diagnosis, treatment and rehabilitation. Sympathy, understanding taking the help of members of his family are available weapons in such cases. Only in case of life saving situations force can be used with ward boys which in no way is inhuman.

Manipulation

In communication, in progress response and in nursing examination, patient may show manipulated tactics. Manipulation is highly dangerous because of its influence in problem solving through data collection, analysis and assessment. Second opinion, re-examination and repeat assessment are available means to overcome manipulation.

Loneliness

This is natural in case of geriatric patients. In them it is reversible with available means of concern, sympathy, constant hearing and psychotherapy. There are selected group of patients who are basically introvert and are not to be confused with loneliness. Good interaction, assurance and building confidentiality help in overcoming loneliness due to introvert nature.

REHABILITATION ASPECT IN NURSING COMPONENT

Definition

The rehabilitation aspect of nursing is coordinated and combined efforts of medical, social, educational and vocational measures to give the patient good functional ability.

Principles

Rehabilitation aspect of nursing include element of social integration. Secondary nursing component should include multidisciplinary approach involving physiotherapy, occupational therapy, speech therapy, psychotherapy, educating, social welfare work, vocational guidance and placement services.

The main nursing aims in rehabilitation are:

- Restoration of function (medical)
- Restore capacity of earn (vocational)
- Restore social relation (social)
- Restore confidence (psychological).

Process

Illness and disability are threat to economic security and involve more suffering than pain connected with illness. Worry over finance, disrupted family relation, unemployment, loss of organ etc., not only delay recovery but also healing of organic lesion.

Nursing component should have a sufficient knowledge of the community resources to enable them to advice the patient and his family.

Their burden will be lightened if specialists in social work and vocational guidance are participating in patient's care.

Team required for rehabilitation aspect is:

- Orthopaedician
- Physiotherapist
- Occupational therapist
- Speech therapist
- Audiologist
- Psychologist
- Psychosocial counsellor (MSW)
- Social worker (MSW)
- Government administrators.

Nursing responsibility as a professional is a wider activity in collaboration with team suggested above. She follows instructions, monitors rehabilitation, records the progress of action and submits report of progress to concerned specialities of rehabilitation team.

Since nursing element is a chemical bond in each act of rehabilitation be it physical, vocational, social or psychological no specific marking can be done as to nursing responsibility. Nurse initiates, implements, monitors, reports and dismisses and thus is a key person in nursing rehabilitations.

CHAPTER SEVENTEEN

Public Health Services in India

PUBLIC HEALTH ADMINISTRATION

HEALTH AND SOCIAL SERVICES IN INDIA

Health Planning Reports

A number of committees starting from pre-independence have given a few recommendations for the health development and social development. A brief review of major committee reports need highlighting.

Bhore Committee 1946

Under the leadership of Sir Joseph Bhore the committee made recommendations for the future development of the country.

The committee quotes:

"If the nation's health is to be built, the health programme should be developed on a foundation of preventive health work and that such activities should proceed side by side with those concerned with the treatment of patients."

The committee recommended the following:

a. Integration of prevention and cure at all levels.
b. Primary Health Centre Development.
   Short term—Rural PHC per 40,000 population with 2 MOH, 4 PHN, one nurse, 4 ANM, 4 Dais, 2 SI, 2 HA, One pharmacist and 15 class IV employees.
   Long term—Called 3 million plan.
   Rural PHC per 20,000 with 75 beds.
c. 3 months rural posting to house surgeons

It is a major document which has provided health planning in India.

Mudaliar Committee 1962

This is called "Health survey and planning committee". This studied the progress of Bhore Committee report and made certain recommendations for health services expansion. They are:

- District hospital must be strengthened with specialist services
- Regional (Divisional) level office to supervise 2 to 3 district health and F.W. offices
- Each PHC should cover 40,000 population
- PHC should provide quality health care
- Integration of medical service and health service
- Development of all India medical service similar to I.A.S. cadre.

Kartar Singh Committee 1973

It is called "Committee on multi purpose workers under health and FP"

Main recommendations made by the committee are:

- ANM are redesigned as MPW (F) /FHW
- BHW Malaria surveillance worker, HE Assistant, FP Assistant are redesignated as MPW (M)/MHW
- In the beginning where Malaria and Smallpox were under control, multipurpose

worker (Male and Female) scheme were to be initiated and later to other areas

- P.H.C. should have 50,000 population
- Each PHC should have 16 sub-centres each with 3000 population
- Each sub centre should have M.P.W (M) and MPW (F)
- Health Supervisor (M) should supervise 3-4 MPW (M)
- Health supervisor (F) should supervise 3-4 female MPW (F)
- MOH of PHC should control all MPW (M) and MPW (F) in the PHC area.

Kartar Singh Committee report is a milestone in the history of public health nursing service administration.

Srivastav Committee 1975

This is called "Group on Medical Education and Support Manpower." Its main recommendations are:

- Male and Female Health Assistant should supervise 2 MPW (M) and 2 MPW (F) and each MPW should cover an area of 5000 population.
- HA (F) and MPW (F) should be located in sub-centre.
- For simple promotive, preventive and curative service a band of para professionals like school teacher, post master, *Gram'sevak* or a literate youth are created.
- Between PHC and community 2 cadre of health workers are created HA's and MPW's. (Health Assistants and Multi Purpose Workers).
- Development of Referral service involving civil hospitals, teaching hospitals etc.

HFA by 2000 AD—Report

As per WHO resolution 1977 HFA is for attainment by all the highest possible level of health along with productive life and good social life. It implies the removal of obstacle to ill health. It is a revolutionary and historic concept by W.H.O.

In 1978 Government of India developed a workable report by a committee for a National Health Policy.

The report is the response of WHO call for H.F.A. and Alma Ata declaration which earmarked the following goals:

- I.M.R. reduction to below 60
- Rising life expectation to 64
- Reducing crude death rate to 9
- Reducing crude birth rate to 21
- To achieve NNR of one
- To provide potable water to entire rural community.

The report implementation is seen through Five Year Plan, Annual plan, Minimum need and 20-point Programmes.

Health Service Organization

Structure, functioning and essentiality of health system in India is unique. Centre makes health policy; States run health care services independent of centre. According to Union List, Concurrent List and State List with assistance for certain schemes.

2001 first stage census drafted 20 million households, 6.5 lakh villages, 5500 towns and cities which function on a 3-tier system of health care services.

Dharwad District in Karnataka State in India is illustrated for Health Service Organisation (Tables 17.1 and 17.2).

Decentralised State Administration

Village

To make health accessible and available, policy was made for the following:

a. **Village Health Guide (V.H.G.):** He is a literate volunteer who can secure people's participation. Scheme of VHG came to existence in 1977. They are chosen from the

Table 17.1: Health system in India

	I District (Dharwad)	
DH & FWO Dharwad Zilla Parishad, Dharwad PHC (6 PHCs) Sub-centre (23 sub-centres)	District Hospital (Dharwad)	City Corporation Health authorities (Hubli Dharwad Municipal Corporation)
State Ministry	II State (Karnataka) Directorate with Dy. Director & Jt. Director	Direct control
	III Centre (G.O.I.)	
Union Ministry	D.G.H.S. (Director General of Health Health)	C.C.H. (Central Council of Services)
Union function	H & FW merged - International Health Regulation	(Chairman and Members) Health Policy Legislation
Concurrent function	- Drug standard - Medical store - PG, Training - Med. Research (ICMR) - CGHS - CHEB - Medical Library (Med Line)	- Grant in Aid - Cooperation with state

Table 17.2: 3 tier system of heath care in India

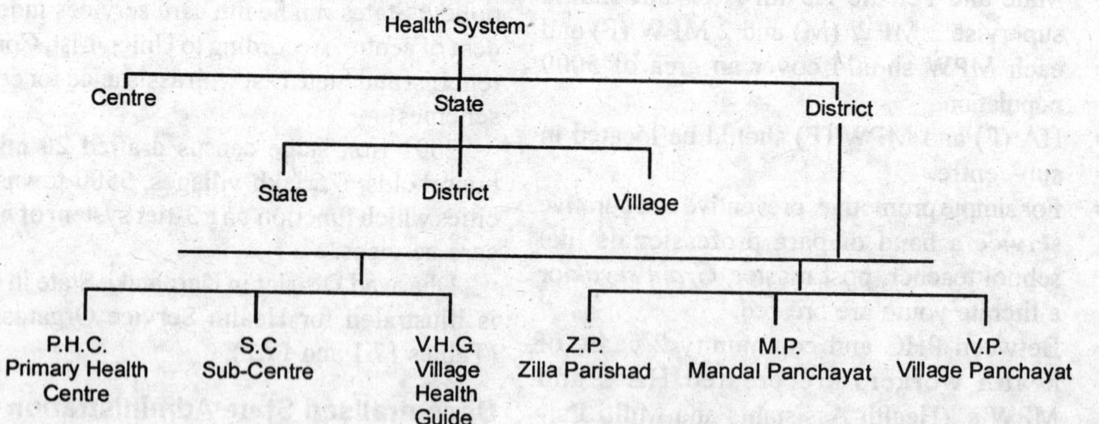

community. They act as a link between PHC and public. Criteria in their selection are:

- Local residents
- Able to read and write (6th or 7th std.)
- Acceptable to community
- Should spare 2-3 hours per day for community work.

They undergo training for 3 months (with stipend) of Rs. 200 per month. After training they receive a working manual and a medicine kit. They spare 2-3 hours, get Rs. 50 stipend per month and drug worth 600.00 per year.

As on today there are about 3,24,000 VHG working in the country. The target is get 1 VHG per village per 1000 rural population.

b. Indigenous dais: They are called TBA (Traditional Birth Attendants). They are given 1 month training with Rs. 300 stipend. After training they are provided with a delivery kit. She gets Rs. 10 for every registered case of pregnancy and Rs. 3 for every registered infant. Total trained Dais are about 7,00,000 in India.

c. Anganwadi worker: Under ICDS an AWW is selected from the community. She undergoes training for 4 months. She is paid Rs. 250 per month honorarium for her service (Rs. 400/- when State Government Assistance is present). She helps in health check up, immunisation, supplementary nutrition, health education, non-formal education and referral services.

Sub-Centre

It is an out post attached to a P.H.C. covering a population of 5000. One MPW(M) and one MPW(F) are posted to work under a sub centre. Mainly RCH, immunisation and F.P. are emphasised. Government is trying to give facility for I.U.D. insertion and urine examination for albumin and sugar. Health assistant female supervises the activity of MPW(F).

Panchayat Raj System

It is a 3-tier health system at 3 levels :

They are:

- *Village panchayat* level.
- *Panchayat samiti* at Block level (Taluka level).
- *Zilla parishad* at district level.

Panchayat at Village Level

Gram panchayat is an executive organ responsible for village development. It has a president (*Sarpanch*), vice president, a secretary. Administration, sanitation, public health, socio-economic development are discussed by them. When they give legal verdict it is called *Nyaya Panchayat.*

Panchayat Samiti at Block Level

About 100 villages of 1,00,000 population has a *samiti* consisting of *sarpanchs* of the block. BDO acts as secretary of *samiti.* It is responsible for community development programme of the block.

Zilla Parishad at District Level

It is rural local self Government of the district. All heads of *panchayat samiti* are members. Deputy Commissioner (Collector) is a non voting member. It will have above 60 members. Health services, family planning service of the district come under *Zilla Parishad.*

Rural Health Services

It contains 3 levels of health service delivery centres namely community health centre, primary health centre and sub-centre.

Community Health Centre

Each CHC covers 1,20,000 population in a community development block. It has 30 beds, specialists in Medicine, Surgery, OBG and paediatrics. It will have X-ray and lab facilities. There are 3076 CHC in the country.

Staff

1 Community health officer (Medical or non-medical)
4 Medical officers
7 Nurse midwives
1 Dresser
1 Pharmacist
1 Lab technician
1 X-ray technician

2 Ward boys
1 *Dhobi*
3 Sweepers
1 *Mali*
1 *Chowkidar*
1 Aya
1 Peon.

C.H.C. refers cases to district hospital or the state level hospital or medical college hospitals (Teaching hospitals).

Primary Health Centre

It is an outcome of Bhore Committee Report. PHC provides integrated health services. We have about 23,000 PHCs in the country.
Staff: (at PHC level which cover 30,000 population)

1 MO
1 Pharmacist
1 Nurse midwife
1 HW(F)
1 BEE
1 HA (M)
1 HA (F)
1 UDC
1 LDC
1 Lab technician
1 Driver
4 Class IV employees.

Functions

- Medial care
- Reproductive and child health
- Family welfare planning
- Water supply and sanitation
- Control of communicable diseases
- Collection of vital statistics
- Health education
- Carry out national health programmes
- Referral service
- Training of health assistants, Health workers, Health guides and local dais
- Basic laboratory services

PHC is equipped to perform with the following:

- Tubectomy
- Vasectomy
- MTP
- Minor OT procedures

Government has proposed and brought into action that each medical college to adopt 3 primary health centres for Re-Orientation of Medical Education (ROME).

Sub-Centre

It covers a population of 5,000 and has following staff:
MPW (M)—1
MPW (F)—1
Voluntary health guide—1
T B A—1

The function is the same as PHC but restricted to the population it covers viz., 5,000 population.

Community Development Programme (CDP)

Community development is a process designed to create conditions of economic and social progress for the whole community with its active participation and the fullest possible reliance upon the community's initiative. Here people are united for their development.

C.D.P. was launched in 1952 for the allround development of rural areas. It is an organised programme by community development blocks, each covering 1,20,000 population. There are about 6100 community development blocks in the country.

It envisages the following programmes:

a. Improvement of agriculture
b. Improvement of communication
c. Education

d. Health
e. Sanitation
f. Housing.

The community development block will work for intensive development for 5 years followed by continued work in second phase of 5 years. It is mainly centrally sponsored programme. By its programme, it is tackling rural poverty and unemployment.

National Planning and Policy

Government of India set up a commission for assessment of human resource, capital and material of the country for drafting the development plans. It is called "Planning Commission". It was further developed with many divisions in 1957.

The Structure of Planning Commission

Functions are:

- Projections for future 25 years development
- Make recommendations to Government
  - On problems
  - On Policies (Legislation)
  - On Economic development.

Present Status

District is a unit for planning by planning commission. It has given importance to developmental planning in health sector.

1. Water and sanitation
2. Control of communicable diseases
3. Medical education, training and research
4. Medical care through:
   - Hospitals
   - Dispensaries
   - PHC's
5. Public health service
6. Family planning
7. Indigenous systems of medicines.

Depending on felt need of the people and technical feasibility, changes are brought out from time to time. The coordinating body between Central Government and State Government is *Bureau of Planning* which was formed in 1965. They are implemented at village level through district planning.

Five Year Plans

Planning commission which gave importance to health programmes has proposed five-year plans to rebuild rural India, to lay foundation of industrial progress and to secure balanced development of all parts of the country viz., 28 states and 7 union territories. The broad objectives of health programme during five year-plans are:

- Control and eradication of major diseases
- Establishing PHC and sub-centre for basic health services
- Population control (FWP)
- Development of health manpower.

Five Year Plan Outlay

First 5-year plan	1951-56
Second 5 year plan	1956-61
Third five-year plan	1961-66
Annual plan	1966-67
Annual plan	1967-68
Annual plan	1968-69
Fourth 5 year plan	1969-74
Fifth five-year plan	1974-79
Annual plan	1979-80
Sixth 5 year plan	1980-85
Seventh five-year plan	1985-90
Annual plan	1990-91
Annual plan	1991-92
Eighth five-year plan	1992-97
Ninth 5 year plan	1997-2002
Tenth 5 year. plan proposed	2002-2007

(Total plan investments = 921291 crores,
Investments for health = 9253 crores,
Investments for family welfare = 27125 crores.)

Annual plan	2002-2003
Annual plan	2004-2005

During 9th five-year plan district level surveillance for diseases was strengthened, appropriate systems for emergency, disaster and accidents were implemented, screening of nutritional deficiencies was implemented, Growth rate reduction policy was targeted and emphasis on RTI/STD surveillance was given.

Following is the achievement of 9th Five year plan (2002) + 10th Five year plan till date upto 2005:

Village health guides trained	3,24,000
H.W. male	73,300
H.W. female	1,38,000
Health visitors	42,900
A.N.M. (MPW (F))	5,11,200
Nurses	8,76,600
Doctors	5,90,000
Dental colleges	142
Medical colleges	222
Total beds	9,90,000
P.H.C.	22,936
Sub-centres	1,38,368

NATIONAL HEALTH PROGRAMME

Various ongoing health programmes are grouped under following categories:

1. *For population problem*
   - A. National FWP Programme
   - B. IPP (India Population Project)
   - C. PPC (Post Partum Programme)
2. *For health care problem*
   - A. HFA (Health for All)
   - B. Primary Health Care
3. *For Environmental sanitation problem*
   - A. NWS and SP (National water supply and sanitation programme)
   - B. Accelerated Rural WS Programme (Rural water supply)
4. *For Nutrition Problem*
   - A. ANP (Applied Nutrition Programme)
   - B. SNP (Special Nutrition Programme)
   - C. BNP (Balwadi Nutrition Programme)
   - D. Mid-day Meal School Programme
   - E. Vitamin A Prophylaxis Programme
   - F. IFA (Iron Folic Acid Supplementation Programme)
     (NNAPP) (National Nutritional Anaemia Prophylaxis Programme)
   - G. NIDDCP (National Iodine Deficiency Disorder Control Programme)
   - H. ICDS (Integrated Child Development Service Scheme)
   - I. IPP (India Population Project)
   - J. Defluoridation of water
   - K. PFA Act (Prevention of Food Adulteration Act)
   - L. National Programme for Control of Blindness.
5. For communicable diseases problem:
   - A. STD Control Programme
   - B. Malaria Action Programme
   - C. NFCP (National Filaria Control Programme)
   - D. NTP (National Tuberculosis)
   - E. MLEC (Modified leprosy elimination Campaign)
   - F. Control of Diarrhoeal Diseases
   - G. ARI Control programme
   - H. AIDS control programme
   - I. Guinea Worm Eradication Programme
   - J. JE control (Japanese Encephalitis)
   - K. Kala Azar Control Programme
   - L. Dengue Fever Control Programme
   - M. UIP (Universal Immunisation).

Some of the major National Health Programmes are discussed in detail:

National Iodine Deficiency Disorder Control Programme

It is discussed under Nutrition (Chapter 6).

National Programme for the Control of Blindness (1976)

It is 100 percent centrally sponsored programme which incorporates old national trachoma control programme of 1968.

The present problem of blindness is 1.49% which is to be reduced to 0.3% through national level programme.

Chalked out programme contained:

- Establishment of regional institute of ophthalmology
- Upgrading medical colleges hospitals
- Upgrading district hospitals
- Development of mobile ophthalmic units
- Recruitment of ophthalmic manpower
- Provision of ophthalmic services.

By improving physical, technical and managerial capabilities of teaching hospitals, district hospitals, community health centres, PHC's and NGO institutions, it is possible to provide high quality cataract treatment.

Ophthalmologists are given special training for the required skills for cataract surgery.

During the year 2002 Government of India has revised the strategy of national programme for the control of blindness. This new strategy includes:

a. NPCB is made more comprehensive by including the following:
   - Fixed facility surgical approach of Lens removal and IOL implantation (Intra Ocular Lens) to get better quality of post operative vision.
   - Refractive error correction in school children
   - Treatment of trachoma infection
   - Treatment of glaucoma
   - Vitamin A prophylaxis
   - Improving follow-up service of cataract operations.

National STD Control Programme

STD control programme started in 1946. Sex related diseases (STDs) is related to health seeking behaviour of patient, STD awareness and its effects on health. Diagnosis and treatment of STD is done at five regional STD referral centres and 510 district hospital and 735 STD clinics across the country. Since HIV/AIDS more easily gets transmitted in presence of STD and RTIs, both are linked together for an effective control. Hence HIV/AIDS control includes diagnosis and treatment of STD as a recently drawn strategy. In 1992 NACO made it an integral part of AIDS control programme.

STD clinics carry out clinical, laboratory and epidemiological components as services under STD control.

Case reporting by STD and RTIs/AIDS, awareness and involvement of general practitioners in STD control.

Contact tracing, cluster testing and special group including high risk behaviour groups screening help in case finding. Medical social worker will help in guidance, counselling and motivating for full treatment.

Condom promotion as prophylaxis against STD is advocated.

Health education for creating awareness about source, transmission and impact in the community is very important in imparting of health seeking behaviour of patients with STD/RTIs.

Other measures include:

- Control of prostitution by legislation
- Control of drug abuse and alcoholism by legislation
- Rehabilitation of CSW (Commercial Sex Workers)
- Family health awareness campaign.

Syndromic Approach

This is a method of management and control of STDs and RTIs where diagnosis and treatment is based on a group of symptoms and signs. Treatment is targeted towards all diseases that could cause that syndrome. It allows diagnosis without extensive laboratory test and treatment with a single visit, or referred after 1 week if treatment fails.

National Antimalaria Programme

National malaria control programme (NMCP) was started in 1953 with DDT spray twice a year. By 1958 the successful result made the programme to eradication called (NMEP) National Malaria Eradication Programme. There was reappearance (resurgence) of malaria in 1976 due to many reasons like (a) Operational defect (b) Technical defect (c) Administrative defect d) Resistance to insecticide. In 1977 MPO (Modified Plan of Operation) was launched which was mainly based on API Zones (Annual Parasite Index) for operational purpose.

During all these periods active surveillance was done, where health workers visited houses, collected blood smear of fever cases and gave treatment. In passive surveillance fever cases come to hospitals and health centres. Health workers are given targets of smear collection in the field.

Two main indicators used in malaria effective control are:

i. $$\text{API} = \frac{\text{Confirmed cases during 1 year}}{\text{Population under surveillance}} \times 1000$$

(Annual Parasite Incidence)

ii. $$\text{ABER} = \frac{\text{No. of slides examined}}{\text{Population under surveillance}} \times 100$$

(Annual Blood Examination Rate)

In 1978 malaria control through primary health care was approved. Because of increase in malaria, in 1994 Malaria Action Programme was initiated as part of unipurpose worker to MPWs to integrate national programme.

Later in 1997 World Bank gave support for Enhanced Malaria Control Project.

In 1998, by roll back malaria programme, the health system got strengthened.

From 1999 malaria control is going on under "National Anti-malaria Programme."

Main activity for Malaria control are as under:

In areas with API above 2:

- Pyrethroids spray 2 rounds at 6 weeks interval if DDT and malathion resistant
- Entomological assessment (Mosquito examination)
- Active and Passive Surveillance (fortnightly for active)
- Treatment of malaria case (PT and RT).

In Areas with API Below 2:

- Spraying–Focal sprays around areas with falciparum malaria severe malaria cases
- Surveillance both active and passive
- Radical treatment of detected cases
- Blood smear follow-up for 12 months (every month) from positive cases
- Epidemiological investigation.

PT (Presumptive treatment):

All fever cases are presumed as malaria and presumptive treatment is given soon after taking blood smear (also refer page 194).

R.T (Radical treatment):

If blood smear is positive, radical treatment is given (also refer page 194).

National Filaria Control Programme

It was started in 1955. Now it is estimated that 500 million people are exposed to the risk of infection in India. In 1978 this programme was combined with malaria control because of uniformity in control measure and for proper effective use of resources. Main activities include antilarval measures and filaria treatment.

At present, there are 210 filaria control units, 30 survey units and 200 Filaria clinics functioning.

W.H.O. recommendation is followed in endemic areas:

"Annual single dose therapy with DEC along with NFCP strategy."

NICD Delhi is conducting training and research on filaria control.

National Tuberculosis Programme

In 1962 with the establishment of NTI (National Tuberculosis Institute) at Bangalore, the control programme was launched with a long-term and short-term objectives.

Long-term – To make tuberculosis no more a public health problem by check at no new case occurrence and reducing prevalence rate to below 1%.

Short-term – Diagnosis and treatment
B.C.G. Vaccination
As an integrated health service.

DTC (District TB Centre) is the nucleus of the programme. Out of existing 600 TB clinics 410 are upgraded to DTC to undertake the control in a district. Planning, organising and implementing DTP through all hospitals, centres and dispensaries, covering rural, suburban and urban areas are the functions of DTC.

In India there are 460 districts and all 466 districts have DTC In available TB clinics about 48,000 beds for TB patients is made available. For training and Demonstration NTI, Bangalore and TCC Chennai (TB chemotherapy centre) are well-known.

Activities of D.T.C.

a. *Case finding*: Detection of cases by sputum examination and tuberculin test. MMR (Mass Miniature Radiography) is discontinued under RNTCP. At DTC Tuberculin Test is done.
b. Treatment is offered by domiciliary care by motivation and treatment (Table 17.3).

In 1992 national TB control was revised with following strategies:

a. To achieve 85% cure rate of infectious cases by directly observed treatment.
b. To achieve 70% detection rate by quality sputum microscopy.
c. To involve NGO for IEC activities.

Table 17.3: Structure and function of DTC

D.T.C. covers (average) 50 health institutions

Staff	*Function*
1. DTO	1. Case finding
1. MO	M.M.R.
2. Lab technicians	Tuberculin test
2. Health visitors	Sputum exam
1 X-ray technician	2. Record maintenance
1. Team leader (Non medical)	3. Treatment by RNTCP (Dots method)
1. Statistician	4. BCG vaccination
1. Pharmacist	5. Preventive treatment
	6. Rehabilitation
	7. Surveillance

RNTCP (Revised National Tuberculosis Control Programme)

All tuberculosis patients receive free treatment under DOTS which is community based treatment. Under supervision of MPW of PHC local voluntary workers like teacher, anganwadi worker, dai, ex-patient, social workers help in DOTS administration. Other workers are DOTS agents. They receive Rs. 150 honorarium per patient after completing treatment. The success of DOTs depends on accountability, good drug supply directly observed treatment by health workers, good quality sputum microscopy and political commitment and patient compliance through health education.

The drugs are supplied in blister packs, separately for intensive phase and continuation phase. They are kept ready in boxes for supply to patients for a full course of treatment. One day's medication in each pack for intensive phase and one week's medication in each pack for continuation phase are kept in boxes.

Detailed drug regimen and specifications are dealt in Chapter 11.

Modified Leprosy Elimination Campaign

NLEP started in 1955 with case detection and DDS drug treatment on ambulatory basis. In 1980

Government felt the possibility of eradication. Since 1983 NLEP with a goal of eradication by reducing case load to below 1 per 10,000 population was considered.

NLEP contained:

- Population survey
- School survey
- Contact examination
- Voluntary referral
- Multi drug regimen (MDT)
- Health education
- Rehabilitation.

For the control and eradication we have about 800 leprosy control units and about 6000 SET centres (Survey education treatment).

Since 1997 MLEC was launched with training to Medical Officers, health workers and volunteers. Two main activities included are:

– House to house search for case
– Health awareness on leprosy.

This MLEC has an objective of elimination of leprosy by 2005 in the world. Research activities are going on in Agra, Chingelput, Orissa, Chhatisgarh and West Bengal, international organisation like SIDA, DANIDA, WHO, Damien Foundation are providing assistance in MLEC.

C.D.D. (Control of Diarrhoeal Disease)

This was started in 1978 to reduce deaths and sufferings occurring due to diarrhoea. Upto 1985, emphasis was on case management. After 1985 O.R.T. was emphasised and knowledge on home available fluids were disseminated. Later in 1992 it got incorporated under CSSM. Presently CDD is taken care of by R.C.H. programme from 1997 which is detailed in Chapter 11.

U.I.P. (Universal Immunisation Programme)

Most powerful and cost effective weapon of disease control is U.I.P. In 1974 E.P.I. (Expanded Programme on Immunisation) was initiated to prevent 6 vaccine preventable disease viz, diphtheria, whooping cough, tetanus, poliomyelitis, tuberculosis and measles. The word expansion meant for extension of services, extension of coverage and extension of vaccines. UIP is assisted mainly by UNICEF. In 1985 EPI was renamed as UCI (Universal Child Immunisation). Since 1985 this is carried out with the name UIP where universal coverage means to cover all aspects of immunisation activity i.e. research and development and delivery system.

Additional force of coverage of UIP has been by IPPI (Intensive Pulse Polio Immunisation), UMC (Urban Measles Campaign) and N.N.T.E. (Neonatal Tetanus Elimination).

Incidentally UIP is a part of CSSM (from 1992) and is a part of RCH (from 1997).

Social Welfare Services

This is highlighted under MCH (Chapter 7).

SPECIAL COMMUNITY HEALTH SERVICES

Community health service is comprehensive health care for giving medical care to the sick and community preventive care for health promotion. Primary health care or first contact care for the family help in diagnosis and treatment of a case, apart from carrying out functions of PHC which is undertaken designed for community health service.

RCH activity covering perinatal, antenatal, intranatal and postnatal services and child care services are major areas accounts for 50% of health care services. They include two more main aspects of family planning and conducting home deliveries.

Immunisation for the prevention of preventable diseases is a full scale health care service.

Assessment of social, environmental and nutritional needs of the community and directing the attention of social workers to such need is an aspect of nursing care service in public health.

Some of the nurses are appointed as district public health nurse to plan, implement and evaluate nursing activities in the district.

Following are the special community health nursing services apart from regular hospital and health centre health care services etc.

Industrial Nursing Service

There is provision for appointment of nursing staff in factories where more than 500 workers are working. The area of nursing in industrial setting is discussed in Chapter 12. They include care of sick, care of injured, preplacement examinations, periodic examinations, sanitation or good housekeeping in industry, first aid, industrial safety, organisation of crèches, counselling, guidance and rehabilitation.

Tuberculosis Nursing Services

Staff at hospitals, dispensaries, PHC, Sub centre –all are functionaries for tuberculosis control programme. Clinical examination, radiological diagnosis, sputum examination, contact examination followed by directly observed therapy to patient under R.N.T.C.P. is specified as a special community health service.

When patient is provided with short course chemotherapy, the drug is administered under direct supervision (DOTS): DOTS is a Community Based Tuberculosis Treatment which combines the benefit of supervised treatment and the benefit of community based care and support.

Domiciliary care of nursing care, guidance, counselling, DOTS, follow-up, contact tracing are added job responsibilities of a health worker.

Leprosy Nursing Services

Leprosy being a social disease and as an elimination campaign has many components of community health services. Training of health workers for diagnosis, treatment, nursing and rehabilitation is first line of action in MLEC.

Secondly, house to house visit for the search of case to detect new leprosy cases is done at a scheduled activity in the community.

Thirdly, creating awareness about leprosy by health education, clarification and clearing misconceptions for the social acceptance of cured cases.

Major community health service is the rehabilitation of a patient who is a burnt out case, for his self-reliance and self-support. This vocational rehabilitation forms major service under special community health services.

Leprosy hospitals and rehabilitation centres where complicated cases are admitted with tropical ulcer, wound, burns, skin lesions etc., which need daily or many times a day care for nursing and treatment.

Health Team

At district level, CHC level, PHC level or sub-centre level, working health group complement each other. They share a common goal. After training, all possess ability and skills to manage any community health problem.

Health team have set objectives formulated by health and family welfare services and postulated by the felt need of the community. Health team follow certain rules, procedures and legal obligations in delivering health goods to the community.

Health team by their organised effort; plan, implement and evaluate health activity and health programmes is based on set of objectives. Team with their mutual cooperation and with the help of community participation render care, prevention and promotion of health to the sick, disabled and handicaps.

Health team of a community centre, of a primary health centre and a sub-centre are listed above under rural health services.

M.O.H. of P.H.C. is the leader who supervises and administers the health activities.

Nursing Personnel

Nursing personnel are a group of auxiliary health workers who go to form members of health team in sub-centre, in PHC, in community health centre, in civil hospital and in teaching hospital. Accordingly categories of nursing personnel fall under following groups:

- Nursing advisor to Central Government.
- Nursing specialist under CHS scheme.
- Nursing tutors in nursing education.
- Nursing administrators like nursing super-intendent, matron, district public health nurse.
- Senior nursing staff like head nurse, health supervisor female.
- Junior nursing staff like staff nurse, ward nurse, MPW(F).
- Student trainees.

Following Table 17.4 provides the achievement in 9th five-year and present estimate 2003 with regard to nursing personnel:

Table 17.4: Nursing personnel

	1997-2002		*2003 March (Estimate)*
Nurse	776,643	Nurse	8,04,000
MPW (F) (ANM)	411,220	HS (F)	49,010
Health visitor HS(F)	35,890	MPW(F)	6,09,000
Health worker (F) MPW(F)	134,086	TBA	4,17,000
Dais TBA/CHG	3,23,000		

Nurse Population Ratio

The norm suggested is 1 per 5000 population (1 : 5600 as per NRHM). Taking all available figures it seems nurse population ratio norm is reached. But when qualified nurse proportion is taken there is still need for the further manpower development in India.

Presently there is a need for promotional training programmes and continued nursing education programmes to update the vast developing nursing education from general nursing care to special nursing care.

LEADERSHIP

IMPORTANCE

As a leader in her group nurse has to maintain the cohesion of the nursing group and guide her group to achieve highest level of achievement. Another aspect of her leadership, external to her nursing group is that, she has to represent nursing profession and has to represent as nurses' spokeswoman for uplifting the nursing organisation. She has to gather information and resources that are necessary to facilitate the work of nursing group. Nurse will be representing this in the community and other agencies in the field.

Characteristics of Leadership

Use of position has given rise to three types of characteristics:

1. Autocratic
2. Democratic
3. Laissez-faire.

In autocratic type, all authority is vested in leader herself. In democratic type, responsibility is delegated. In laissez-faire type, there is no demarcation of authority and responsibility.

Leadership depends on successful channels of communication which are available in a system or organisation (Fig. 17.1).

Group Activities in Indian Villages

There are many health activities which need group participation. Almost all national health programmes are carried out as group activity and hence their understanding is a requirement for an effective health programme.

Immunisation of children, a tubectomy camp, an O.T.C. camp (Orientation Training Camp to village leaders for health awareness), a school health check-up programme, a cancer screening

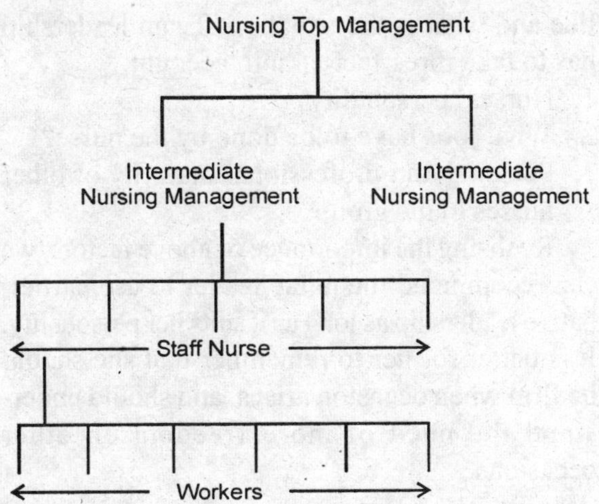

Fig. 17.1: Communication system in nursing

programme, a blood donation camp are examples of group activities. Following are basics in group activities:

- Need people's involvement.
- Need people's participation.
- Need to work through community leaders.
- Village leaders are to be trained before a health activity.
- Social acceptance is required.
- It needs interdepartmental co-ordination (Inter-sectoral coordination).

Leadership in Nursing

Whenever nursing profession embark on a joint project, some form of leadership is required. In case of play or conversation in a group where no specific purpose exist, we see that one person assumes leadership. Sometimes leader is appointed.

Leadership qualities exist in all, but suitable education help to acquire skills of leadership. Interactions with members make the type of leadership.

Leader seated high away from others clearly demarcate a barrier, which is an obstacle to the function of a leader.

There are advantages and disadvantages in both types of leadership. Most committee procedure is formal and all remarks are addressed to the chair. Committees are meant to settle issues efficiently and fairly rapidly after preliminary discussion has already taken place. Hospital with large staff and complex problems may need both types of leadership on different occasions. Both need practice for successful use.

UNDERSTANDING OF OTHERS (IN LEADERSHIP)

There are many patterns a leader may adopt to understand others and to get work done by them. They are:

a. *Telling:* The leader makes a plan, announces decision and follows through.
b. *Selling:* The leader makes a plan, persuade others to assist him in implementing the plan.
c. *Consulting:* The leader asks the group to make a plan from subordinates, tests the essential parts of the plan with them and is responsive to their inputs.
d. *Joining:* The leader encourages the subordinates to begin making plan, but joins with them later.

Nurses as leaders tend to do better when using the pattern of leadership that is more natural for them. But a leader should also understand that subordinates have different personalities, varied problems and situations. Such diverse group calls for a variety of leadership pattern.

Thus telling, selling, consulting and joining are known as: "group dynamics". This attitude where organizational or professional prestige is given importance over the leadership or activity performance is called "group morale". Group morale is one of the influencing characters that builds group dynamics and understanding of others.

LEADERSHIP TRAITS

Research conducted by social scientists has shown that leadership is made up of a number of traits and that there is no single type of personality that can be labelled as a leadership type. Certain traits, if are on pronounced degree; they can understand the need and desire of a group. Traits help in gaining group confidence.

Most common traits are:

- Intelligence
- Self-confidence
- Formal education
- Adaptability
- Emotional stability
- Enthusiasm
- Conceptual ability
- Human relations skills.

Now traits can be learnt by trial and error and can be made suitable to a given group.

FUNCTIONS OF LEADER

- Finding out human behaviour in social interactions as a group activity.
- Taking decision for practical approach
- Plan, organise and direct the efforts of others
- Relate social actions for human benefits.

LEADERSHIP DEVELOPMENT

Leadership development is a developed style, is an appropriation, is dependable on workers and situation. It is not a static, but goes on modifying according to season, people and situation.

When workers (staff) are insecure in position and in an unstructured situation, the leadership developed will be an authoritative or a directive type. The best for all seasons is participatory type.

An effective leader is the pride of a group. This is one thumb-rule test one can apply in assessing one's own leadership effectiveness.

Nurse as a Leader

What is the best way to lead nurses by a nurse? There can be no readymade answer to this question. Much will depend on what the nurse is like and what is the situation. Team leadership has to take three factors into account:

1. Nurses' personality.
2. What jobs have to be done by the nurse?
3. Personal and professional maturity of other nurses in the group.

Realising the importance of above factors, we can recommend the nurse leader to use participative leadership as long as it suits her personality. It is better for her to remember that she should be firm when occasion arises, and should understand the need of more freedom on other occasions.

VOLUNTARY HEALTH AGENCIES IN INDIA (NGOs)

INTRODUCTION

Nurse as a member of community Health team need orientation and information on such agencies which are helping human community by their welfare programmes. It is voluntary agencies that have pioneered the health development in any country. They have missionary zeal and an organisation consisting of an administrative body, a committee to raise funds through membership and all actions are carried out on a voluntary basis.

FUNCTIONS

Services by Voluntary Health Agencies (Functions):

It can be represented in a diagram to depict its vast encroachment in the welfare of the people (Fig. 17.2). If there are any new ways of approach or ways of doing, it is always by a voluntary health organisation.

Pioneering health service activity and legislation on matters of health have always been from voluntary health agencies.

General functions of voluntary Health agencies in India:

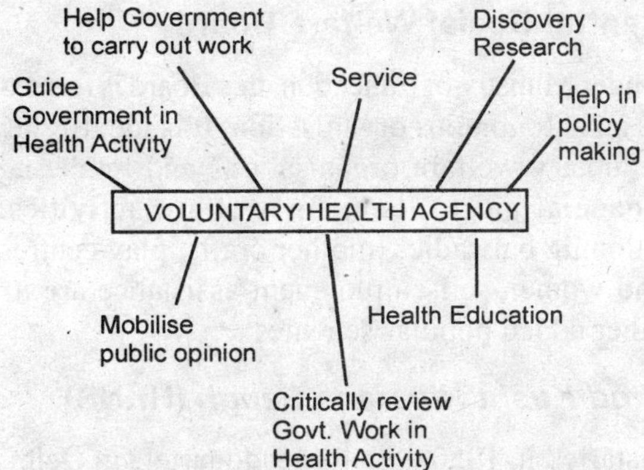

Fig. 17.2: Functions of a voluntary health agency

- Medical relief
- Initiation of measures according to their objectives
- Supplementing Government effort
- Development of manpower, media and methods for health education
- Evaluation of health activities in India
- Reporting—Helps in policy making.

HISTORY

In India, at the beginning of past century voluntary service worked for rehabilitation of war raged community. Lepers' rehabilitation help and care for women by gram sevikas have been recorded.

After independence, India has seen well developed network of voluntary health associations which functioned for the welfare of mankind. Major agencies which are worth mentioning are under following heads:

1. *Relief operation*
   - Indian Red Cross Society
   - *Bharath Sevak Samaj*
   - All India Blind Relief Society
2. *Specific disease control*
   - *Hind Kusht Nivaran Sangh*
   - Tuberculosis Association of India
   - Indian Cancer Society
3. RCH
   - Indian Council of Child Welfare
   - The *Kasturba* Memorial Fund
   - FPAI
   - All India Women's Conference
4. *Professional bodies*
   - The Trained Nurses' Association
   - IMA
   - Indian Dental Association
   - General Practitioners' Association
   - Geriatric Association of India
5. *Social welfare*
   - Central Social Welfare Board
   - State Social Welfare Board.

AGENCIES

Trained Nurses Association of India

Before 1946 trained birth attendants used to gather in a forum which never made any group activities. When Delhi and Vellore started graduate education, nursing care took a different direction to establish themselves as an organised group. By 1952 we could see an organised effort of grouping among trained nurses but without any registered body. Of late, various specialized courses are being made available such as community health nursing, midwifery, operating assistant and rehabilitation nursing. By sixties an organised group called Trained Nurses Association has formed with the objective of involvement into community welfare activities such as:

- Nursing care of children.
- Nursing care of elderly.
- Blood donation campaign and camps.
- First aid facility.
- Vocational rehabilitation.
- Relief work with Red Cross, I.M.A. and General Practitioners.

Indian Red Cross Society

There are many branches across the country executing relief work during earthquake, floods, drought and disease epidemics disaster, natural calamity management. It is providing assistance to fetch milk and medical supplies to many hospitals, R.C.H. centres and orphanages. The primary obligation of the Red Cross is to take care of wounded, sick or injured armed forces. For permanent disabled and ex-service men Red Cross has initiated "Red Cross Homes".

Recently, great attention of Indian Red Cross has fallen on First Aid, blood donation (voluntary) and family planning clinic which can bring medical relief and social relief to the society.

General Practitioners' Association

Thousands of branches are doing yeomen service in bringing medical relief to vulnerable groups. It has its members from all systems of medicine Allopathy, *Ayurveda, Unani*, Homoeopathy, *Siddha* and other Indian systems of medicine. Over hundreds of health check-up camps, health awareness camps, Blood donation camps, screening camps are conducted every year thus providing access to health and welfare to common man.

All India Women's Conference

Started in 1976, is running ANC clinics, PNC clinic, child guidance clinics, adult education centres, milk distribution centres and family planning clinics.

All India Blind Relief Society

Started in 1946, is associated with eye camps for identification of preventable blindness and conducting cataract surgery camps with post-operative follow-ups and free spectacles for refractory corrections. Recently AIBRS has introduced cataract surgery with I.O.L. implantation which otherwise is not affordable by a common man.

Bharat Sevak Samaj

Started in 1952 it is helping people to achieve health by their own effort and actions. Village sanitation is given priority by BSS workers.

Central Social Welfare Board

Under Ministry of Education, this Board is formed as an autonomous organisation. It is identifying voluntary welfare organisations and rendering financial aid to them for welfare activities. Running balwadies, mother crafts, play centres and women self-employment assistance are its other added popular schemes.

Hind Kusht Nivarana Sangh (HKNS)

It started in 1950 with its headquarters in Delhi. Financial assistance to leprosy homes, health education by posters and training of physiotherapists are main activities of HKNS.

Indian Council for Child Welfare

It started in 1952. It has a network of state councils in India. Its main objectives are to provide social and economic security to child by legislative means through right of the child.

IMA

It is a professional body which is guiding Medical Council of India. I.M.A. is helping in setting up Quality Standards in professional education in medical profession and health science profession. It is also involved in organising relief camps and medical relief during natural calamities. It coordinates with Indian Red Cross Society. Also conduct CME for doctors. It actively participates in national programme.

The *Kasturba* Memorial Fund

It started in 1944. It aims at helping rural women through *Gram Sevikas.*

Tuberculosis Association of India (TAI)

It started in 1939 and has many branches in India. It mobilises fund through "TB seal campaign", trains medical and paramedical staff in treatment. There are many leading tuberculosis institutions in India which are run by TAI.

CHAPTER EIGHTEEN

International Health

IMPORTANCE

The boom in science and technology during the last century has resulted in all-round socio-economic development of transport, communication, education, industry, trade and commerce around the globe. This has brought people closer with cross-culture, around the world. Cutting across distances and culture, people travel long distances for the purpose of trade, commerce and education. This kind of a situation has thrown challenges on international health status. In this event, infections and communicable diseases, which were earlier restricted to selected countries are becoming global problems.

In the early centuries in order to avoid spread of such infections and communicable diseases, all ships, crew travellers and cargoes were to be detained for about 40 days at the dock, thus putting hardships to travellers, but with little benefit. This early practice "Quarantine" later become an international health measure against major diseases like cholera, yellow fever, plague, relapsing fever etc.

HISTORY

First Sanitary Conference was held in Paris in 1851. Pan American Sanitary Bureau set up in 1902, later produced a code popularly called "The Pan American Sanitary Code". During 1907 Paris office was created (office International d' Hygiene Publique) which shifted its responsibility to WHO in 1950.

First World War gave an arena for an organisation of League of Nations in 1923.

During Second World War (1943) UNRRA (United Nations Relief Rehabilitation Administration) was set up which lost its shape when WHO was born in 1945.

MAJOR INTERNATIONAL HEALTH ORGANISATIONS

WHO

On April 7, 1948, WHO came into force as an international organisation under United Nations. Each year WHO Day is celebrated on 7th April and a theme is selected to focus and to project light on international health problems. WHO day themes of current century are:

2000 Safe blood starts with me—blood saves lives
2001 Stop exclusion—dare to care
2002 Move for health
2003 Shape the future of life – Healthy environment for children.
2004 Road safety is no accident
2005 Make every mother and child count
2006 Working together for health

WHO has given definition for health; has its own constitution, own governing bodies, own membership and budget. Alma Ata conference in primary health care and health for all by 2000 made good impact on global health care system.

WHO has about 200 country membership and has following functions which are being carried out successfully:

- Collaboration with all other international and national organisations.
- Literature and information on health and disease are released to the world.
- Stimulates all research for human benefit.
- Reports, records, ICD are made available as Health statistics.
- Taken up family health as a major project.
- Environmental health activities like water for all, environmental health monitoring and development of environmental health criteria are undertaken.
- Promotes and supports comprehensive health programmes.

S.E.A.R.O.

The South East Asia Regional Office in New Delhi is a Regional Office with the membership of 11 countries (India, Indonesia, Bangladesh, Myanmar, Korea, Thailand, Nepal, Sri Lanka, Bhutan, Mangolia and Maldives).

U.N.I.C.E.F.

It was established in 1946 and now is called UNICF [E = emergency is removed] (United Nations International Children Fund). This works with other international organisations in covering RCH, nutrition, provision of potable water supply, disposal of night soil of older children leading to "country health programming" for the children.

Functions of UNICEF include:

- Family and child welfare
- Child nutrition
- Child health
- Child education
- GOBI campaign (Growth monitoring, oral rehydration, breastfeeding, immunisation)
- UBS (Urban Basic Service).

CARE

It is a major relief organisation called Co-operative for Assistance and Relief Everywhere. Till 1980 it was mainly helping in projects on food to 6-11 age children. Now it is helping in projects like I.C.D.S. Anaemia control, Adolescent girls project and Associated R.C.H. projects.

Colombo Plan

It is a co-operative economic development plan mooted in 1950 as an outcome of the meeting at Colombo. Industrial development, agricultural developments are aimed at the plan. Major outcome in India are, establishment of AIIMS in Delhi and cobalt therapy units in medical colleges.

DANIDA

It is assistance by Government of Denmark for the prevention of blindness, for the veterinary health (Dairy Development) and for higher studies in M.Sc. ophthalmology for developing countries.

FAO

It looks after several areas of world co-operation since 1945 for efficient farming, raising living standard and nutritional improvement. It has organised FFHC (Freedom From Hunger Campaign) in 1960 for the world. It is disseminating and providing information and education in the field of food, agriculture and nutrition.

Ford Foundation

It is responsible for the development of family planning and rural health. Most important projects of Ford Foundation are:

(a) Establishment of NIHAE (National Institute of Health Administration and Education) in Delhi, (b) Gandhigram Rural health service project at Gandhigram, (c) Sanitary Latrine projects, (d) Orientation training centres for the Public Health Training, (e) Kolkata Water Supply and Drainage Scheme, and (f) Research on reproductive Biology.

International Red Cross

It is a product of appeal by A Swiss, Dunant, for relief to help the wounded in times of war by means of volunteers. Initiated in 1859, formed a committee in 1864. Now Red Cross symbol denotes its services anywhere for wounded, co-ordinated through 90 countries.

ILO

Since working and living conditions of working population needed attention, International Labour Organisation was formed in 1919. It looks into social justice, improving labour conditions through social stability and health and welfare. Standard working conditions were formulated to the working force and ILO is collaborating this all over the world.

Rockefellers Foundation

Internationally famous philanthropist John D Rockefeller founded this in 1913 to promote the well-being of mankind at global net. Public Health and Medical Education are two pillars of foundation, on which other advancement like life science, social science, humanities and agriculture science developed. Establishment of AIIH & PH (All India Institute of Hygiene and Public Health) at Kolkata, NIV (National Institute of Virology) at Pune and several field demonstration centres hallmark the focused attention of Foundation.

SIDA (The Swedish International Development Agency)

By procurement of X-ray unit, microscopes, anti TB drugs, SIDA is supporting tuberculosis control all over the globe.

USAID

It is an extended U.S. aid to many countries since 1961. United States agency for international development is helping to improve nursing education in developing countries. Other areas of USAID assistance are: (a) Malaria (b) Health education (c) Family planning (d) Water supply and sanitation.

UNFPA

The United Nations Fund for Population Activities is helping countries for the development of national capability for the manufacture of contraceptives and developing population education programmes.

UNDP

United Nations Development Programme in short UNDP was started in 1966 to help poor nations to develop their own resources in social and economic areas. Assistance is offered in the development of agriculture, industry, education, science, health and social welfare of developing countries through aid from UNDP for their development.

World Bank

It is a specialized agency of UN; through Board of Governors, World Bank is helping developing countries to raise their living standards. IPP, Roadways, Power, Water, World Food and Population Control are assisted wholly by World Bank.

Index

N

O

P